## Arthritis Sourcebook

*Basic Information about Specific Forms of Arthritis and Related Rheumatic Disorders, Including Rheumatoid Arthritis, Osteoarthritis, Gout, Polymyalgia Rheumatica, Psoriatic Arthritis, Spondyloarthropathies, Juvenile Rheumatoid Arthritis, and Juvenile Ankylosing Spondylitis; Along with Information about Medical, Surgical, and Alternative Treatment Options and Including Strategies for Coping with Pain, Fatigue, and Stress*

Edited by Allan R. Cook. 600 pages. 1998. 0-7808-0201-2. $78.

■

## Back & Neck Disorders Sourcebook

*Basic Information about Disorders and Injuries of the Spinal Cord and Vertebrae, Including Facts on Chiropractic Treatment, Surgical Interventions, Paralysis, and Rehabilitation, Along with Advice for Preventing Back Trouble*

Edited by Karen Bellenir. 548 pages. 1997. 0-7808-0202-0. $78.

**"The strength of this work is its basic, easy-to-read format. Recommended."**
— *Reference and User Services Quarterly, Winter '97*

■

## Blood & Circulatory Disorders Sourcebook

*Basic Information about Blood and Its Components, Anemias, Leukemias, Bleeding Disorders, and Circulatory Disorders, Including Aplastic Anemia, Thalassemia, Sickle-Cell Disease, Hemochromatosis, Hemophilia, Von Willebrand Disease, and Vascular Diseases; Along with a Special Section on Blood Transfusions and Blood Supply Safety, a Glossary, and Source Listings for Further Help and Information*

Edited by Karen Bellenir and Linda M. Shin. 575 pages. 1998. 0-7808-0203-9. $78.

■

## Burns Sourcebook

*Basic Information about Various Types of Burns and Scalds, Including Flame, Heat, Electrical, Chemical, and Sun; Along with Short- and Long-Term Treatments, Tissue Reconstruction, Plastic Surgery, Prevention Suggestions, and First Aid*

Edited by Allan R. Cook. 600 pages. 1998. 0-7
7. $78.

■

## Cancer Sourcebook, 1st Edi

*Basic Information on Cancer Types, Sympto... nostic Methods, and Treatments, Including Statistics on Cancer Occurrences Worldwide and the Risks Associated with Known Carcinogens and Activities*

Edited by Frank E. Bair. 932 pages. 1990. 1-55888-888-8. $78.

**"Written in nontechnical language. Useful for patients, their families, medical professionals, and librarians."**
— *Guide to Reference Books, '96*

**"Designed with the non-medical professional in mind. Libraries and medical facilities interested in patient education should certainly consider adding the *Cancer Sourcebook* to their holdings. This compact collection of reliable information . . . is an invaluable tool for helping patients and patients' families and friends to take the first steps in coping with the many difficulties of cancer."**
— *Medical Reference Services Quarterly, Winter '91*

**"Specifically created for the nontechnical reader . . . an important resource for the general reader trying to understand the complexities of cancer."**
— *American Reference Books Annual, '91*

**"This publication's nontechnical nature and very comprehensive format make it useful for both the general public and undergraduate students."** — *Choice, Oct '90*

■

## New Cancer Sourcebook, 2nd Edition

*Basic Information about Major Forms and Stages of Cancer, Featuring Facts about Primary and Secondary Tumors of the Respiratory, Nervous, Lymphatic, Circulatory, Skeletal, and Gastrointestinal Systems, and Specific Organs; Statistical and Demographic Data; Treatment Options; and Strategies for Coping*

Edited by Allan R. Cook. 1,313 pages. 1996. 0-7808-0041-9. $78.

**"This book is an excellent resource for patients with newly diagnosed cancer and their families. The dialogue is simple, direct, and comprehensive. Highly recommended for patients and families to aid in their understanding of cancer and its treatment"**
— *Booklist Health Sciences Supplement, Oct '97*

**"The amount of factual and useful information is extensive. The writing is very clear, geared to general readers. Recommended for all levels."** — *Choice, Jan '97*

■

## Cancer Sourcebook for Women

*Basic Information about Specific Forms of Cancer That Affect Women, Featuring Facts about Breast Cancer, Cervical Cancer, Ovarian Cancer, Cancer of the Uterus and Uterine Sarcoma, Cancer of the Vagina,*
*...tical and Demographic*
*...nagement Suggestions,*
*...es*

Peter D. Dresser. 524
.

**...tandable, non-technical ...blic libraries or hospital and academic libraries that collect patient education or consumer health materials."**
— *Medical Reference Services Quarterly, Spring '97*

**Cancer Sourcebook for Women** *(Continued)*

**"Would be of value in a consumer health library. . . . written with the health care consumer in mind. Medical jargon is at a minimum, and medical terms are explained in clear, understandable sentences."**

— *Bulletin of the MLA, Oct '96*

**"The availability under one cover of all these pertinent publications, grouped under cohesive headings, makes this certainly a most useful sourcebook."**

— *Choice, Jun '96*

**"Presents a comprehensive knowledge base for general readers. Men and women both benefit from the gold mine of information nestled between the two covers of this book. Recommended."**

— *Academic Library Book Review, Summer '96*

**"This timely book is highly recommended for consumer health and patient education collections in all libraries."** — *Library Journal, Apr '96*

## Cardiovascular Diseases & Disorders Sourcebook

*Basic Information about Cardiovascular Diseases and Disorders, Featuring Facts about the Cardiovascular System, Demographic and Statistical Data, Descriptions of Pharmacological and Surgical Interventions, Lifestyle Modifications, and a Special Section Focusing on Heart Disorders in Children*

Edited by Karen Bellenir and Peter D. Dresser. 683 pages. 1995. 0-7808-0032-X. $78.

**". . . comprehensive format provides an extensive overview on this subject."** — *Choice, Jun '96*

**". . . an easily understood, complete, up-to-date resource. This well executed public health tool will make valuable information available to those that need it most, patients and their families. The typeface, sturdy non-reflective paper, and library binding add a feel of quality found wanting in other publications. Highly recommended for academic and general libraries."**

— *Academic Library Book Review, Summer '96*

## Communication Disorders Sourcebook

*Basic Information about Deafness and Hearing Loss, Speech and Language Disorders, Voice Disorders, Balance and Vestibular Disorders, and Disorders of Smell, Taste, and Touch*

Edited by Linda M. Ross. 533 pages. 1996. 0-7808-0077-X. $78.

**"This is skillfully edited and is a welcome resource for the layperson. It should be found in every public and medical library."**

— *Booklist Health Sciences Supplement, Oct '97*

## Congenital Disorders Sourcebook

*Basic Information about Disorders Acquired during Gestation, Including Spina Bifida, Hydrocephalus, Cerebral Palsy, Heart Defects, Craniofacial Abnormalities, Fetal Alcohol Syndrome, and More, Along with Current Treatment Options and Statistical Data*

Edited by Karen Bellenir. 607 pages. 1997. 0-7808-0205-5. $78.

**"Recommended reference source."** — *Booklist, Oct '97*

## Consumer Issues in Health Care Sourcebook

*Basic Information about Health Care Fundamentals and Related Consumer Issues, Including Exams and Screening Tests, Physician Specialties, Choosing a Doctor, Using Prescription and Over-the-Counter Medications Safely, Avoiding Health Scams, Managing Common Health Risks in the Home, Care Options for Chronically or Terminally Ill Patients, and a List of Resources for Obtaining Help and Further Information*

Edited by Karen Bellenir. 592 pages. 1998. 0-7808-0221-7. $78.

## Contagious & Non-Contagious Infectious Diseases Sourcebook

*Basic Information about Contagious Diseases like Measles, Polio, Hepatitis B, and Infectious Mononucleosis, and Non-Contagious Infectious Diseases like Tetanus and Toxic Shock Syndrome, and Diseases Occurring as Secondary Infections Such as Shingles and Reye Syndrome, Along with Vaccination, Prevention, and Treatment Information, and a Section Describing Emerging Infectious Disease Threats*

Edited by Karen Bellenir and Peter D. Dresser. 566 pages. 1996. 0-7808-0075-3. $78.

## Diabetes Sourcebook, 1st Edition

*Basic Information about Insulin-Dependent and Noninsulin-Dependent Diabetes Mellitus, Gestational Diabetes, and Diabetic Complications, Symptoms, Treatment, and Research Results, Including Statistics on Prevalence, Morbidity, and Mortality, Along with Source Listings for Further Help and Information*

Edited by Karen Bellenir and Peter D. Dresser. 827 pages. 1994. 1-55888-751-2. $78.

**. . . very informative and understandable for the layperson without being simplistic. It provides a comprehensive overview for laypersons who want a general understanding of the disease or who want to focus on various aspects of the disease."** — *Bulletin of the MLA, Jan '96*

*Second Edition*

# Health Reference Series

AIDS Sourcebook, 1st Edition
AIDS Sourcebook, 2nd Edition
Allergies Sourcebook
Alternative Medicine Sourcebook
Alzheimer's, Stroke & 29 Other Neurological Disorders Sourcebook
Alzheimer's Disease Sourcebook, 2nd Edition
Arthritis Sourcebook
Back & Neck Disorders Sourcebook
Blood & Circulatory Disorders Sourcebook
Burns Sourcebook
Cancer Sourcebook, 1st Edition
New Cancer Sourcebook, 2nd Edition
Cancer Sourcebook for Women
Cardiovascular Diseases & Disorders Sourcebook
Communication Disorders Sourcebook
Congenital Disorders Sourcebook
Consumer Issues in Health Care Sourcebook
Contagious & Non-Contagious Infectious Diseases Sourcebook
Diabetes Sourcebook, 1st Edition
Diabetes Sourcebook, 2nd Edition
Diet & Nutrition Sourcebook, 1st Edition
Diet & Nutrition Sourcebook, 2nd Edition
Ear, Nose & Throat Disorders Sourcebook
Endocrine & Metabolic Disorders Sourcebook
Environmentally Induced Disorders Sourcebook
Fitness & Exercise Sourcebook
Food & Animal Borne Diseases Sourcebook
Gastrointestinal Diseases & Disorders Sourcebook
Genetic Disorders Sourcebook
Head Trauma Sourcebook
Health Insurance Sourcebook
Immune System Disorders Sourcebook
Kidney & Urinary Tract Diseases & Disorders Sourcebook
Learning Disabilities Sourcebook
Men's Health Concerns Sourcebook
Mental Health Disorders Sourcebook
Ophthalmic Disorders Sourcebook
Oral Health Sourcebook
Pain Sourcebook
Pregnancy & Birth Sourcebook
Public Health Sourcebook
Rehabilitation Sourcebook
Respiratory Diseases & Disorders Sourcebook
Sexually Transmitted Diseases Sourcebook
Skin Disorders Sourcebook
Sleep Disorders Sourcebook
Sports Injuries Sourcebook
Substance Abuse Sourcebook
Women's Health Concerns Sourcebook

Health Reference Series

*Second Edition*

# Diabetes SOURCEBOOK

*Basic Consumer Health Information about Type 1 Diabetes (Insulin-Dependent or Juvenile-Onset Diabetes), Type 2 Diabetes (Noninsulin-Dependent or Adult-Onset Diabetes), Gestational Diabetes, and Related Disorders, Including Diabetes Prevalence Data, Management Issues, the Role of Diet and Exercise in Controlling Diabetes, Insulin and Other Diabetes Medicines, and Complications of Diabetes, Such as Eye Diseases, Periodontal Disease, Amputation and End-Stage Renal Disease; Along with Reports on Current Research Initiatives, a Glossary, and Resource Listings for Further Help and Information*

**Edited by**
**Karen Bellenir**

*Omnigraphics, Inc.*

**Penobscot Building / Detroit, MI 48226**

## Bibliographic Note



Beginning with books published in 1999, each new volume of the *Health Reference Series* will be individually titled and called a "First Edition." Subsequent updates will carry sequential edition numbers. To help avoid confusion and to provide maximum flexibility in our ability to respond to informational needs, the practice of consecutively numbering each volume will be discontinued.

Edited by Karen Bellenir

Peter D. Dresser, Managing Editor, *Health Reference Series*

Omnigraphics, Inc.

Tamekia Nichole Ashford, *Production Associate*
Matthew P. Barbour, *Manager, Production and Fulfillment*
Laurie Lanzen Harris, *Vice President, Editorial Director*
Peter E. Ruffner, *Vice President, Administration*
James A. Sellgren, *Vice President, Operations and Finance*
Jane J. Steele, *Marketing Consultant*

Robert R. Tyler, Executive Vice President and Associate Publisher
Frederick G. Ruffner, Jr., Publisher





Library of Congress Cataloging-in-Publication Data

Diabetes sourcebook : basic consumer health information about Type 1 diabetes (insulin-dependent or juvenile-onset diabetes), Type 2 diabetes (noninsulin-dependent or adult-onset diabetes), gestational diabetes, and related disorders . . . / edited by Karen Bellenir. -- 2nd ed.
p. cm. -- (Health reference series ; v. 3)
Includes bibliographical references and index.
ISBN 0-7808-0224-1 (lib. bdg. ; alk. paper)
1. Diabetes--Popular works. I. Bellenir, Karen. II. Series. (DNLM: 1. Diabetes Mellitus popular works. WK 801 D5408 1999 / W1 HE506R v.3 1999)
RC660.4.D56 1999
616.4'62--dc21
DNLM/DLC
for Library of Congress

98-45983
CIP

∞

This book is printed on acid-free paper meeting the ANSI Z39.48 Standard. The infinity symbol that appears above indicates that the paper in this book meets that standard.

Printed in the United States

# Table of Contents

## Part III: Diabetes Management



## Part IV: The Role of Diet and Exercise in Diabetes Management



## Part V: Insulin and Other Diabetes Medicines

## *Part VI: Complications of Diabetes*



## *Part VII: Research Initiatives*



## *Part VIII: Additional Help and Information*

# Preface

## About This Book

Since the publication of *Diabetes Sourcebook, First Edition* (1994), many changes have occurred in the field of diabetes care. New dietary guidelines have been published by the American Diabetes Association, new lower fasting plasma glucose levels have been recommended for use in diagnosing diabetes, and an international expert committee advocated a change in the names of the two main types of diabetes. Because the former names often caused confusion, the type of diabetes that was known as juvenile-onset diabetes, or insulin-dependent diabetes (IDDM), is now type 1 diabetes. The type of diabetes that was known as adult-onset diabetes, or noninsulin-dependent diabetes (NIDDM), is now type 2 diabetes. The new names reflect an effort to move away from basing the names on the treatment or the age of onset.

Experts also now suggest that all adults age 45 and older be tested for diabetes and that people under 45 be tested if they are at high risk. In 1995, the National Institute of Diabetes and Digestive and Kidney Diseases estimated that 16 million Americans had diabetes. Of these, eight million remained undiagnosed. Long term complications of untreated diabetes include:

- *Heart disease*—people with diabetes experience heart disease two to four times more commonly than the general population.
- *Stroke*—the risk of stroke is 2.5 times higher in people with diabetes.

- *High blood pressure*—60 to 64 percent of people with diabetes have high blood pressure.
- *Blindness*—diabetes is the leading cause of new cases of blindness among adults 20 to 74 years of age.
- *Kidney disease*—diabetes accounts for 36 percent of new cases of end-stage renal disease.
- *Nerve disease*—between 60 and 70 percent of people with diabetes experience nerve damage.
- *Amputations*—more than half of lower limb amputations in the U.S. occur among people with diabetes.
- *Dental disease*—periodontal disease occurs with greater frequency and severity in people with diabetes.

This sourcebook provides necessary information to help people understand the risk factors for diabetes, recognize the symptoms, and obtain appropriate care. It updates Omnigraphics' *Diabetes Sourcebook, First Edition*; 95% of the material presented has either been revised or is new to this edition.

## How to Use This Book

This book is divided into parts and chapters. Parts focus on broad areas of interest. Chapters are devoted to single topics within a part.

*Part I: Diabetes Prevalence* provides statistical information about diabetes and diabetic complications in the United States. Individual chapters highlight specific minority populations experiencing a high incidence of diabetes.

*Part II: Types of Diabetes and Related Disorders* describes the risk factors for and symptoms of type 1 diabetes (insulin-dependent or juvenile-onset diabetes), type 2 diabetes (noninsulin-dependent or adult-onset diabetes), and gestational diabetes. Information is also provided about pre-existing diabetes in pregnant women, hypoglycemia, and syndrome X—a constellation of disorders that may lead to type 2 diabetes.

*Part III: Diabetes Management* offers practical help to people with diabetes. It describes the day-to-day routines that can help manage the disease and reduce the possibility of complications. A special chapter is devoted to the concerns frequently expressed by parents of diabetic children.

*Part IV: The Role of Diet and Exercise in Diabetes Management* explores the relationship between diabetes management and the lifestyle factors of diet and exercise. It includes specific recommendations and offers guidance on implementing food and exercise plans. Additional information on these important topics can be found in *Diet and Nutrition Sourcebook* and *Fitness and Exercise Sourcebook*. Both volumes are part of Omnigraphics' *Health Reference Series.*

*Part V: Insulin and Other Diabetes Medicines* provides information about different types of insulin, insulin delivery systems, and other diabetes medications including sulfonylureas, biguanides, alpha-glucosidase inhibitors, and thiazolidinediones. A chapter explaining drug interactions of special concern to diabetics is also included.

*Part VI: Complications of Diabetes* describes some of the major complications of diabetes, explains how they develop, and offers information about their treatment.

*Part VII: Research Initiatives* reports on some important findings in diabetes research and describes promising avenues for further investigation.

*Part VIII: Additional Help and Information* provides a dictionary of diabetes-related terminology, bibliographic information for diabetic cookbooks and other resources, suggestions on locating sources of financial help for diabetes care, and a directory of diabetes organizations.

## Bibliographic Note

This volume contains documents and excerpts from publications issued by the following U.S. government agencies: Centers for Disease Control and Prevention (CDC); National Center for Research Resources (NCRR); National Diabetes Information Clearinghouse (NDIC); National Eye Institute (NEI); National Institute of Child Health and Human Development (NICHD); National Institute of Dental Research (NIDR); National Institute of Diabetes and Digestive and Kidney Diseases (NIDDK); U.S. Department of Health and Human Services (DHHS); and the U.S. Food and Drug Administration (FDA).

In addition, this volume contains copyrighted documents from the following organizations: American Academy of Family Physicians; American Diabetes Association; Diabetes Prevention Program at the University of Washington; Diabetes Research Institute at the University of Miami School of Medicine; Juvenile Diabetes Foundation International; National Kidney Foundation; and the University of Colorado Health Sciences Center. Copyrighted articles from *Diabetes Care*, *Diabetes Forecast*, and *Diabetes Self-Management* are also included. Full citation information is provided on the first page of each chapter.


## Acknowledgements

In addition to the many organizations listed above who provided the material presented in this volume, special thanks are due to researchers Margaret Mary Missar and Jenifer Swanson, permissions specialist Maria Franklin, verification assistant Dawn Matthews, and to Bruce Bellenir, whose contributions far exceed the confines of any title or label.


## Note from the Editor

This book is part of Omnigraphics' *Health Reference Series*. The series provides basic consumer health information about a broad range of medical concerns. It is not intended to serve as a tool for diagnosing illness, in prescribing treatments, or as a substitute for the physician/patient relationship. All persons concerned about medical symptoms or the possibility of disease are encouraged to seek professional care from an appropriate health care provider.

## Health Reference Series *Update Policy*

The inaugural book in the *Health Reference Series* was the first edition of *Cancer Sourcebook* published in 1992. Since then, the *Series* has been enthusiastically received by librarians and in the medical community. In order to maintain the standard of providing high-quality health information for the lay person, the editorial staff at Omnigraphics felt it was necessary to implement a policy of updating volumes when warranted.

Medical researchers have been making tremendous strides, and the challenge to stay current with the most recent advances is one our editors take seriously. Each decision to update a volume will be made on an individual basis. Some of the considerations will include how much new information is available and the feedback we receive from people who use the books. If there's a topic you would like to see added to the update list, or an area of medical concern you feel has not been adequately addressed, please write to:

Editor
*Health Reference Series*
Omnigraphics, Inc.
2500 Penobscot Bldg.
Detroit, MI 48226

The commitment to providing on-going coverage of important medical developments has also led to some technical changes in the *Health Reference Series*. Beginning with books published in 1999, each new volume will be individually titled and called a "First Edition." Subsequent updates will carry sequential edition numbers. To help avoid confusion and to provide maximum flexibility in our ability to respond to informational needs, the practice of consecutively numbering each volume will be discontinued.

# Part One

# Diabetes Prevalence

## Chapter 1

# *Diabetes Overview*

Almost every one of us knows someone who has diabetes. An estimated 16 million people in the United States have diabetes mellitus—a serious, lifelong condition. About half of these people do not know they have diabetes and are not under care for the disorder. Each year, about 650,000 people are diagnosed with diabetes.

Although diabetes occurs most often in older adults, it is one of the most common chronic disorders in children in the United States. About 127,000 children and teenagers age 19 and younger have diabetes.

### *What Is Diabetes?*

Diabetes is a disorder of metabolism—the way our bodies use digested food for growth and energy. Most of the food we eat is broken down by the digestive juices into a simple sugar called glucose. Glucose is the main source of fuel for the body.

After digestion, the glucose passes into our bloodstream where it is available for body cells to use for growth and energy. For the glucose to get into the cells, insulin must be present. Insulin is a hormone produced by the pancreas, a large gland behind the stomach.

When we eat, the pancreas is supposed to automatically produce the right amount of insulin to move the glucose from our blood into

---

National Institute of Diabetes and Digestive and Kidney Diseases (NIDDK), NIH Pub. No. 96-3873, October 1995.

our cells. In people with diabetes, however, the pancreas either produces little or no insulin, or the body cells do not respond to the insulin that is produced. As a result, glucose builds up in the blood, overflows into the urine, and passes out of the body. Thus, the body loses its main source of fuel even though the blood contains large amounts of glucose.

## What Are the Different Types of Diabetes?

The three main types of diabetes are:

- Insulin-dependent diabetes mellitus (IDDM) or Type I diabetes
- Noninsulin-dependent diabetes mellitus (NIDDM) or Type II diabetes
- Gestational diabetes.

### Insulin-Dependent Diabetes

Insulin-dependent diabetes is considered an autoimmune disease. An autoimmune disease results when the body's system for fighting infection (the immune system) turns against a part of the body. In diabetes, the immune system attacks the insulin-producing beta cells in the pancreas and destroys them. The pancreas then produces little or no insulin.

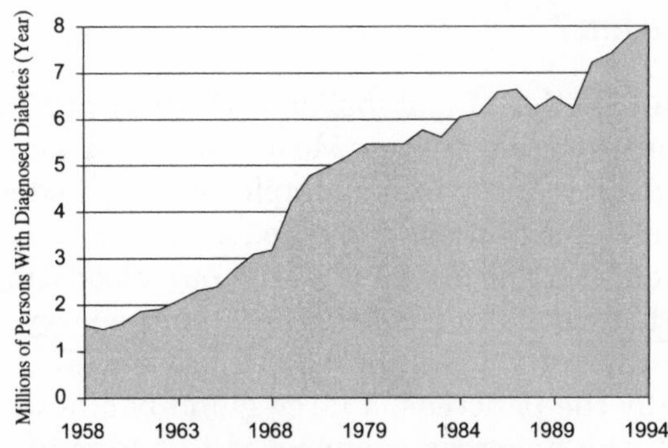


***Figure 1.1.** Prevalence of Diagnosed Diabetes. Source: The data for this chart comes from* Diabetes in America. *2nd Edition (p. 63) by National Institutes of Health, National Institute of Diabetes and Digestive and Kidney Diseases, 1995.*

Someone with IDDM needs daily injections of insulin to live. At present, scientists do not know exactly what causes the body's immune system to attack the beta cells, but they believe that both genetic factors and viruses are involved. IDDM accounts for about 5 to 10 percent of diagnosed diabetes in the United States.

IDDM develops most often in children and young adults, but the disorder can appear at any age. Symptoms of IDDM usually develop over a short period, although beta cell destruction can begin months, even years, earlier.

Symptoms include increased thirst and urination, constant hunger, weight loss, blurred vision, and extreme tiredness. If not diagnosed and treated with insulin, a person can lapse into a life-threatening coma.

### *Noninsulin-Dependent Diabetes*

The most common form of diabetes is noninsulin-dependent diabetes. About 90 to 95 percent of people with diabetes have NIDDM. This form of diabetes usually develops in adults over the age of 40 and is most common among adults over age 55. About 80 percent of people with NIDDM are overweight.

In NIDDM, the pancreas usually produces insulin, but for some reason, the body cannot use the insulin effectively. The end result is the same as for IDDM—an unhealthy buildup of glucose in the blood and an inability of the body to make efficient use of its main source of fuel.

The symptoms of NIDDM develop gradually and are not as noticeable as in IDDM. Symptoms include feeling tired or ill, frequent urination (especially at night), unusual thirst, weight loss, blurred vision, frequent infections, and slow healing of sores.

### *Gestational Diabetes*

Gestational diabetes develops or is discovered during pregnancy. This type usually disappears when the pregnancy is over, but women who have had gestational diabetes have a greater risk of developing NIDDM later in their lives.

## *What Is the Scope and Impact of Diabetes?*

Diabetes is widely recognized as one of the leading causes of death and disability in the United States. According to death certificate data, diabetes contributed to the deaths of more than 169,000 persons in 1992.

Diabetes is associated with long-term complications that affect almost every major part of the body. It contributes to blindness, heart disease, strokes, kidney failure, amputations, and nerve damage. Uncontrolled diabetes can complicate pregnancy, and birth defects are more common in babies born to women with diabetes.

Diabetes cost the United States $92 billion in 1992. Indirect costs, including disability payments, time lost from work, and premature death, totaled $47 billion; medical costs for diabetes care, including hospitalizations, medical care, and treatment supplies, totaled $45 billion.

## Who Gets Diabetes?

Diabetes is not contagious. People cannot "catch" it from each other. However, certain factors can increase one's risk of developing diabetes. People who have family members with diabetes (especially NIDDM), who are overweight, or who are African American, Hispanic, or Native American are all at greater risk of developing diabetes.

IDDM occurs equally among males and females, but is more common in whites than in nonwhites. Data from the World Health Organization's Multinational Project for Childhood Diabetes indicate that IDDM is rare in most Asian, African, and Native American populations. On the other hand, some northern European countries, including Finland and Sweden, have high rates of IDDM. The reasons for these differences are not known.

NIDDM is more common in older people, especially older women who are overweight, and occurs more often among African Americans, Hispanics, and Native Americans. Compared with non-Hispanic whites, diabetes rates are about 60 percent higher in African Americans and 110 to 120 percent higher in Mexican Americans and Puerto Ricans. Native Americans have the highest rates of diabetes in the world. Among Pima Indians living in the United States, for example, half of all adults have NIDDM. The prevalence of diabetes is likely to increase because older people, Hispanics, and other minority groups make up the fastest growing segments of the U.S. population.

## How Is Diabetes Managed?

Before the discovery of insulin in 1921, all people with IDDM died within a few years after the appearance of the disease. Although insulin is not considered a cure for diabetes, its discovery was the first major breakthrough in diabetes treatment.

Today, daily injections of insulin are the basic therapy for IDDM. Insulin injections must be balanced with meals and daily activities, and glucose levels must be closely monitored through frequent blood sugar testing.

Diet, exercise, and blood testing for glucose are also the basis for management of NIDDM. In addition, some people with NIDDM take oral drugs or insulin to lower their blood glucose levels.

People with diabetes must take responsibility for their day-to-day care. Much of the daily care involves trying to keep blood sugar levels from going too low or too high. When blood sugar levels drop too low—a condition known as hypoglycemia—a person can become nervous, shaky, and confused. Judgment can be impaired. Eventually, the person could pass out. The treatment for low blood sugar is to eat or drink something with sugar in it.

On the other hand, a person can become very ill if blood sugar levels rise too high, a condition known as hyperglycemia. Hypoglycemia and hyperglycemia, which can occur in people with IDDM or NIDDM, are both potentially life-threatening emergencies.

People with diabetes should be treated by a doctor who monitors their diabetes control and checks for complications. Doctors who specialize in diabetes are called endocrinologists or diabetologists. In addition, people with diabetes often see ophthalmologists for eye examinations, podiatrists for routine foot care, dietitians for help in planning meals, and diabetes educators for instruction in day-today care.

The goal of diabetes management is to keep blood glucose levels as close to the normal (nondiabetic) range as safely possible. A recent Government study, sponsored by the National Institute of Diabetes and Digestive and Kidney Diseases (NIDDK), proved that keeping blood sugar levels as close to normal as safely possible reduces the risk of developing major complications of diabetes.

The 10-year study, called the Diabetes Control and Complications Trial (DCCT), was completed in 1993 and included 1,441 people with IDDM. The study compared the effect of two treatment approaches—intensive management and standard management—on the development and progression of eye, kidney, and nerve complications of diabetes. Researchers found that study participants who maintained lower levels of blood glucose through intensive management had significantly lower rates of these complications. Researchers believe that DCCT findings have important implications for the treatment of NIDDM, as well as IDDM.

## What Is the Status of Diabetes Research?

NIDDK supports basic and clinical research in its own laboratories and in research centers and hospitals throughout the United States. It also gathers and analyzes statistics about diabetes. Other institutes at the National Institutes of Health also carry out research on diabetes-related eye diseases, heart and vascular complications, pregnancy, and dental problems.

Other Government agencies that sponsor diabetes programs are the Centers for Disease Control and Prevention, the Indian Health Service, the Health Resources and Services Administration, the Bureau of Veterans Affairs, and the Department of Defense.

Many organizations outside of the Government support diabetes research and education activities. These organizations include the American Diabetes Association, the Juvenile Diabetes Foundation International, and the American Association of Diabetes Educators.

In recent years, advances in diabetes research have led to better ways to manage diabetes and treat its complications. Major advances include:

- New forms of purified insulin, such as human insulin produced through genetic engineering
- Better ways for doctors to monitor blood glucose levels and for people with diabetes to test their own blood glucose levels at home
- Development of external and implantable insulin pumps that deliver appropriate amounts of insulin, replacing daily injections
- Laser treatment for diabetic eye disease, reducing the risk of blindness
- Successful transplantation of kidneys in people whose own kidneys fail because of diabetes
- Better ways of managing diabetic pregnancies, improving chances of successful outcomes
- New drugs to treat NIDDM and better ways to manage this form of diabetes through weight control
- Evidence that intensive management of blood glucose reduces and may prevent development of microvascular complications of diabetes

- Demonstration that antihypertensive drugs called ACE-inhibitors prevent or delay kidney failure in people with diabetes.

## What Will the Future Bring?

In the future, it may be possible to administer insulin through nasal sprays or in the form of a pill or patch. Devices that can "read" blood glucose levels without having to prick a finger to get a blood sample are also being developed.

Researchers continue to search for the cause or causes of diabetes and ways to prevent and cure the disorder. Scientists are looking for genes that may be involved in NIDDM and IDDM. Some genetic markers for IDDM have been identified, and it is now possible to screen relatives of people with IDDM to see if they are at risk for diabetes.

The new Diabetes Prevention Trial—Type I, sponsored by NIDDK, identifies relatives at risk for developing IDDM and treats them with low doses of insulin or with oral insulin-like agents in the hope of preventing IDDM. Similar research is carried out at other medical centers throughout the world.

Transplantation of the pancreas or insulin-producing beta cells offers the best hope of cure for people with IDDM. Some pancreas transplants have been successful. However, people who have transplants must take powerful drugs to prevent rejection of the transplanted organ. These drugs are costly and may eventually cause serious health problems.

Scientists are working to develop less harmful drugs and better methods of transplanting pancreatic tissue to prevent rejection by the body. Using techniques of bioengineering, researchers are also trying to create artificial islet cells that secrete insulin in response to increased sugar levels in the blood.

For NIDDM, the focus is on ways to prevent diabetes. Preventive approaches include identifying people at high risk for the disorder and encouraging them to lose weight, exercise more, and follow a healthy diet. The Diabetes Prevention Program, another new NIDDK project, will focus on preventing the disorder in high-risk populations.

## Points to Remember

### *What is diabetes?*

- A disorder of metabolism—the way the body digests food for energy and growth.

### *What are the different types of diabetes?*

- Insulin-dependent diabetes (IDDM)
- Noninsulin-dependent diabetes (NIDDM)
- Gestational diabetes.

### *What is the scope and impact of diabetes?*

- Affects 16 million people
- A leading cause of death and disability
- Costs $92 billion per year.

### *Who gets diabetes?*

- People of any age
- More common in older people, African Americans, Hispanics, and Native Americans.

Chapter 2

# National Diabetes Fact Sheet

## What Is Diabetes?

Diabetes mellitus is a group of diseases characterized by high levels of blood glucose resulting from defects in insulin secretion, insulin action, or both. Diabetes can be associated with serious complications and premature death, but persons with diabetes can take measures to reduce the likelihood of such occurrences.

## The Four Types of Diabetes

- **Type 1 diabetes** was previously called insulin-dependent diabetes mellitus (IDDM) or juvenile-onset diabetes. Type 1 diabetes may account for 5% to 10% of all diagnosed cases of diabetes. Risk factors are less well defined for type 1 diabetes than for type 2 diabetes, but autoimmune, genetic, and environmental factors are involved in the development of this type of diabetes.
- **Type 2 diabetes** was previously called non-insulin dependent diabetes mellitus (NIDDM) or adult-onset diabetes. Type 2 diabetes may account for about 90% to 95% of all diagnosed cases of diabetes. Risk factors for type 2 diabetes include older age,

---

Centers for Disease Control and Prevention (CDC). National Diabetes Fact Sheet: National Estimates and general information on diabetes in the United States. Atlanta, GA: U.S. Department of Health and Human Services, Centers for Disease Control and Prevention, 1997.

obesity, family history of diabetes, prior history of gestational diabetes, impaired glucose tolerance, physical inactivity, and race/ethnicity. African Americans, Hispanic/Latino Americans, American Indians, and some Asian Americans and Pacific Islanders are at particularly high risk for type 2 diabetes.

- **Gestational diabetes** develops in 2% to 5% of all pregnancies but disappears when a pregnancy is over. Gestational diabetes occurs more frequently in African Americans, Hispanic/Latino Americans, American Indians, and persons with a family history of diabetes. Obesity is also associated with higher risk. Women who have had gestational diabetes are at increased risk for later developing type 2 diabetes. In some studies, nearly 40% of women with a history of gestational diabetes developed diabetes in the future.
- **"Other specific types"** of diabetes result from specific genetic syndromes, surgery, drugs, malnutrition, infections, and other illnesses. Such types of diabetes may account for 1% to 2% of all diagnosed cases of diabetes.

## New Diagnostic Criteria for Diabetes

The new diagnostic criteria for diabetes include the following changes. (For further information about the new diagnostic criteria for diabetes, please refer the Report of the Expert Committee on the Diagnosis and Classification of Diabetes Mellitus. *Diabetes Care* 1997 July;20(7): 1183-97.

- The routine diagnostic test for diabetes is now a fasting plasma glucose test rather than the previously preferred oral glucose tolerance test. (However, in certain clinical circumstances, physicians may still choose to perform the more difficult and costly oral glucose tolerance test.)
- A confirmed (except in certain specified circumstances, abnormal tests must be confirmed by repeat testing on another day) fasting plasma glucose value of greater than or equal to 126 milligrams/deciliter (mg/dL) indicates a diagnosis of diabetes. Previously, a value of greater than or equal to 140 mg/dL had been required for diagnosis.
- In the presence of symptoms of diabetes, a confirmed (except in certain specified circumstances, abnormal tests must be confirmed

by repeat testing on another day) nonfasting plasma glucose value of greater than or equal to 200 mg/dL indicates a diagnosis of diabetes.

- When a doctor chooses to perform an oral glucose tolerance test (by administering 75 grams of anhydrous glucose dissolved in water, in accordance with World Health Organization standards, and then measuring the plasma glucose concentration 2 hours later), a confirmed (except in certain specified circumstances, abnormal tests must be confirmed by repeat testing on another day) glucose value of greater than or equal to 200 mg/dL indicates a diagnosis of diabetes.
- In pregnant women, different requirements are used to identify the presence of gestational diabetes.

## *Treatment of Diabetes*

Diabetes knowledge, treatment, and prevention strategies advance daily. Treatment is aimed at keeping blood glucose near normal levels at all times. Training in self-management is integral to the treatment of diabetes. Treatment must be individualized and must address medical, psychosocial, and lifestyle issues.

- **Treatment of type 1 diabetes:** Lack of insulin production by the pancreas makes type 1 diabetes particularly difficult to control. Treatment requires a strict regimen that typically includes a carefully calculated diet, planned physical activity, home blood glucose testing several times a day, and multiple daily insulin injections.
- **Treatment of type 2 diabetes:** Treatment typically includes diet control, exercise, home blood glucose testing, and in some cases, oral medication and/or insulin. Approximately 40% of people with type 2 diabetes require insulin injections.

## *Impaired Fasting Glucose*

Impaired fasting glucose is a new diagnostic category in which persons have fasting plasma glucose values of 110-125 mg/dL. These glucose values are greater than the level considered normal but less than the level that is diagnostic of diabetes. It is estimated that 13.4 million persons, 7.0% of the population, have impaired fasting glucose. Scientists are trying to learn how to predict which of these persons will go on to develop diabetes and how to prevent such progression.

## National Diabetes Information Clearinghouse

National Diabetes Information Clearinghouse
1 Information Way
Bethesda, MD 20892-3560
E-mail: ndic@info.niddk.nih.gov

The National Diabetes Information Clearinghouse (NDIC) is a service of the National Institute of Diabetes and Digestive and Kidney Diseases (NIDDK). NIDDK is part of the National Institutes of Health under the U.S. Public Health Service. Established in 1978, the clearinghouse provides information about diabetes to people with diabetes and their families, health care professionals, and the public. NDIC answers inquiries; develops, reviews, and distributes publications; and works closely with professional and patient organizations and government agencies to coordinate resources about diabetes.

Publications produced by the clearinghouse are reviewed carefully for scientific accuracy, content, and readability.

## Chapter 3

# *Diabetes Statistics*

### *Prevalence of Diabetes*

**Total:** 15.7 million people—5.9% of the population—have diabetes.
**Diagnosed:** 10.3 million people
**Undiagnosed:** 5.4 million people

For further information on prevalence, see the Appendix section in this chapter.

### *Incidence of Diabetes*

**New cases diagnosed per year:** 798,000

### *Deaths Among Persons with Diabetes*

- Studies have found death rates to be twice as high among middle-aged people with diabetes as among middle-aged people without diabetes.
- Based on death certificate data, diabetes contributed to187,800 deaths in 1995.
- Diabetes was the seventh leading cause of death listed on U.S. death certificates in 1995, according to CDC's National Center for Health Statistics.

---

NIH Publication No. 98-3926, last updated February 18, 1998.

- Diabetes is believed to be underreported on death certificates, both as a condition and as a cause of death.

## Prevalence of Diabetes by Age

**Age 65 years or older:** 6.3 million. *18.4% of all people in this age group have diabetes.*

**Age 20 years or older:** 15.6 million. *8.2% of all people in this age group have diabetes.*

**Under age 20: 123,000.** *0.16% of all people in this age group have diabetes.*

## Prevalence of Diabetes by Sex in People 20 Years or Older

**Men:** 7.5 million. *8.2% of all men have diabetes.*

**Women:** 8.1 million. *8.2% of all women have diabetes.*

These figures do not include the approximately 123,000 cases of diabetes in children and teenagers in the United States.

## Prevalence of Diabetes by Race/Ethnicity in People 20 Years or Older

**Non-Hispanic whites:** 11.3 million. 7.8% of all non-Hispanic whites have diabetes.

**Non-Hispanic blacks:** 2.3 million. 10.8% of all non-Hispanic blacks have diabetes. On average, non-Hispanic blacks are 1.7 times as likely to have diabetes as non-Hispanic whites of similar age.

**Mexican Americans:** 1.2 million. 10.6% of all Mexican Americans have diabetes. On average, Mexican Americans are 1.9 times as likely to have diabetes as non-Hispanic whites of similar age.

**Other Hispanic/Latino Americans:** On average, Hispanic/Latino Americans are almost twice as likely to have diabetes as non-Hispanic whites of similar age. (Sufficient data are not currently available to derive more specific estimates for 1997.)

**American Indians and Alaska Natives:** Prevalence varies among tribes, bands, pueblos, and villages, and ranges from <5% to

50% for diagnosed diabetes. There are more than 550 federally recognized tribes, bands, pueblos, and villages in the United States.

**Asian Americans and Pacific Islanders:** Prevalence data for diabetes among Asian Americans and Pacific Islanders are limited. Some groups within this population are at increased risk for diabetes. For example, data collected from 1988 to 1995 suggest that Native Hawaiians are twice as likely to have diagnosed diabetes as white residents of Hawaii.

These figures do not include the approximately 123,000 cases of diabetes in children and teenagers in the United States.

## Complications of Diabetes

### *Heart Disease*

- Heart disease is the leading cause of diabetes-related deaths. Adults with diabetes have heart disease death rates about 2 to 4 times as high as that of adults without diabetes.

### *Stroke*

- The risk of stroke is 2 to 4 times higher in people with diabetes.

### *High Blood Pressure*

- An estimated 60% to 65% of people with diabetes have high blood pressure.

### *Blindness*

- Diabetes is the leading cause of new cases of blindness in adults 20 to 74 years old.
- Diabetic retinopathy causes from 12,000 to 24,000 new cases of blindness each year.

### *Kidney Disease*

- Diabetes is the leading cause of end-stage renal disease, accounting for about 40% of new cases.
- 27,851 people with diabetes developed end-stage renal disease in 1995.

- In 1995, a total of 98,872 people with diabetes underwent dialysis or kidney transplantation.

### Nervous System Disease

- About 60% to 70% of people with diabetes have mild to severe forms of nervous system damage (which often includes impaired sensation or pain in the feet or hands, slowed digestion of food in the stomach, carpal tunnel syndrome, and other nerve problems).
- Severe forms of diabetic nerve disease are a major contributing cause of lower extremity amputations.

### Amputations

- More than half of lower limb amputations in the United States occur among people with diabetes.
- From 1993 to 1995, about 67,000 amputations were performed each year among people with diabetes.

### Dental Disease

- Periodontal disease (a type of gum disease that can lead to tooth loss) occurs with greater frequency and severity among people with diabetes. Periodontal disease has been reported to occur among 30% of people aged 19 years or older with type 1 diabetes.

### Complications of Pregnancy

- The rate of major congenital malformations in babies born to women with preexisting diabetes varies from 0% to 5% among women who receive preconception care to 10% among women who do not receive preconception care.
- Between 3% to 5% of pregnancies among women with diabetes result in death of the newborn; the rate for women who do not have diabetes is 1.5%.

### Other Complications

- Diabetes can directly cause acute life-threatening events, such as diabetic ketoacidosis and hyperosmolar nonketotic coma.

(Diabetic ketoacidosis and hyperosmolar nonketotic coma are medical conditions that can result from biochemical imbalance in uncontrolled diabetes.)

- People with diabetes are more susceptible to many other illnesses. For example, they are more likely to die of pneumonia or influenza than people who do not have diabetes.

## Cost

**Total (direct and indirect):** $98.2 billion (United States, 1992)
**Direct medical costs:** $44.1 billion
**Indirect costs:** $54.1 billion (disability, work loss, premature mortality)

## Appendix

### *How were the estimates in this fact sheet derived?*

Periodically, the federal government conducts surveys to determine the health of Americans. Such surveys involve questionnaires and medical tests. The diabetes prevalence and incidence estimates presented in this fact sheet were developed by analyzing the newest available national survey data and then adjusting for changes in the population based on 1997 census estimates. The prevalence of diagnosed diabetes represents the number who said they had diabetes. The prevalence of undiagnosed diabetes represents the number of people who said they did not have diabetes, but when given a fasting plasma glucose test, they did in fact have abnormally elevated blood glucose levels (defined as fasting plasma glucose levels greater than or equal to 126 mg/dL). Other estimates presented in this fact sheet were based on individual surveys, research projects, and registry data. A listing of references and additional data sources are at the end of this chapter.

### *Has the number of persons with diabetes changed since the previous National Diabetes Fact Sheet, which was issued in 1995?*

Between the 1995 and 1997 fact sheets, the number of persons with diagnosed diabetes increased from 8 million to10.3 million, but the number of persons with undiagnosed diabetes decreased. For the 1995 National Diabetes Fact Sheet, the number of persons with undiagnosed diabetes was estimated from research using the oral glucose tolerance test to identify undiagnosed diabetes. In contrast, for the 1997 National Diabetes Fact Sheet, the number of persons with undiagnosed diabetes was estimated from research using the fasting plasma glucose test, according to recently enacted recommendations. These tests are not equivalent, however, and fewer cases of undiagnosed diabetes are identified using the fasting plasma glucose test under current recommendations.

An enhanced national effort to identify previously undiagnosed persons may also have contributed to a decrease in the number of persons with undiagnosed diabetes. Continued efforts to identify persons with undiagnosed diabetes, the implementation of new guidelines for screening, and the use of an easier and less expensive diagnostic test are all likely to lead to even further decreases in the number of persons with undiagnosed diabetes and increases in the number of persons with diagnosed diabetes.

## References

American Diabetes Association. Economic Consequences of Diabetes Mellitus in the U.S. in 1997. *Diabetes Care* 1998;21(2):296-309.

National Diabetes Data Group, National Institutes of Health. *Diabetes in America*, 2nd Edition. Bethesda, MD: National Institutes of Health, 1995. NIH Publication No. 95-1468.

Report of the Expert Committee on the Diagnosis and Classification of Diabetes Mellitus. *Diabetes Care* 1997 July; 20(7):1183-97.

Valway S, Freeman W, Kaufman S, Welty T, Helgerson SD, Gohdes D. Prevalence of diagnosed diabetes among American Indians and Alaska Natives, 1987. *Diabetes Care* 1993;16 (Suppl 1):271-276.

U.S. Department of Health and Human Services. *Physical activity and health: a report of the Surgeon General*. Atlanta, GA: U.S. Department of Health and Human Services, Centers for Disease Control and Prevention, National Center for Chronic Disease Prevention and Health Promotion, 1996.

U.S. Renal Data System. *USRDS 1997 Annual Data Report*. Bethesda, MD: National Institutes of Health, National Institute of Diabetes and Digestive and Kidney Disease, 1997.

## Additional Sources

Calculations were performed by the National Institutes of Health and the Centers for Disease Control and Prevention using data from various surveys including the Third National Health and Nutrition Examination Survey (NHANES III), the National Health Interview Survey (NHIS), and U.S. Census estimates for current population. The national prevalence estimates for diabetes were based on Harris MI et al., *Diabetes Care* 1998; 21: 514-524.

Information about Native Hawaiians was provided by the Hawaii Diabetes Control Program and is based on Wen M, Unpublished Analysis of Data from the Behavioral Risk Factor Surveillance System (BRFSS) from 1988-1995.

## Acknowledgments

The following organizations collaborated in compiling the information for this text:

**American Association of Diabetes Educators**
http://www.diabetesnet.com/aade.html

**American Diabetes Association**
http://www.diabetes.org

**Centers for Disease Control and Prevention**
http://www.cdc.gov/diabetes

**Department of Veterans Affairs**
http://www.va.gov/health/diabetes/

**Health Resources and Services Administration**
http://www.hrsa.dhhs.gov

**Indian Health Service**
http://www.ihs.gov/IHSMAIN.html

**Juvenile Diabetes Foundation International**
http://www.jdfcure.com

**National Diabetes Education Program**
http://www.niddk.nih.gov/health/diabetes/ndep/ndep.htm

**National Institute of Diabetes and Digestive and Kidney Disease of the National Institutes of Health**
http://www.niddk.nih.gov

U.S. Department of Health and Human Services
**Office of Minority Health**
http://www.omrhc.gov

## Chapter 4

# *Diabetes in African Americans*

Today, diabetes mellitus is one of the most serious health challenges facing the more than 30 million African Americans. The following statistics illustrate the magnitude of this disease among African Americans.

- In 1993, 1.3 million African Americans were known to have diabetes. This is almost three times the number of African Americans who were diagnosed with diabetes in 1963. The actual number of African Americans who have diabetes is probably more than twice the number diagnosed because previous research indicates that for every African American diagnosed with diabetes there is at least one undiagnosed case.
- For every white American who gets diabetes, 1.6 African Americans get diabetes.
- One in four black women, 55 years of age or older, has diabetes. (Among African Americans, women are more likely to have diabetes than men.)
- Twenty-five percent of blacks between the ages of 65 and 74 have diabetes.
- African Americans with diabetes are more likely to develop diabetes complications and experience greater disability from the complications than white Americans with diabetes.

---

National Institute of Diabetes and Digestive and Kidney Diseases (NIDDK), NIH Pub. No. 97-3266, March 1997.

## How Many African Americans Have Diabetes?

National Health Interview Surveys (NHIS) conducted between 1963 and 1990 show that African Americans have a rising prevalence of diabetes. (Prevalence is the percentage of cases in a population.) Most African Americans with diabetes have Type 2, or noninsulin-dependent diabetes. Type 2 diabetes usually develops after age 40. However, in high-risk populations, susceptible people may develop it at a younger age. A small number of African Americans have Type 1 or insulin-dependent diabetes, which usually develops before age 20.

NHIS conducted from 1991 to 1992 indicate higher rates of diabetes among African Americans than among white Americans. At age 45 or older, the prevalence of diabetes is 1.4 to 2.3 times as frequent in blacks as in whites. The greatest difference seen in NHIS was among people aged 65 to 74. Figure 4.1 details these 1991-92 NHIS statistics. Statistics collected in 1993 indicate that in this age group, 17.4 percent of black Americans had diagnosed diabetes, compared to 9.5 percent of white Americans.

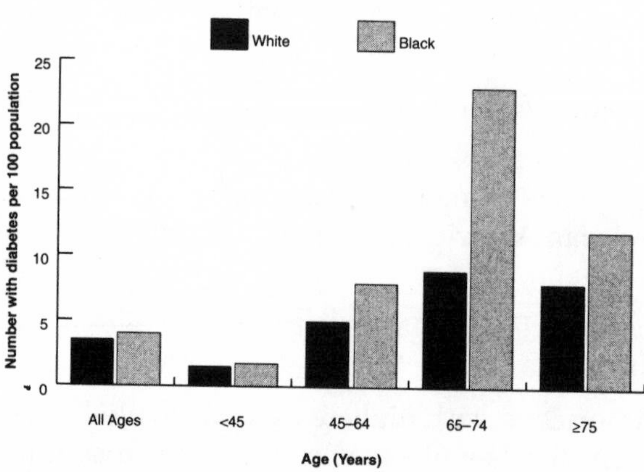


***Figure 4.1.** Prevalence of Diagnosed Diabetes Among Blacks and Whites, U.S., 1991-92. Source:* Diabetes in America, *616.*

## What Risk Factors Increase the Chance of Developing Type 2 Diabetes?

The frequency of diabetes in black adults is influenced by the same risk factors that are associated with Type 2 diabetes in other populations. Three categories of risk factors increase the chance of developing Type 2 diabetes in African Americans. The first is genetics, which includes inherited traits and group ancestry. The second is medical risk factors, including impaired glucose tolerance, hyperinsulinemia and insulin resistance, and obesity. The third is lifestyle risk factors, including physical activity.

### *Genetic Risk Factors*

**Inherited Traits.** Researchers suggest that African Americans—and recent African immigrants to America—have inherited a "thrifty gene" from their African ancestors. Years ago, this gene enabled Africans, during "feast and famine" cycles, to use food energy more efficiently when food was scarce. Today, with fewer "feast and famine" cycles, the thrifty gene that developed for survival may instead make weight control more difficult. This genetic predisposition, along with impaired glucose tolerance (IGT), often occurs together with the genetic tendency toward high blood pressure.

**Group Ancestry.** African-American ancestry is also an important predictor of the development of diabetes. To understand how rates of diabetes vary among African Americans, it is important to look at the historical origins of black populations in America. Genetic predisposition to diabetes is based, in part, on a person's lineage. The African-American population formed from a genetic admixture across African ethnic groups and with other racial groups, primarily European and North American Caucasian.

### *Medical Risk Factors*

**Impaired Glucose Tolerance (IGT).** People with IGT have higher-than-normal blood glucose levels—but not high enough to be diagnosed as diabetes. Some argue that IGT is actually an early stage of diabetes. African-American men and women differ in their development of IGT. As black men grow older, they develop IGT at about the same rates as white American men and women. African-American women, who have higher rates of diabetes risk factors, convert more rapidly from IGT to overt diabetes than black men and white women and men.

**Hyperinsulinemia and Insulin Resistance.** Higher-than-normal levels of fasting insulin, or hyperinsulinemia, are associated with an increased risk of developing Type 2 diabetes. It is known that hyperinsulinemia often predates diabetes by several years. One study showed a higher rate of hyperinsulinemia in African-American adolescents in comparison to white American adolescents. To date, insufficient information is available on the relationship between insulin resistance or hyperinsulinemia and the development of Type 2 diabetes in African Americans.

**Obesity.** Obesity is a major medical risk factor for diabetes in African Americans. The National Health and Nutrition Survey (NHANESII), conducted between 1976 and 1980, showed substantially higher rates of obesity in African Americans aged 20 to 74 years of age who had diabetes, compared to those who did not have diabetes. NHANESII also showed higher rates of obesity among African-American women and men than white Americans without diabetes. (See Figure 4.2.)

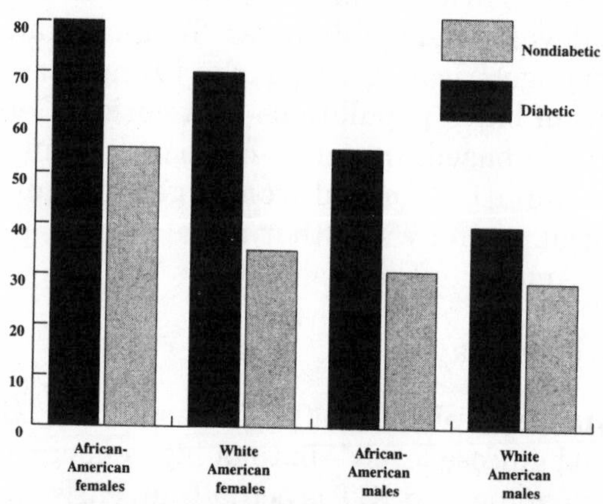


African-American men and women in the United States have higher rates of obesity, with or without diabetes. Obesity is a risk factor for Type 2 and many of its complications. (NHANES)

***Figure 4.2.*** *Obesity in African Americans and White Americans, Males and Females, With and Without Diabetes (Percent of Population).*

Some recent evidence shows that the degree to which obesity is a risk factor for diabetes may depend on the location of the excess weight. Truncal, or upper body obesity, is a greater risk factor for Type 2 diabetes, compared to excess weight carried below the waist. One study showed that African Americans have a greater tendency to develop upper-body obesity, which increased their risk of Type 2.

Although African Americans have higher rates of obesity, researchers do not believe that obesity alone accounts for their higher prevalence of diabetes. Even when compared to white Americans with the same levels of obesity, age, and socioeconomic status, African Americans still have higher rates of diabetes. Other factors, yet to be understood, appear to be at work.

### *Lifestyle Risk Factors*

**Physical Activity.** Physical activity is a strong protective factor against Type 2 diabetes. Researchers suspect that a lack of exercise is one factor contributing to the unusually high rates of diabetes in older African-American women.

## *How Does Diabetes Affect African-American Young People?*

African-American children have lower rates of Type 1 diabetes than white American children. The prevalence of Type 1 diabetes in white American children aged 15 and younger is nearly twice as high as in African American children of the same age.

Researchers tend to agree that genetics probably makes Type 1 diabetes more common among children with European ancestry. In fact, African-American children with some European ancestry have slightly higher prevalence of Type 1 diabetes. This incidence is also influenced by environmental and lifestyle factors.

## *How Does Diabetes Affect African-American Women During Pregnancy?*

Gestational diabetes, which develops in about 2 to 5 percent of all pregnant women, usually resolves after childbirth. Several studies have shown that African-American women have a higher rate of gestational diabetes. An Illinois study showed an 80 percent higher incidence of gestational diabetes in African Americans compared with white women. Once a woman has had gestational diabetes, she has an increased risk of developing gestational diabetes in future pregnancies. In addition, experts estimate that about half of women with gestational diabetes—regardless of race—develop Type 2 diabetes within 20 years of the pregnancy.

## How Do Diabetes Complications Affect African Americans?

Compared to white Americans, African Americans experience higher rates of three diabetes complications—blindness, kidney failure, and amputations. They also experience greater disability from these complications. Some factors that influence the frequency of these complications, such as delay in diagnosis and treatment of diabetes, denial of diabetes, abnormal blood lipids, high blood pressure, and cigarette smoking, can be influenced by proper diabetes management.

### Kidney Failure

African Americans experience kidney failure, also called end-stage renal disease (ESRD), from 2.5 to 5.5 times more often than white Americans. Interestingly though, hypertension, not diabetes, is the leading cause of kidney failure in black Americans. Hypertension accounts for almost 38 percent of ESRD cases in African Americans, whereas diabetes causes 32.5 percent. In spite of their high rates of the disease, African Americans have better survival rates from kidney failure than white Americans.

### Visual Impairment

The frequency of severe visual impairment is 40 percent higher in African Americans with diabetes than in white Americans. Blindness caused by diabetic retinopathy is twice as common in blacks as in whites. Compared to white women, black women are three times more likely to become blind from diabetes. African-American men have a 30 percent higher rate of blindness from diabetes than white American men. Diabetic retinopathy may occur more frequently in black Americans than whites because of their higher rate of hypertension.

### Amputations

African Americans undergo more diabetes-related lower-extremity amputations than white or Hispanic Americans. One study of 1990 U.S. hospital discharge figures showed amputation rates for African

Americans with diabetes were 19 percent higher than for white Americans. In a 1991 California study, however, African Americans were 72 percent more likely to have diabetes-related amputations than white Americans, and 117 percent more likely than Hispanic Americans.

## Does Diabetes Cause Excess Deaths in African Americans?

Diabetes was an uncommon cause of death among African Americans at the turn of the century. By 1993, however, according to the Centers for Disease Control and Prevention's National Center for Health Statistics, death certificates listed diabetes as the fifth leading cause of death for African Americans aged 45 to 64, and the third leading cause of death for those aged 65 and older in 1990. Diabetes is more dangerous for African-American women, for whom it was the third leading cause of death for all ages in 1990.

Diabetes death rates may actually be higher than these studies show for two reasons. First, diabetes might not have been diagnosed. Second, many doctors do not list diabetes as a cause of death, even when the person was known to have diabetes.

## How Is NIDDK Addressing the Problem of Diabetes in African Americans?

Within many African-American communities around the country, NIDDK supports centers that provide nutrition counseling, exercise, and screening for diabetes complications. These centers are called Diabetes Research and Training Centers.

### *Prevention*

In 1996, NIDDK launched its Diabetes Prevention Program (DPP). The goal of this research effort is to learn how to prevent Type 2 diabetes in people with impaired glucose tolerance (IGT) and in women with a history of gestational diabetes. As mentioned, both are strong risk factors for Type 2 diabetes.

About 4,000 volunteers are needed to participate in DPP. The study will be conducted at 25 centers throughout the United States and will seek to enroll volunteers from groups at high risk for developing Type 2 diabetes. Because of the propensity toward diabetes among some ethnic groups, about half of the DPP participants will be African American, Hispanic American, and Native American. Other at-risk participants will be elderly, overweight people and women with a previous history of gestational diabetes.

DPP will evaluate three interventions to prevent Type 2: an intensive healthy eating and exercise program and the use of two diabetes medications—metformin and troglitazone. Researchers will tailor interventions to the cultural needs of individuals in the program. Beginning in 1996, DPP will follow participants for about 5 years, with findings to be released before 2005.

## Points to Remember

- In 1993, 1.3 million African Americans were known to have diabetes. This is almost three times the number of African Americans who were diagnosed with diabetes in 1963.
- For every white American who gets diabetes, 1.6 African Americans get diabetes.
- The highest incidence of diabetes in blacks occurs between 65 and 74 years of age. Twenty-five percent of these individuals have diabetes.
- Obesity is a major medical risk factor for diabetes in African Americans, especially for women. Some diabetes may be prevented with weight control through healthy eating and regular exercise.
- African Americans have higher incidence of and greater disability from diabetes complications such as kidney failure, visual impairment, and amputations.
- If African Americans can prevent, reverse, or control diabetes, their risk of complications will decrease.
- Healthy lifestyles, such as eating healthy foods and getting regular exercise, are particularly important for people who are at increased risk of diabetes.

## Sources

Harris, M. I., Hadden, W. C., Knowler, W. C., & Bennett, P. H. (1987). Prevalence of diabetes and impaired glucose tolerance and plasma glucose levels in U.S. population aged 20-74 years. *Diabetes*, 36, 523-34.

National Center for Health Statistics. (1992). Current estimates from the National Health Interview Survey, 1992. *Vital and Health Statistics*, Series 10, 184.

National Center for Health Statistics. (1994). Current estimates from the National Health Interview Survey, 1992. *Vital and Health Statistics*, Series 10, 189.

Tull, E. S., & Roseman, J. M. (1995). Diabetes in African Americans. In National Institute of Diabetes and Digestive and Kidney Diseases (Ed.), *Diabetes in America*. 2nd Edition (NIH Publication No. 95-1468, pp. 613-630). Bethesda, MD: National Institutes of Health.

## Additional Resources

**National Diabetes Information Clearinghouse**
1 Information Way
Bethesda, MD 20892-3560
Tel: (301) 654-3327
Fax: (301) 907-8906
E-mail: ndic@aerie.com

The National Diabetes Information Clearinghouse (NDIC) offers additional information about diabetes and African Americans, including the following:

- Diabetes and African Americans: Search-on-File (annotated bibliography)
- *Noninsulin-Dependent Diabetes* (booklet)
- *The Diabetes Dictionary* (booklet available in English and Spanish)
- *Do Your Level Best: Start Controlling Your Blood Sugar Today* (booklet, limited literacy).

Single copies of all four publications are free. Bulk orders are available for health care professionals. In addition, these publications are available on the World Wide Web at <http://www.niddk.nih.gov>. For more information about diabetes and African Americans and to order publications, contact NDIC.

**Weight-control Information Network**
1 Win Way
Bethesda, MD 20892-3665
Tel: (301) 951-1120 or (800) WIN-8098
Fax: (301) 951-1107
E-mail: WINNIDDK@aol.com

**American Diabetes Association**
**National Service Center**
1660 Duke Street
Alexandria, VA 22314
Tel: (800) 232-3472
Fax: (703) 549-6995
Home page: http://www.diabetes.org

## Additional Readings

National Institute of Diabetes and Digestive and Kidney Diseases. (1995). *Diabetes in America*, 2nd Edition. (NIH Publication No. 95-1468). Bethesda, MD: National Institutes of Health.

Centers for Disease Control and Prevention, Office of Surveillance and Analysis. (1994). *Chronic Disease in Minority Populations: African-Americans, American Indians and Alaska Natives, Asians and Pacific Islanders, Hispanic Americans*. (pp. 2-1 to 2-34). Atlanta, GA.

U.S. Department of Health and Human Services, Public Health Service. (1990). *Healthy People 2000: National Health Promotion and Disease Prevention Objectives*. (DHHS Publication No. 91-50212), Washington, DC: Department of Health and Human Services.

## Chapter 5

# *Diabetes in Hispanic Americans*

Diabetes in Hispanic Americans is a serious health challenge because of the increased prevalence of diabetes in this group, the greater number of risk factors for diabetes, greater incidence of several diabetes complications, and the growing population of people of Hispanic ethnicity in the United States.[1] Estimates of the prevalence of Type 2 diabetes, far more common than Type 1 diabetes, are between 9 and 11 percent of the population, compared with 6 percent in non-Hispanic white Americans.[2]

Hispanic Americans are the second-largest and fastest-growing minority group in the Nation. In 1993, there were 27 million Hispanics in the United States, representing 10 percent of the population.[3] By the year 2050, Hispanics will constitute 21 percent of the U.S. population. The following statistics illustrate the magnitude of this disease among Hispanic Americans.

- About 5 percent of Hispanic Americans between the ages of 20 and 44 years and 20 percent of those between the ages of 45 and 74 years have diabetes.[1] These data translate to 1.8 million Hispanic American adults with diabetes. About half of these people have been diagnosed, but the other half remain undiagnosed.
- Diabetes is two to three times more common in Mexican-American and Puerto Rican adults than in non-Hispanic whites.[4] The

---

National Institute of Diabetes and Digestive and Kidney Diseases (NIDDK), NIH Pub. No. 97-3266, April 1997.

prevalence of diabetes in Cuban Americans is lower, but still higher than that of non-Hispanic whites.

- As in all populations, medical risk factors such as impaired glucose tolerance, hyperinsulinemia, insulin resistance, being overweight, central obesity, and a history of gestational diabetes increase the risk of Type 2 diabetes in Hispanic Americans.
- Higher rates of the diabetes complications nephropathy, retinopathy, and peripheral vascular disease have been documented in several studies with Mexican-Americans, whereas lower rates of myocardial infarctions (heart attacks) have been found.

According to the Bureau of the Census, 1990, the majority of Hispanic Americans live in the southcentral and southwestern United States.

## Major Studies of Diabetes in Hispanic Americans

Four population studies conducted in the past 15 years provide the majority of information that exists about the incidence and progression of diabetes among Hispanic Americans. The four studies are briefly described below and citations are provided in the references:

- *The Starr County Study* (Texas) conducted in 1981 assessed the prevalence of severe hyperglycemia in almost 2,500 people 15 years of age and older.[5]
- *The Hispanic Health and Nutrition Examination Survey (HHANES)* of 1982-84 is the only survey to provide information on the prevalence of diabetes in national samples of the three major Hispanic subgroups—Mexican-Americans in the southwestern United States, Puerto Ricans in the New York City area, and Cuban Americans in south Florida. Approximately 6,600 people were involved.[4]
- *The San Antonio Heart Study* (Texas), begun in 1979, assessed diabetes in over 3,000 Mexican-Americans and almost 2,000 non-Hispanic whites between the ages of 25 and 64.[6]
- *The San Luis Valley Diabetes Study* (Colorado), begun in 1984, estimated the prevalence of diabetes in Hispanics and non-Hispanic whites in two counties in southern Colorado.[7]

## How Many Hispanic Americans Have Diabetes?

Mexican-Americans represent the largest Hispanic American subgroup with 64 percent of the Hispanic population. Central and South Americans represent the second largest Hispanic American subgroup, with 13 percent of the Hispanic population.

Table 5.1 provides a list of Hispanic subgroups, the percent of the Hispanic population they each represent, and the percent of the population that has diabetes for two age ranges.

According to HHANES data, for the age range from 45 to 74 years, 26 percent of Puerto Ricans, 24 percent of Mexican-Americans, and 15 percent of Cuban Americans have Type 2 diabetes. The rates are significantly lower for ages 20 to 44.

**Table 5.1.** Hispanic American populations in the United States and percent with diabetes.

| Hispanic American population[3] | % of total Hispanic population[3] | % with diabetes ages 20–44[4] | % with diabetes ages 45–74[4] |
|---|---|---|---|
| Mexican-Americans | 64.0% | 3.8% | 23.9% |
| Central/South Americans | 13.4% | n/a | n/a |
| Puerto Ricans | 10.5% | 4.1% | 26.1% |
| Cuban Americans | 4.7% | 2.4% | 15.8% |
| Other Hispanic subgroups | 7.0% | n/a | n/a |

SOURCE: References 3 and 4

## What Risk Factors Increase the Chance of Hispanics Developing Type 2 Diabetes?

The same risk factors that increase the chance of diabetes in other populations also operate in the Hispanic population.

### Genetic Risk Factors

A family history of diabetes increases the chance that people will develop diabetes. The San Antonio Heart Study showed that the prevalence of diabetes among people who have first-degree relatives (e.g., parents) with diabetes was twice as great as for Mexican-Americans with no family history of diabetes.

Admixture with genes of Americans Indians and Africans (populations with high prevalence of diabetes) is also thought to be a factor for higher rates of diabetes in Hispanics. Hispanics, like members of all subpopulations, inherit their susceptibility to diabetes from their ancestors. Hispanics have three groups of ancestors—Spaniards, American Indians, and Africans. Both American Indians and Africans have high rates of diabetes. Figure 5.2 shows the genetic origins of major Hispanic subgroups.[8]

Although Cuban Americans have both American Indian and African ancestry, neither of these genetic roots contributes more than 20 percent to the current Cuban American gene pool. This fact may explain why Cuban Americans have a higher prevalence of Type 2 diabetes than non-Hispanic white Americans, yet not as high as the other Hispanic groups.

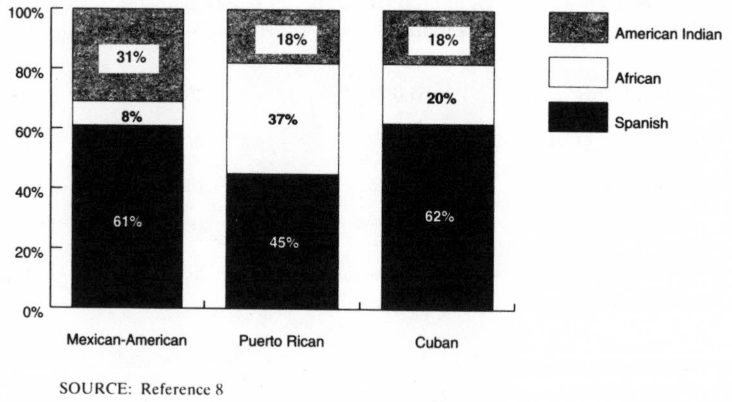


***Figure 5.2.*** *Genetic origins of the major Hispanic subgroups. (Source: reference 8)*

## *Medical Risk Factors*

**Impaired Glucose Tolerance.** One of the best predictors—or risk factors—of Type 2 diabetes is impaired glucose tolerance (IGT). People with IGT have higher-than-normal blood glucose levels—but not high enough to be diagnosed with diabetes. Most experts believe that IGT is an early stage in the natural history of diabetes. As with Type 2 diabetes, IGT is very prevalent among Hispanic Americans.

**Hyperinsulinemia and Insulin Resistance.** Higher than normal levels of fasting insulin (called hyperinsulinemia) and insulin resistance (an inability to use the body's own insulin to properly control blood glucose) are both hallmarks of an increased risk for Type 2 diabetes.

**Obesity.** Obesity is a major risk factor for Type 2 diabetes, and Hispanics are more likely than non-Hispanic whites to be overweight. It is known that the prevalence of obesity is higher in Mexican-Americans and they are known to be two to four times more likely to have Type 2 diabetes than non-Hispanic white Americans of similar weight. Figure 5.3 compares the prevalence of Type 2 diabetes between Mexican-Americans and non-Hispanic whites by the level of obesity.

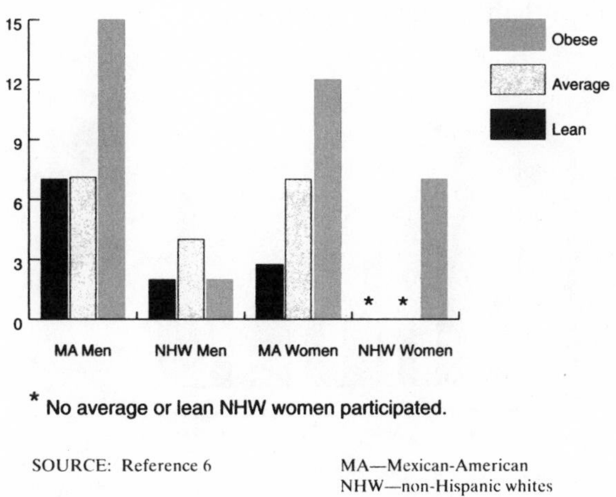


***Figure 5.3.*** *Prevalence of Type 2 diabetes by ethnicity and body weight.*

The degree to which obesity is a risk factor for diabetes depends not just on overall weight, but also on the location of the excess weight. Central, or upper body, obesity is a greater risk factor for Type 2 diabetes, compared to excess weight carried below the waist. Mexican-Americans with upper body obesity have increased risk of Type 2 diabetes.

### Lifestyle Risk Factors

HHANES data showed that fewer men with high levels of work-related physical activity developed diabetes. The San Antonio Heart Study also found that decreased levels of leisure-time physical activity was related to higher incidence of diabetes. Consuming more than twice the alcohol intake per week and having a higher body mass index (an indication of being overweight) also lead to a higher incidence of diabetes. In women, the lifestyle factors were being older, being from lower socioeconomic strata, avoiding sugar more often, and being 40 percent or more above desirable body weight. Leisure-time physical activity and alcohol consumption were not predictors of Type 2 diabetes as they were in men.

## How Does Diabetes Affect Hispanic Young People?

Hispanic children, both male and female, have lower rates of Type 1 diabetes than non-Hispanic white children. Figure 5.4 shows the incidence of Type 1 diabetes by age group.[9]

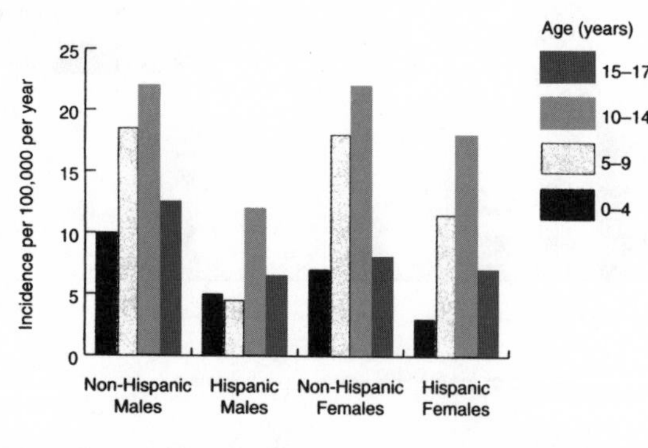


**Figure 5.4.** *Incidence of Type 1 diabetes in Colorado by age.*

## How Does Diabetes Affect Hispanic Women During Pregnancy?

Gestational diabetes is a form of diabetes that develops in about 2 to 5 percent of all pregnant women and usually resolves after childbirth.

Mexican-American women, especially when they are overweight, have higher rates of gestational diabetes than non-Hispanic white women.

## How Do Diabetes Complications Affect Hispanic Americans?

### Kidney Disease

The San Antonio Heart study showed that the prevalence of clinical evidence of kidney damage (proteinuria) was more frequent in Mexican-Americans with diabetes than in non-Hispanic whites. A higher incidence of microalbuminuria, an early indicator of diabetic nephropathy, was also seen in the San Antonio Heart study comparing Mexican-Americans to non-Hispanic whites. However, the San Luis Valley study showed no difference when comparing the incidence of diabetic nephropathy between Hispanics and non-Hispanic whites or an excess of nephropathy in non-Hispanic whites.

Mexican-Americans who develop kidney failure fare better than others on kidney dialysis. According to a report from Texas, Mexican-Americans survived longer on renal dialysis than non-Hispanic white Americans.

### Eye Disease

In the San Antonio Heart Study, the rate of diabetic retinopathy among Mexican-Americans was more than twice that of non-Hispanic white Americans. The Third National Health and Nutrition Survey (NHANES III) also found that Mexican-Americans had higher rates of diabetic retinopathy. However, the San Luis Valley study found lower rates of retinopathy in Hispanics. The results of both the San Antonio Heart Study and the San Luis Valley study indicated that insulin use and level of glycemia were significantly associated with retinopathy.

### Nerve Disease

In the San Luis Valley Diabetes Study there was no significant difference in the prevalence of diabetic neuropathy when comparing Hispanics and non-Hispanic whites.

### Peripheral Vascular Disease

In the San Antonio Heart Study, Mexican-Americans with Type 2 diabetes had a higher rate of peripheral vascular disease when compared with non-Hispanic whites; however, this increased incidence was not statistically significant.

### *Heart Disease*

Heart disease is the most common cause of death in people with diabetes, especially Type 2 diabetes. However, in the Texas and Colorado studies, Mexican-Americans had lower rates of myocardial infarctions than non-Hispanic white Americans.

## *How Is NIDDK Addressing the Problem of Diabetes in Hispanic Americans?*

In 1996, NIDDK launched its Diabetes Prevention Program (DPP) to learn how to prevent Type 2 diabetes in people with impaired glucose tolerance (IGT) and in women with a history of gestational diabetes.

About 4,000 volunteers will be enrolled in DPP, and the study will be conducted at 25 centers throughout the United States. Because of the propensity for diabetes among some minority groups, about half of the DPP participants will be Hispanic American, African American, Native American, and Pacific Islanders. Other high-risk participants will be elderly and overweight people.

DPP will evaluate three interventions to preventing Type 2: an intensive healthy eating and exercise program, and the use of two diabetes medications—metformin and troglitazone. Researchers will tailor interventions to the cultural needs of individuals in the program. Beginning in 1996, DPP will follow participants for about 5 years, with findings to be released before 2005.

## *Points to Remember*

- Hispanic Americans, especially Mexican-Americans and Puerto Ricans, develop Type 2 diabetes at higher rates than non-Hispanic white Americans.
- 1.8 million Hispanic American adults (more than 1 in 10) have Type 2 diabetes. Half of these individuals are diagnosed and the other half remain undiagnosed.
- Different Hispanic groups have different rates of diabetes. In the 45 to 74 age group, about 26 percent of Puerto Ricans, 24 percent of Mexican-Americans, and 15 percent of Cuban Americans have diagnosed diabetes.

- Genetic risk factors for Type 2 diabetes are diabetes in first degree family members, significant American Indian or African ancestry or both.
- Medical risk factors for Type 2 diabetes are impaired glucose tolerance, hyperinsulinemia and insulin resistance, overall obesity, central obesity, and a history of gestational diabetes.
- Higher rates of the diabetes complications nephropathy, retinopathy, and peripheral vascular disease have been documented in several studies with Mexican-Americans, whereas lower rates of myocardial infarctions (heart attacks) have been found.

## References

This fact sheet, *Diabetes in Hispanic Americans*, draws on statistics reported in *Diabetes in America*, 2nd Edition, Chapter 32, Diabetes in Hispanic Americans, published by the National Institute of Diabetes and Digestive and Kidney Diseases; NIH Publication No. 95-1468, 1995. Several other citations are provided in the references that follow.


1. National Institutes of Health. (1995). *Diabetes in Hispanic Americans*, Chapter 32. In *Diabetes in America*, 2nd Edition, National Institute of Diabetes and Digestive and Kidney Diseases (NIH Publication No. 95-1468). Bethesda, MD.
2. National Institutes of Health. (1995). *Diabetes Statistics*, National Diabetes Information Clearinghouse, National Institute of Diabetes and Digestive and Kidney Diseases. (NIH Publication No. 96-3926). Bethesda, MD.
3. U.S. Bureau of the Census. (1993, March). *Hispanic Populations in the United States*. (Publication #T20 #475). Washington, DC.
4. Flegal, K. M., Ezzati, T. M., Harris, M. I., Haynes, S. G., Juarez, R. Z., Knowler, W. C., Perez-Stable, E. J., & Stern, M. P. (1991). Prevalence of diabetes in Mexican Americans, Cubans, and Puerto Ricans from the Hispanic Health and Examination Survey, 1982-84. *Diabetes Care*, 14 (Suppl. 3), 628-638.
5. Hanis, C. L., Ferrell, R. E., Baron, S. A., Aguilar, L., Garza-Ibarra, A., Tulloch, B. R., Garcia, C. A., & Schull, W. J. (1983). Diabetes among Mexican-Americans in Starr County, Texas. *American Journal of Epidemiology*, 118, 659-672.

6. Stern, M. P., Gaskill, S. P., Hazuda, H. P., Gardner, L. I, & Haffner, S. M. (1983). Does obesity explain excess prevalence of diabetes among Mexican Americans? Results of the San Antonio Heart Study. *Diabetologia*, 24, 272-277.

7. Hamman, R. F., Marshall, J. A., Baxter, J., Kahn, L. B., Mayer, E. J., Orleans, M., Murphy, J. R., & Lezotte, D. C. (1989). Methods and prevalence of non-insulin-dependent diabetes mellitus in a biethnic Colorado population: The San Luis Valley Diabetes Study. *American Journal of Epidemiology*, 129, 295-311.

8. Hanis, C. L., Hewett-Emmett, D., Bertin, T. K, & Schull, W. J. (1991). Origins of U.S. Hispanics: Implications for diabetes. *Diabetes Care*, 14 (suppl. 3), 618-627.

9. Kostraba, J., Gay, E. C., Cai, Y., Cruikshanks, K. J., Rewers, M. J., Klingensmith, G. J., Chase, H. P., Hamman, R. F. (1992). Incidence of insulin-dependent diabetes mellitus in Colorado. *Epidemiology*, 3, 232-38.

## Resources from the NDIC

The National Diabetes Information Clearinghouse (NDIC), a service of NIDDK, provides Spanish-language diabetes education materials and information on diabetes in Hispanic Americans including the following titles:

- *Diabetes and Hispanics: Search-on-File*. An annotated bibliography of current Spanish-language diabetes education materials from other institutions.
- *Diabetes Statistics*. A descriptive review of the prevalence and treatment of diabetes in the United States.
- *Diccionario de la Diabetes* (*The Diabetes Dictionary* in Spanish).
- *Insuficiencia renal crónica terminal: elección del tratamiento que le conviene a usted (End-Stage Renal Disease: Choosing a Treatment That's Right for You).*

Single copies of these publications are free. Bulk orders are available for health care professionals. For more information about diabetes and Hispanic Americans and to order publications, contact: National Diabetes Information Clearinghouse, 1 Information Way, Bethesda, MD 20892-3560, Tel: (301) 654-3327, Fax: (301) 907-8906, E-mail: ndic@aerie.com

# Chapter 6

# *Diabetes in Asian and Pacific Islander Americans*

## *Introduction*

Asian and Pacific Islander Americans, although constituting less than 3% of the total U.S. population in 1990, comprise a very diverse group, with more than 20 population groups. The majority (about 95%) are Asian, with the major categories being Chinese, Filipino, Japanese, Asian Indian, Korean, and Vietnamese. These numbered almost 7 million in the 1990 U.S. Census. The major categories of Pacific Islanders are Hawaiian, Samoan, and Guamanian, numbering about 323,000 in the same census. Fifty-six percent of the Asian and Pacific Islander population lived in the West in 1990, and about 73% lived in just seven states (California, New York, Hawaii, Texas, Illinois, New Jersey, and Washington).

Insulin-dependent diabetes mellitus (IDDM) is relatively rare in this population. Among Japanese, a lower frequency of those genes that are associated with IDDM has been offered as possible explanation for the low incidence of the disease. Limited data suggest, however, that IDDM may be higher in migrant Japanese and Asian-Indian children.

Diabetes in the Asian and Pacific Islander population is predominantly of the non-insulin-dependent type (NIDDM). Among Asian Americans, data on prevalence of NIDDM are available only for Japanese, Chinese, Korean, and Filipino populations. Information is

---

Excerpted from "Diabetes in Asian and Pacific Islander Americans," by Wilfred Y. Fugimoto, MD in *Diabetes in America, second edition* NIH Publication No. 95-1468; 1995.

available, however, for migrant Asian populations in other countries (Singapore, Mauritius, Brazil, South Africa, Fiji, Trinidad, and England). Information is also available for several native nonmigrant Asian populations (Japanese, Chinese, Asian Indian, Korean, and Filipino). Taken together, these data show prevalence of NIDDM to be higher in migrant Asians than in native nonmigrant Asians. For Pacific Islanders, the limited data available for Hawaiians and Samoans show prevalence rates for NIDDM to be high in these groups.

Data compiled on estimates of abnormal glucose tolerance in adults from diverse populations worldwide have shown diabetes in adults to be a global health problem. The risk for development of diabetes, however, is not uniform among populations. At greatest risk appear to be minority populations living in industrialized countries. This increase is especially troubling since many high-risk migrant populations have been traditionally believed to have low diabetes prevalence in their homelands.

## *IDDM in Asian and Pacific Islander Populations*

The age-adjusted annual incidence rates (per 100,000 persons per year) of childhood-onset (onset at less than 15 years) IDDM in the United States, although ranging from 9.4 in San Diego, CA, to 20.8 in Rochester, MN, are considerably greater than rates reported in Japan. A nationwide survey in Japan reported a rate of 0.6, while in a survey of Hokkaido, Japan, the incidence rate was 1.7, the lowest incidence of

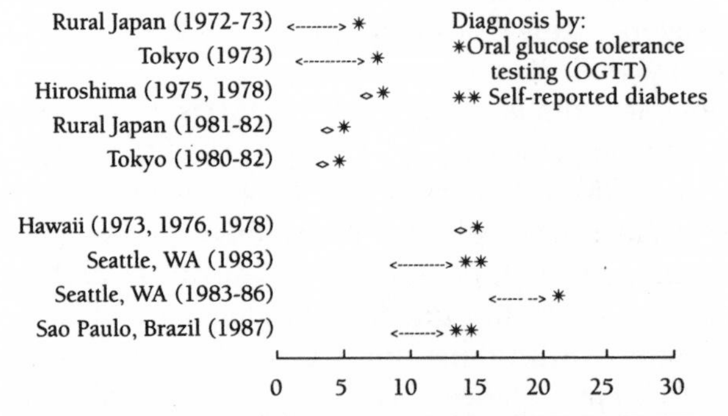


Diagnosis of diabetes was based on either self-report or oral glucose tolerance testing. Age range was ~40-75 years.

***Figure 6.1.*** *Prevalence of Diabetes in Selected Japanese Populations*

IDDM reported by a diabetes registry having virtually complete ascertainment. A lower frequency of those genes that are associated with IDDM has been offered as a possible explanation for the low frequency of the disease among Japanese.

Reliable incidence rates for IDDM in other Asian populations are not available, nor are they available for Pacific Islander populations. However, for the incidence of IDDM in the different Asian and Pacific Islander groups in the United States, an epidemiologic study of IDDM patients age 0-19 years in San Diego, CA, has reported IDDM incidence rates in Asians, as well as in Mexicans and blacks, to be significantly less than among Caucasians. This suggests that among multiple racial groups living in the same environment, Caucasians may be at higher risk of developing IDDM than Asians.

## NIDDM in Asian and Pacific Islander Populations

### *Asian*

Diabetes mellitus is less frequent in Asian than in western countries and is usually of the noninsulin-dependent type. Since NIDDM is considered to be one of the diseases associated with the lifestyle changes seen with westernization, research among immigrant Asian populations may lead to better understanding of factors mediating this association.

Various methods have been used to diagnose diabetes, often making direct comparisons of diabetes rates among studies difficult. None-

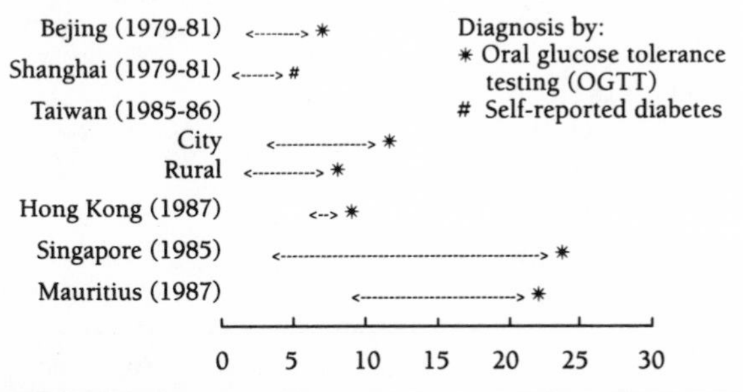


Diagnosis of diabetes was based on oral glucose tolerance testing. Age range was ~50-70 years.

***Figure 6.2.*** *Prevalence of Diabetes in Selected Chinese Populations*

theless, differences in diabetes rates between native Asian populations and migrant Asian populations are quite striking. Some of the data illustrating these differences are given for Japanese (Figure 6.1), Chinese (Figure 6.2), and Asian Indians (Figure 6.3).

*Asian Americans*

Within the United States, Hawaii has the highest percentage of individuals of Asian ancestry. Hawaii offers an excellent opportunity to examine the effects of lifestyle change on the frequency of diabetes among different racial groups. From a survey conducted in 1958 and 1959, age-adjusted prevalence rates, both for total cases and for newly diagnosed diabetes, were at least twofold greater in each of the four major Asian groups (Chinese, Filipino, Japanese, and Korean) than in Caucasians (Sloan, NR. Ethnic distribution of diabetes mellitus in Hawaii, *JAMA* 183:419-24, 1963).

**Japanese.** The data collected in Hawaii showed an increased age-adjusted prevalence of diabetes in Japanese when compared with Caucasians, 20.1% versus 7.3% for total cases and 12.6% versus 4.8% for new cases. Several other studies have also reported an increased prevalence of NIDDM in Japanese Americans.

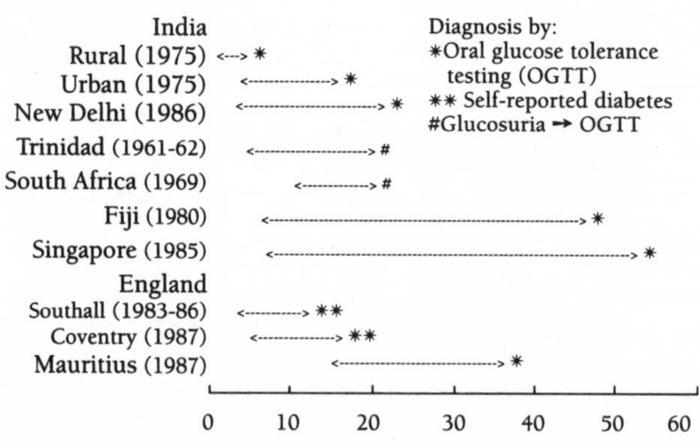


***Figure 6.3.*** *Prevalence of Diabetes in Selected Asian-Indian Populations*

From an examination of death certificates, mortality rates attributed to diabetes have been ascertained for Japanese and Caucasians in Hawaii from 1952–1979. Over this period, there was a marked secular increase in diabetes death rates in Japanese while diabetes death rates fell in Caucasians.

**Chinese.** Sloan showed the age-adjusted diabetes prevalence to be 10.3% for new cases and 14.6% for total cases among Chinese in Hawaii. Diabetes as cause of death has been reported to be increased among Chinese Americans, not only when compared with Caucasians in the United States, but also when compared with Chinese in Taiwan, Hong Kong, and Singapore. Diabetes has been shown to be a more frequent underlying cause of death in Chinese men than in Caucasian men in New York City (Figure 6.4). The prevalence of diagnosed diabetes was high among elderly Chinese Americans 60 years of age and older in Boston, MA, ascertained in 1981-83 to be 12.5% among men and 13.3% among women.

**Korean.** Sloan reported the age-adjusted prevalence of total cases of diabetes in Koreans in Hawaii to be 19.7% and for new cases of diabetes to be 11. 7%.

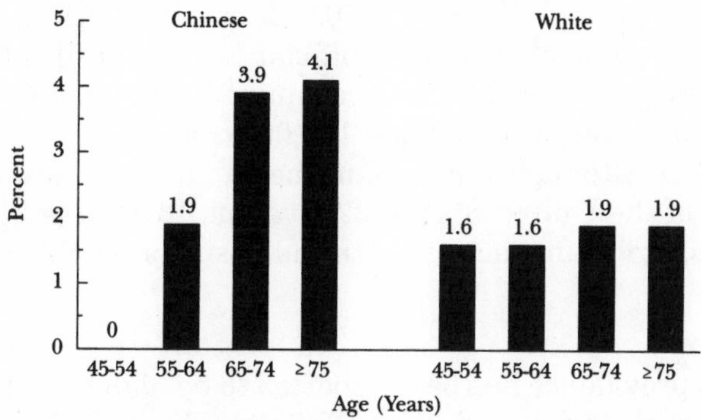


***Figure 6.4.*** *Percent of Deaths Attributed to Diabetes Among Chinese and White Men in New York City, 1968-72.*

**Filipino.** The age-adjusted prevalence of total cases of diabetes in Filipinos in Hawaii was 21.8% and for new cases of diabetes 15.5%. Filipinos had the highest prevalence of both total cases and new cases of diabetes among the four largest ethnic Asian groups in Hawaii (Chinese, Filipino, Japanese, and Korean).

### *Pacific Islanders*

In 1990 the two largest Pacific Islander groups in the United States were Hawaiians and Samoans, both of Polynesian origin. Diabetes prevalence in isolated Polynesian populations is low. In Funafuti, Tuvalu, prevalence of diabetes was 1.1% in males and 7.2% in females in 1976. The large gender difference was attributed to differing levels of physical activity, men being engaged in manual labor while women were almost completely sedentary. Furthermore, caloric intake by women was inappropriately high in relation to their level of physical activity.

In Western Samoa, home to the world's largest Polynesian population, age- and sex-adjusted diabetes prevalence in the rural population was less than half that in the urban (3.4% versus 8.7%). This difference was still present after adjusting for body weight. In contrast to the urban areas, daily activities in the rural areas involved heavy labor and gave access to basic traditional foods. In rural subjects, prevalence of diabetes was about threefold greater in women than in men, a finding similar to that in Tuvalu. Since diet was similar between rural men and women, greater physical activity in men may have had a protective effect.

American Samoa, a traditionally agricultural island, experienced rapid modernization in the late 1950s. Correlated with this has been an increase in adiposity. In 1976, official death records of American Samoa for the years 1962-74 were examined. The Samoan diabetes-related mortality rate was 13.9 per 100,000 compared with a U.S. rate of 15.9 in 1959. After age adjustment, the Samoan rate was more than double that of the United States (32.2 versus 13.4). It is likely that a significant contributing factor was the adiposity of the Samoan people.

#### *Hawaiians*

Diabetes prevalence has been reported to be high in full- and part-Hawaiians on the Island of Oahu. The age-adjusted diabetes prevalence was 4.9% in Hawaiians and 2.7% in part-Hawaiians in the survey for years 1958 and 1959, compared with 0.7% in Caucasians (Figure 6.5). Data on self-reported diabetes prevalence were also obtained for

1974-76 through questionnaires administered by the Health Surveillance Unit of the Hawaii State Department of Health. Hawaiians and part-Hawaiians had intermediate diabetes prevalence rates (men 2.0% and women 2.2%, compared with 4.5% in Chinese men and 2.8% in Chinese women, and 1.3% in Caucasian men and 1.5% in Caucasian women). There were, however, possible errors in these data related to the method of sampling and respondent errors that could not be corrected by verification. One study reported age-adjusted diabetes prevalence rates during 1980-86 of 3.0% for native Hawaiian men and 3.1% for native Hawaiian women in Hawaii (compared with 1.4% for Caucasian men and 1.5% for Caucasian women). Diagnostic criteria were not described, however. In another study, diabetes prevalence was greatly increased in Hawaiians age 20-59 years on the Island of Molokai, particularly in the age groups 40-49 years (greater than 15%) and 50-59 years (greater than20%). Approximately 65% of those participating were 20% or more above the average body mass index for Caucasians, and 45% were 40% or more overweight by these standards.

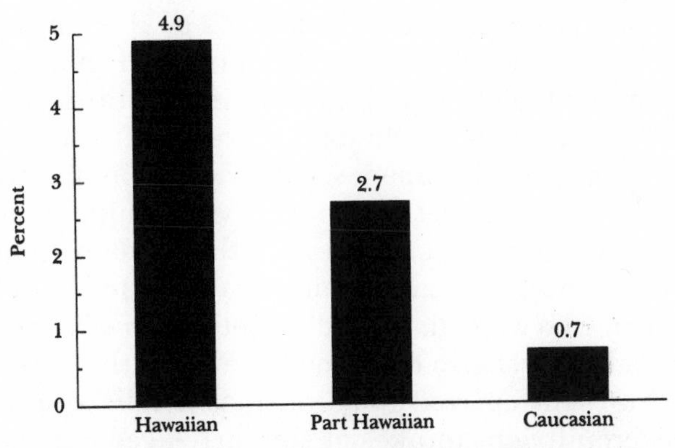


Capillary blood samples were obtained at 2-2.5 hours after a meal containing at least 50 g carbohydrate, and persons with blood glucose >130 mg/dl were referred to their physicians, who were asked to determine whether the person was diabetic and whether the diagnosis had been previously known.

***Figure 6.5.*** *Age-Adjusted Prevalence of Diabetes in Full- and Part-Hawaiians and Caucasians in Hawaii, 1958-59.*

*Samoans*

Obesity is highly prevalent in migrant Samoan populations. In an urbanized Samoan community living in the San Francisco Bay area, about 50% of the sample exceeded the 95th percentile for weight, although average height was between the 25th and 50th percentile of the U.S. population. Weight of Samoans in California exceeded that of their counterparts in Hawaii and Samoa. Obesity was accompanied by elevated blood pressure, and in women, by elevated fasting plasma glucose. Although the number of fasting plasma glucose samples was too small for detailed analysis, 18% of the male fasting sample and 9% of the female had plasma glucose levels that exceeded the 95th percentile for fasting plasma glucose in the U.S. population.

### Potential Causal Risk Factors

*Lifestyle*

Studies in Asian and Pacific Islander populations have suggested that dietary changes and reduction in physical activity are lifestyle changes that may be important in the etiology of NIDDM. A possible explanation of this is the "thrifty" genotype hypothesis, which proposes that in populations that were subject to periods of famine, a survival advantage was given to those with a metabolism that stored energy with maximum efficiency. In periods of abundance, however, this leads to obesity. It has been further proposed that such populations may be prone to developing the insulin resistance syndrome, or "Syndrome X" under lifestyle changes of westernization.

Research in the Seattle Japanese-American Community Diabetes Study has shown that diabetic men were consuming a significantly greater amount of animal fat and protein than men with normal glucose tolerance, even when total kilocalories were similar. Self-reported nondiabetic men who were diagnosed diabetic from a 75-g OGTT (Oral Glucose Tolerance Test) also consumed significantly more animal fat and protein than self-reported and confirmed nondiabetic men. A comparison of macronutrient intakes of similarly-aged Japanese-American men in Seattle and Japanese men in Japan showing much lower intake of fat in Japan, is of interest in view of the lower prevalence of diabetes in Japan. Furthermore, the increase in prevalence of diabetes in Japan is associated with a change between 1960 and 1985 in the dietary pattern of the Japanese towards the consumption of proportionally greater amounts of fat and saturated fat and lesser amounts of carbohydrate.

As regards physical activity, there is evidence that urbanization and movement away from heavy manual labor has been associated with increased diabetes prevalence in Asian and Pacific Islander populations.

*Weight Gain*

In westernizing migrants, weight gain, a powerful risk factor for NIDDM, probably plays an important role. It has been postulated that westernizing migrants with the "thrifty" genotype are susceptible to develop central obesity as a consequence of both reduced physical activity and consumption of a diet high in saturated fat. In some Asian populations, the amount of weight gain may not be large. Central obesity is in turn associated with insulin resistance and hyperinsulinemia and other adverse metabolic consequences, such as dyslipidemia. NIDDM, however, occurs only when a significant islet beta-cell secretory defect develops.

*—by Wilfred Y. Fujimoto, MD*

Dr. Wilfred Y. Fujimoto is Professor, Division of Metabolism, Endocrinology, and Nutrition, Department of Medicine, University of Washington School of Medicine, Seattle, WA.

## Chapter 7

# Diabetes in Native Americans

### Summary

The epidemic of non-insulin-dependent diabetes mellitus (NIDDM) in Native American communities has occurred primarily during the second half of this century. Although NIDDM has a genetic component, with rates highest in full-blooded Native Americans, the incidence and prevalence of the disease have increased dramatically as traditional lifestyles have been abandoned in favor of westernization, with accompanying increases in body weight and diminished physical activity. Anthropologic studies have shown that several tribes perceive diabetes as an assault from outside the community. Diabetes was once described as benign in American Indians; now, diabetes and its complications are major contributors to morbidity and mortality in all Native American populations, except the isolated Arctic groups whose lifestyles remain relatively unchanged. Insulin-dependent diabetes mellitus (IDDM) is rare in Native Americans and most cases of IDDM are found in individuals with significant non-Native American ancestry.

Much of our understanding of the natural history of NIDDM in North American Indians is derived from the longitudinal epidemiologic studies of the Pima Indians in southern Arizona. The relationship of obesity to subsequent diabetes as described in studies of the

---

Excerpted from "Diabetes in North American Indians and Alaska Natives," by Dorothy Gohdes, MD in *Diabetes in America, Second Edition*, NIH Publication No. 95-1468; 1995.

Pimas is present in all Native American populations. Native American communities experience high rates of microvascular complications from diabetes, although the rates of cardiovascular disease differ from tribe to tribe. The differences may reflect genetically based variations in lipid metabolism or other coronary risk factors or, alternatively, differences in lifestyle. The extent of diabetes in Native American communities today demands public health programs that incorporate specific psychosocial and cultural adaptations for individual tribes.

## Introduction

Native Americans are a diverse group of people whose ancestors lived in North America before the European settlement. In the United States alone, there are more than 500 tribal organizations. In addition to their tribal affiliations, Native Americans are often distinguished by language and/or cultural groups, some of which extend across both the United States and Canada. Contemporary Native American populations live in urban areas and on reservations or reserves in both countries. In the United States, about 1.9 million individuals identified themselves in the 1990 Census as American Indian or Alaska Native, but only 1.2 million of these resided in the 33 reservation states served by the Indian Health Service (IHS), an agency of the U.S. Public Health Service. Few data exist on the health of urban Native Americans in either the United States or Canada. Overall, the Native American populations of North America are young, with a median age in 1990 of 26 years, compared with 33 years for all races in the United States. In addition, Native Americans are disadvantaged both economically and educationally compared with the general U.S. population.

## Prevalence

Because American Indians living on reservations are not included in U.S. national health surveys, data on the prevalence of diabetes in Native Americans residing in the United States are limited. Rates have been estimated from case registries maintained at health facilities, glucose testing at a community level, and surveys of self-reported diabetes. In the United States and Canada, prevalence estimates for diagnosed diabetes are available from health care facilities where care is provided at no charge to Native Americans. The IHS estimated the rates of diagnosed diabetes from ambulatory care visits that covered 86% of the estimated 1 million American Indians served through the

IHS in 1987. Duplicate records were excluded by using unique patient identifiers. A similar estimate covering 76% of the Inuit and Canadian Natives living on reserves was also undertaken in 1987, using cases known to the Medical Services Branch of the Department of National Health and Welfare in Canada. Crude and age-adjusted rates of diabetes from these two surveys are shown in Table 7.1. The rates decreased toward the north and west in Canada. Although a similar trend was not apparent in the United States, rates in the far northwest were relatively low in both countries. Rates of diabetes were higher in women than in men in all Canadian provinces, a trend also

**Table 7.1.** Diagnosed Diabetes in Native American Communities in the U.S. and Canada, All Ages, 1987.

| | Crude prevalence per 1,000 | Age-adjusted prevalence per 1,000 |
|---|---|---|
| *United States* | | |
| Tucson | 76 | 119 |
| Aberdeen | 60 | 105 |
| Phoenix | 65 | 104 |
| Albuquerque | 55 | 94 |
| Bemidji | 53 | 92 |
| Nashville | 63 | 87 |
| Billings | 50 | 86 |
| Oklahoma | 49 | 60 |
| Navajo | 32 | 56 |
| Portland | 29 | 49 |
| Alaska | 9 | 15 |
| All IHS | 45 | 69 |
| *Canada* | | |
| Atlantic | 43 | 87 |
| Quebec | 29 | 48 |
| Ontario | 46 | 76 |
| Manitoba | 28 | 57 |
| Saskatchewan | 17 | 39 |
| Alberta | 22 | 51 |
| Yukon | 7 | 12 |
| NW Terr. Indian | 5 | 8 |
| NW Terr. Inuit | 3 | 4 |
| British Columbia | 9 | 16 |

U.S. rates are age-adjusted to the 1980 U.S. population; Canada's rates are age-adjusted to the 1985 Canadian population.

found for the United States in current diabetes estimates by the IHS. Women had higher rates of diabetes (13.2%) than men (11.0%) in a special medical expenditure survey of American Indians eligible for IHS services conducted in 1987. In the survey, the age- and sex-adjusted diabetes rate in individuals aged 19 years and older was 12.2%, compared with 5.2% in the general U.S. population. These studies used criteria of the World Health Organization (WHO) and the U.S. National Diabetes Data Group (NDDG) for diagnosis of NIDDM.

Striking increases in the prevalence of diabetes in recent years have been described in Pima Indians and other tribes. Because the incidence of diabetes has also increased in Pimas, and presumably in other tribes, the increased prevalence in many tribes is probably due to an increased incidence and cannot be attributed solely to longer survival of diabetic individuals.

## Determinants of Diabetes

The longitudinal studies of diabetes conducted in Pima Indians since 1965 have provided extensive information about NIDDM and its natural history in American Indians. The form of diabetes that affects Pimas is characterized biochemically and immunologically as NIDDM, an observation that confirms the paucity of IDDM also noted in other tribes.

### Genetics

Diabetes rates are highest in full-blooded Native Americans, as first observed in Choctaw Indians in 1965 and subsequently in other tribes. The prevalence of diabetes in residents of the Pima community is highest in individuals of full Native American heritage. In Pimas, diabetes rates are highest in the offspring of parents who themselves developed diabetes at a young age. Diabetes is also familial in Oklahoma Indians, an observation suggesting that genetics and/or family lifestyles predispose individuals to NIDDM. Although the precise genetic components of NIDDM have not been completely described in American Indians, a genetic marker linked with insulin resistance, a major factor in the pathogenesis of NIDDM, has been described in Pimas.

### Obesity

Obesity is a major risk factor for diabetes in Pimas and is widespread in many tribes, with increasing rates of obesity measured in several communities in the United States and Canada. A striking increase in obesity has occurred in Pimas in recent years. In addition, longer duration of obesity has been shown to increase the risk of diabetes.

Central obesity was characteristic of Canadian Indians studied in Manitoba and Ontario. In young Pimas, waist-to-hip ratio, a measure of central obesity, was more strongly associated with diabetes than body mass index, a measure of overall obesity. In Navajo women, a small study found an increased waist-to-hip ratio associated with a statistically significant increased risk of diabetes, but a similar association was not significant in Navajo men 45.

## *Lifestyle*

Both diet patterns and physical activity have changed markedly in Native American communities over recent decades. Although detailed longitudinal surveys are not available for most tribes, the disruption of traditional agriculture and hunting has resulted in increased consumption of fat—typical of the contemporary western diet. In Pimas, a high-calorie diet has been associated with the development of diabetes. Carbohydrate intake was the single strongest predictor of NIDDM but was closely related to total calorie and fat consumption.

Physical activity has decreased as individuals have acquired motorized transportation and sedentary occupations. Diabetic Pimas reported less lifetime and current physical activity than nondiabetic individuals. A recent case-control study in Zuni Indians showed the risk of presenting with diabetes decreased significantly with increasing physical activity, even after adjusting for obesity, suggesting that physical activity itself decreased the risk of NIDDM independently of body weight.

## *Pathogenesis*

Studies of the pathogenesis of NIDDM in Pimas indicate that insulin resistance, as measured by nonoxidative glucose disposal, is an early metabolic defect. Longitudinal studies have found that insulin secretion and insulin resistance increase as individuals develop impaired glucose tolerance. Insulin levels then fall as frank NIDDM develops, often at a relatively young age.

Energy metabolism and obesity have been studied in an attempt to characterize a “thrifty gene.” Although the exact causes of obesity have not been explained, studies in Pimas have found energy expenditure to be familial and a low metabolic rate to be predictive of subsequent weight gain. Detailed metabolic studies have not been conducted in other tribes, but a propensity to obesity and NIDDM is widespread, as has been the change from traditional high-carbohydrate diets to modern high-fat diets. Contemporary high-fat diets are associated with deterioration of carbohydrate metabolism in both Pimas and Caucasians. Although our understanding of the current "epidemic" of NIDDM in Native Americans is based on studies of Pimas, the interaction between environmental changes and genetic susceptibility to NIDDM is not limited to Pimas but appears to be widespread in all indigenous North Americans, as well as other populations throughout the world.

## Mortality

The mortality from diabetes in Native Americans is striking, yet it is seriously underestimated in U.S. vital statistics data. The figures published for diabetes death rates in 1986-88 showed the age-adjusted American Indian death rate was 2.7 times the rate for the

**Table 7.2.** Age-Adjusted Mortality Rates for Deaths Due to Diabetes, American Indian and Alaska Native Population, 1984-89.

| | Rate per 100,000 population | | | |
|---|---|---|---|---|
| IHS Service Area | 1984-86 | 1985-87 | 1986-88 | 1987-89 |
| Total | 24.5 | 25.2 | 26.2 | 29.1 |
| Aberdeen | 44.7 | 41.3 | 35.6 | 50.1 |
| Alaska | 5.7 | 5.9 | 5.8 | 7.6 |
| Albuquerque | 25.0 | 32.4 | 33.1 | 32.8 |
| Bemidji | 32.9 | 29.4 | 28.6 | 39.0 |
| Billings | 24.8 | 27.8 | 23.6 | 40.1 |
| California | 10.4 | 15.2 | 15.5 | 15.3 |
| Nashville | 30.5 | 30.4 | 39.5 | 45.0 |
| Navajo | 21.2 | 23.8 | 23.6 | 27.4 |
| Oklahoma | 21.3 | 20.1 | 20.6 | 21.1 |
| Phoenix | 54.0 | 51.4 | 53.9 | 53.2 |
| Portland | 15.5 | 18.3 | 24.2 | 25.4 |
| Tucson | 52.9 | 59.0 | 69.6 | 68.1 |

Data are for populations residing in the IHS service areas and are age-adjusted to the 1940 U.S. Census; Alaska rates are based on <20 deaths.

general U.S. population. These figures reflect only cases in which diabetes was the underlying cause of death, not those in which it was a contributing cause or those in which diabetes was not listed on the death certificate. Mortality rates by IHS Area are shown in Table 7.2. During 1984-86, there were 1,252 Native American deaths with diabetes listed as a contributing cause of death and 708 deaths with diabetes listed as the underlying cause. In addition, the National Mortality Followback Study found that Native American heritage was underreported on death certificates by 65%. When the 1986-88 relative mortality rates are adjusted for underreporting of heritage, the diabetes mortality for Native Americans is 4.3 times the rate for whites. In a New Mexico study, American Indians experienced 3.6 times the diabetes death rates of whites. Over a 30-year period in New Mexico, diabetes death rates in American Indians increased 550% in women and 249% in men. A mortality study on Canadian Indian reserves in seven provinces found the risk of death from diabetes to be 2.2 times higher for native men and 4.1 times higher for native women than the rates for the Canadian population as a whole.

Detailed mortality studies in Pimas during 1975-84 found that the age- and sex-adjusted death rate from diabetes was 11.9 times greater than the 1980 death rate for all races in the United States. Diabetic nephropathy was the leading cause of death in diabetic Pimas, followed by ischemic heart disease. Longer duration of diabetes and proteinuria were both associated with increased mortality. A 10-year followup of a cohort of diabetic Oklahoma Indians also showed striking death rates: 5% annually for men and 4% for women, which were three and four times the rates expected for men and women in the general Oklahoma population. Circulatory disease causes of death in this cohort exceeded those attributed to diabetes as the underlying cause. Although the contributions of diabetic renal disease and atherosclerotic heart disease to overall diabetes-related mortality vary among tribes, both clearly contribute to the very significant mortality from diabetes in North American Indian communities.

*—by Dorothy Gohdes, MD*

Dr. Dorothy Gohdes is Director, Indian Health Service Diabetes Program, Albuquerque, NM.

# *Part Two*

# *Types of Diabetes and Related Disorders*

## Chapter 8

# *Are You at Risk for Diabetes?*

Find out if you are at high risk of getting diabetes by answering and scoring the following statements.

1. **I had a baby weighing more than nine pounds at birth or had diabetes during pregnancy.**
   If you answered Yes give yourself a score of 6.
   If you answered No give yourself a score of 0.

2. **I have a parent(s), sister, or brother with diabetes.**
   If you answered Yes add 3 to your score.
   If you answered No add 0.

3. **I consider myself Hispanic, African American, American Indian, Asian American, or Pacific Islander.**
   If you answered Yes add 3 to your score.
   If you answered No add 0.

4. **I am overweight.**
   If you answered Yes add 3 to your score.
   If you answered No add 0.

---

Diabetes Risk Analysis, an undated document produced by the Diabetes Prevention Program at the University of Washington, (206) 764-2768, e-mail: uwdpp@u.washington.edu; reprinted with permission granted in June 1998.

5. **I have been told I have a high blood sugar level.**
   If you answered Yes add 6 to your score.
   If you answered No add 0.

6. **I am between 45 and 64 years of age.**
   If you answered Yes add 1 to your score.
   If you answered No add 0.

7. **I am under 65 years of age AND I get little or no exercise during a usual day.**
   If you answered Yes add 3 to your score.
   If you answered No add 0.

8. **I am 65 years old or older.**
   If you answered Yes add 3 to your score.
   If you answered No add 0.

Now, add up your total score from items 1-8.

If you scored **1-5 points, you are probably at low risk** for having diabetes now. But don't forget about it —especially if you are Hispanic, African American, Native American, Asian American or a Pacific Islander.

If you scored **6 or more points, you are at high risk** for having or getting diabetes. Only a doctor can determine if you have diabetes. Receive a free screening by the Diabetes Prevention Program at the University of Washington or see a doctor and find out for sure.

Chapter 9

# Diabetes: Clearer Names and a Lower Number for Diagnosis

An international expert committee recently recommended a change in the names of the two main types of diabetes because the former names caused confusion. The type of diabetes that was known as Type I, juvenile-onset diabetes, or insulin-dependent diabetes (IDDM) is now *type 1 diabetes*. The type of diabetes that was known as Type II, noninsulin-dependent diabetes (NIDDM), or adult-onset diabetes is now *type 2 diabetes*. The new names reflect an effort to move away from basing the names on the treatment or age of onset.

## A Lower Number to Diagnose Diabetes

The expert committee recommended a lower fasting plasma glucose (FPG) number to diagnose diabetes. The new FPG number is greater than or equal to 126 milligrams per deciliter (mg/dl), rather than greater than or equal to 140 mg/dl. This recommendation was based on a 2-year review of more than 15 years of research. This research showed that when blood glucose was consistently over 126 mg/dl the prevalence of diabetes complications, such as heart disease and loss of sight, increased dramatically and developed before the diagnosis of diabetes. The experts believe the earlier diagnosis and treatment can prevent or delay the costly and burdensome complications of diabetes.

For the first time, these experts suggest that adults age 45 and older be tested for diabetes. If their blood glucose is normal at the first

National Diabetes Information Clearinghouse, February 1998.

test, they should be tested at 3-year intervals. People under 45 should be tested if they are at high risk for diabetes. Risk factors include

- Being more than 20 percent above ideal body weight or having a body mass index (BMI) of greater than or equal to 27 kgm/m$^2$.
- Having a first-degree relative with diabetes (mother, father, or sibling).
- Being a member of a high-risk ethnic group (African American, Hispanic, Asian, or Native American).
- Delivering a baby weighing more than 9 pounds or having diabetes during a pregnancy.
- Having blood pressure at or above 140/90 mm/Hg.
- Having abnormal blood fat levels, such as high density lipoproteins (HDL) less than or equal to 35 mg/dl or triglycerides greater than or equal to 250 mg/dl.
- Having impaired glucose tolerance when previously tested for diabetes.

The committee states a diagnosis of diabetes is warranted for any of three positive tests, with a second positive test on a different day:

- A fasting plasma glucose of greater than or equal to 126 mg/dl.
- A casual plasma glucose (taken any time of day) of greater than or equal to 200 mg/dl with the symptoms of diabetes.
- An oral glucose tolerance test (OGTT) value of greater than or equal to 200 mg/dl in the blood measured at the 2-hour interval. (The OGTT is given over a 3-hour timespan and administered by a physician or medical laboratory. The person comes in fasting and a blood sample is taken. He or she drinks a glucose syrup. Then a blood sample is taken from the person to measure glucose once an hour for 3 hours.)

The committee recommended that the fasting plasma glucose is preferable to OGTT because it is less expensive, easier to administer, and more acceptable to the person being tested.

A new category for glucose intolerance—impaired fasting glucose (IFG)—was defined as having a fasting plasma glucose value of greater than or equal to 110 mg/dl but less than 126 mg/dl. The existing category, impaired glucose intolerance (IGT), is now defined as results of an OGTT greater than or equal to 140 mg/dl but less than 200 mg/dl in the 2-hour sample.

## *Testing for Diabetes During Pregnancy*

The expert panel also suggested a change in the testing for diabetes during pregnancy, stating that women at low risk for gestational diabetes do not need to be tested. This group includes women who are

- Younger than 25 years of age.
- At normal body weight.
- Without family history of diabetes.
- Not members of a high-risk ethnic group.

All women who do not fall into the low-risk category should continue to be tested for gestational diabetes during the 24th to 28th weeks of pregnancy.

The National Diabetes Information Clearinghouse (NDIC) has more free information on diabetes. Contact NDIC at:

**National Diabetes Information Clearinghouse (NDIC)**
1 Information Way
Bethesda, MD 20892-3560
fax: (301) 907-8906
e-mail: ndic@niddk.nih.gov.

To learn whether you have diabetes and what type of diabetes you have, ask your health care provider.

# Chapter 10

# Type 1 Diabetes: Insulin-Dependent Diabetes

## What Is Diabetes?

Diabetes is a group of conditions in which glucose (sugar) levels are abnormally high. Diabetes occurs when the pancreas stops making enough insulin, which is necessary for the proper metabolism of digested foods.

About 14 million people in the United States have some form of diabetes, although only half are diagnosed. The three main types of diabetes are insulin-dependent, also known as Type I diabetes; noninsulin-dependent, also called Type II diabetes; and gestational diabetes, which occurs during pregnancy.

Insulin-dependent diabetes mellitus (IDDM) most often develops in children and young adults. Sometimes people over age 40 get IDDM, but it usually begins at younger ages. For this reason, IDDM used to be known as "juvenile" diabetes. IDDM is one of the most common chronic disorders in U.S. children. Each year, from 11,000 to 12,000 children are diagnosed with IDDM. Among the more than 7 million people in the United States who are being treated for diabetes, about 5 to 10 percent have IDDM.

Noninsulin-dependent diabetes mellitus (NIDDM) is the most common type of diabetes. It accounts for 90 to 95 percent of diagnosed diabetes and almost all of undiagnosed diabetes. NIDDM usually

---

U.S. Department of Health and Human Services, National Institute of Diabetes and Digestive and Kidney Diseases (NIDDK), NIH Pub. No. 95-2098, September 1994.

develops in adults over age 40 and is most common in those who are overweight. People with NIDDM usually produce some insulin, but the body cells cannot use it efficiently because the cells are resistant to the insulin. By losing weight, exercising, or taking oral medications, most people with NIDDM can overcome this resistance to insulin. However, some people with NIDDM require daily insulin injections.

Gestational diabetes occurs in some women during pregnancy. It usually ends after the baby is born, but women with gestational diabetes may develop NIDDM when they get older. Gestational diabetes results from the body's resistance to the action of insulin. This resistance is caused by hormones the placenta produces during pregnancy. The condition develops about midway through the pregnancy. Gestational diabetes is usually treated with diet. Some women may need insulin. Gestational diabetes cannot be treated with pills that lower blood glucose as these medicines can cause harm to the baby.

### Note about Terminology in This Chapter

This chapter is about insulin-dependent diabetes, or IDDM for short. The word "diabetes" in the text refers to insulin-dependent diabetes unless otherwise noted. This chapter does not replace the advice of a doctor. However, it can help you learn about diabetes and suggest questions to ask a doctor. Local diabetes organizations and clinics that sponsor meetings and educational programs about diabetes can also be helpful. Groups that have information about diabetes programs are listed in Chapter 67.

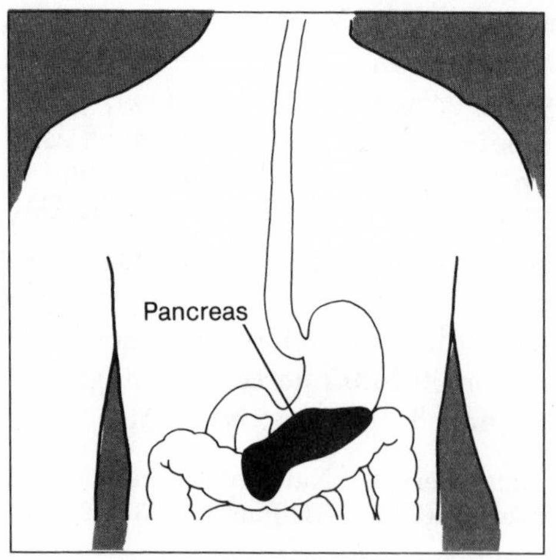


**Figure 10.1.** *The pancreas.*

## What Causes Diabetes?

When we eat, foods containing proteins, fats, and carbohydrates are broken down into simpler, easily absorbed chemicals. One of these is a form of simple sugar called glucose. Glucose circulates in the blood stream where it is available for body cells to use. The body relies on glucose as a source of fuel for important organs such as the brain.

The pancreas, a large gland located behind the stomach, produces the hormone insulin. In people without diabetes, the pancreas makes the correct amount of insulin needed to allow glucose to enter body cells. In people with diabetes, however, not enough insulin is produced. As a result, glucose builds up in blood, overflows into the urine, and passes out of the body unused. Thus, the body loses an important source of fuel—even though the blood contains large amounts of glucose.

Insulin also allows the body to store excess glucose as fat, proteins as muscle protein, and important enzymes that control metabolism. A severe deficiency of insulin causes excess breakdown of stored fats and proteins.

## What Are the Causes and Symptoms of IDDM?

### Causes of IDDM

In people with insulin-dependent diabetes (IDDM), the pancreas produces too little or no insulin at all. The pancreas is not able to produce insulin because the body's immune system has destroyed the insulin-producing cells.

Scientists do not know why the body's immune system, which allows it to fight disease and other "foreign" substances that may invade the body, attacks and destroys insulin-producing cells. A combination of factors may be involved, including exposure to common viruses or other substances early in life, as well as an inherited risk for IDDM.

Researchers can now test family members of people with IDDM to identify those at increased risk for diabetes. Scientists hope to find a way to prevent the disease through a study called the Diabetes Prevention Trial—Type 1. This study is described in the research section of this chapter.

### Early Symptoms of IDDM

The early symptoms of IDDM can be gradual or sudden. They include frequent urination (particularly at night), increased thirst, unexplained weight loss (in spite of increased appetite), and extreme tiredness. These symptoms are caused by the build-up of sugar in the blood and its loss in the urine.

To eliminate sugar in the urine, the kidney "borrows" water from the body. The loss of this extra sugar and water in the urine results in dehydration, which causes increased thirst.

In addition to causing high blood glucose, the lack of insulin causes the body to break down stored fats and proteins. As fats are broken down, the body can convert these fats into waste products called ketones. If ketone production is excessive, abnormal amounts of ketones in the blood can spill into the urine. If blood ketone levels rise too high, a life-threatening condition called ketoacidosis can develop, which requires immediate medical attention. Symptoms of ketoacidosis include abdominal pain, vomiting, rapid breathing, extreme tiredness, and drowsiness.

### *Points to Remember*

The symptoms of IDDM include:

- Frequent urination
- Increased thirst
- Increased hunger
- Unexplained weight loss
- Extreme tiredness

## How Does a Person Live with Diabetes?

Diabetes requires constant attention and daily care to keep blood sugar levels in balance. Injecting insulin, following a diet, exercising, and testing blood sugar are some of the day-to-day requirements. To feel good and stay healthy, a person with IDDM must follow a daily management routine. For this reason, diabetes is often referred to as a "24-hour" disease. This section provides general guidelines for diabetes management and explains the roles of various health care professionals who can help you manage your diabetes. The treatment recommendations are based on a 10-year study recently completed by the Federal Government called the Diabetes Control and Complications Trial (DCCT).

### *The Diabetes Control and Complications Trial*

Diabetes can affect many parts of the body. Over time, it can damage a person's kidneys, eyes, nerves, and heart. These long-term complications can result in kidney disease, vision loss, nerve damage, heart attack, and other problems. The DCCT proved that lowering blood sugar levels delayed or prevented diabetes complications by 50 to 80 percent.

The DCCT compared two approaches to managing IDDM: intensive and standard treatment. People in the intensive treatment group learned how to adjust their insulin according to food intake and exercise. They injected insulin three to four times a day or used an insulin pump and tested their blood sugar at least four times a day and once a week at 3 a.m. They also followed a diet and exercise plan and met once a month with a health care team composed of a physician, nurse educator, dietitian, and mental health professional.

People in the standard treatment group followed a plan that was not as strict. They took one or two insulin injections a day, tested sugar levels once or twice a day, and met with the doctor or nurse every 3 months.

At the end of the DCCT, volunteers on intensive treatment had lower rates of kidney, eye, and nerve damage than volunteers in the standard treatment group. The study showed that efforts to improve control of blood sugar made a major difference. In fact, the study found that any long-term lowering of blood sugar levels will reduce the risk of complications, even in people with poor control of their diabetes and early complications of diabetes. For this reason, people with IDDM are encouraged to do the best they can to keep their blood sugar levels as close to the normal range as possible.

However, intensive treatment does increase the risk of low blood sugar episodes, or hypoglycemia, and is not recommended for everyone, particularly older adults, children under age 13, people with heart problems or advanced complications, and people with a history of frequent severe hypoglycemia. Your doctor should help you decide if intensive control is right for you.

*Points to Remember*

The DCCT showed that intensive control of blood sugar levels can help reduce the risk of complications associated with diabetes. The study showed that any sustained lowering of blood sugar levels is helpful.

### Health Care Providers

Diabetes requires daily attention, and you need to learn how to care for your diabetes. A number of people can help you:

**A doctor experienced in treating diabetes.** These doctors are called endocrinologists or diabetologists. They will work with you to develop an individualized management routine and help you determine your ideal blood sugar range and ways to stay within that range.

"People with IDDM should be under the care of, or have regular contact with, a diabetes specialist who is up to date on diabetes and its management," advises Dr. Julio Santiago, an endocrinologist with the DCCT Center at Washington University in St Louis. "During the last 10 years, diabetes care has greatly improved and become more complex. Services offered by diabetes specialists help people with IDDM learn the nuts and bolts of modern care and its benefits," he says.

**A diabetes educator.** Diabetes educators specialize in teaching people how to manage their diabetes. Most are registered nurses, pharmacists, dietitians, or physician assistants with advanced training and experience. They help you and your physician develop a management plan based on your age, school or work schedule, daily activities, and eating habits. They can teach you the importance of good nutrition, exercising regularly, and testing your blood sugar. These professionals can also help you adjust to having diabetes. Diabetes educators who use the initials C.D.E. (Certified Diabetes Educator) after their names have passed an examination qualifying them to provide health education to people with diabetes.

**A nutritionist or dietitian.** Nutritionists or dietitians trained in diabetes care provide diet guidelines and meal planning advice. They can teach you how to balance food intake and insulin requirements and how to handle special situations such as low blood sugar (hypoglycemia) and sick days. Some dietitians are also C.D.E.s.

**A mental health professional.** A person with diabetes can never take a vacation from daily management chores. For this and other reasons, diabetes can affect the way a person feels. If you need advice on managing diabetes during stressful or difficult times, or if having diabetes makes you feel sad or depressed, talking to a social worker, psychologist, or psychiatrist may be helpful.

"These professionals are trained to help people cope with chronic conditions that require constant care," says Dr. Alan Jacobson, a psychiatrist at the Joslin Diabetes Center in Boston. Dr. Jacobson, who counseled volunteers at the DCCT center at Joslin, says "Discussing their problems and anxieties with a professional helped DCCT volunteers feel emotionally and physically in control."

If a mental health professional is not available to you, Dr. Jacobson suggests joining a local diabetes support group. "Talking with someone else who has IDDM may help," he advises. Information about support groups is available from your physician or C.D.E. and local offices of the American Diabetes Association (ADA) and Juvenile Diabetes Foundation (JDF) International. These organizations also can provide suggestions on how to form a support group if one does not exist in your community. The addresses of these organizations are located in Chapter 67.

## Daily Insulin

People with IDDM must give themselves insulin every day. Insulin cannot be taken in pill form. It can be injected, which involves use of a needle and syringe, or it can be given by an insulin pump. Insulin pumps are worn outside the body on a belt or in a pocket. They deliver a steady supply of insulin through a tube that connects to a needle placed under the skin. Extra amounts of insulin are taken before meals, depending on the blood glucose level and food to be eaten.

Another injection aid is an insulin pen. This device contains a replaceable insulin cartridge and a sterile, disposable needle. Insulin pens are handy because they eliminate the need for carrying extra syringes and insulin bottles. Jet injectors can also be used to give insulin, but these devices are expensive. A jet injector uses high pressure rather than a needle to propel insulin through the skin and into the tissue. Researchers are exploring the use of implantable pumps and other devices for giving insulin. Talk to your doctor about the insulin delivery system that is best for you.

The amount of insulin you need depends on your height, weight, age, food intake, and activity level. Insulin doses must be balanced with meal times and activities, and dosage levels can be affected by illness, stress, or unexpected events. Your doctor or diabetes educator will calculate how much insulin you should take each day to keep your blood sugar levels from rising too high or falling too low. They also will advise you about handling special situations. Most people with newly diagnosed IDDM can begin to inject their own insulin and estimate their insulin dosage needs within the first few days after instruction by a diabetes educator.

### *Points to Remember*

All people with IDDM need insulin. Ways to give insulin include:

- A needle and syringe
- An insulin pump
- An insulin pen
- A jet injector

### Blood Glucose Monitoring

Since the early 1980's, self-monitoring of blood glucose (SMBG) has been shown to be the best way to determine if the blood sugar levels of a person with IDDM are too high or too low. The measurement helps you monitor your diabetes control to determine if adjustments in diet, insulin, or exercise are needed. Although SMBG may at first seem difficult and adds to the expense of treatment, diabetes management has improved greatly since this testing method became widely available.

SMBG involves taking a drop of blood, usually from the tip of a finger, and placing it on a specially coated strip. Strips are "read" either visually or by a meter. Visually read strips change color according to the amount of sugar in the blood. The color is then compared to a color chart provided with the strips. To use a glucose meter, you insert the strip into the meter and it gives a digital reading of your blood sugar level, usually within a minute.

Using a blood glucose meter is a more accurate way to test blood sugar. SMBG meters available since the early 1990s offer many features. Some are small and lightweight, and some can store blood sugar readings for a few days or weeks. Meters are sold in drug stores or in diabetes supply stores. You should consult your diabetes educator about which meter would be most appropriate for your lifestyle. Before using a meter, you should receive instructions from a health care professional on how to operate and maintain the device. Correct use of the meter is necessary to obtain accurate readings.

It is important to follow the manufacturer's recommendations for testing the accuracy of your meter (called calibrating the meter). Failure to do so could cause inaccurate test readings, leading to errors in management.

Results of blood sugar measurements should be recorded in a diabetes diary available through pharmacies and doctors' offices. The books have space for recording events such as extra activities or sickness that may affect blood sugar levels. This information will help you and your doctor adjust insulin doses or make other changes in care, if necessary. Sometimes the diary may show patterns in blood sugar levels that indicate a need to contact a health professional between office visits.

Frequent SMBG was an important tool in the DCCT. "For volunteers in the intensive management group, blood glucose testing results served as a guidepost to making decisions about food intake and insulin doses in order to achieve better control," says Ms. Patricia Callahan, a DCCT diabetes nurse educator at the International Diabetes Center in Minneapolis. "Blood glucose testing should be done at least four times a day or as often as necessary to achieve optimal control," she advises. "The idea is to use your SMBG to make adjustments in your food, exercise, and insulin so that your blood sugar stays in a range that is best for you."

Another blood test, the hemoglobin A1c test, shows the average level of blood sugar for the past 2 to 3 months. Your blood sample is sent to a laboratory for analysis. You should have a hemoglobin A1c test at least every 3 months. Based on the results, you and your physician will know how well you have been doing in controlling your diabetes over the last few months.

*Points to Remember*

Blood glucose testing is very important for monitoring daily care.

- SMBG shows current blood sugar levels.
- Hemoglobin A1c tests average blood sugar levels over the past 2 to 3 months.

### Meal Plans

Like everyone else, people with IDDM should follow a healthy eating plan. Your meal plan should be low in fat and cholesterol because these foods have been linked to heart disease, a common problem in people with diabetes. Children and pregnant women with diabetes may have additional nutritional needs. Guidelines for nutrition are available from your dietitian, diabetes educator, or the ADA. Organizations that can help you find resources for nutritional guidance are listed in Chapter 67.

Different foods have different effects on blood sugar. Therefore, you should try to be as consistent as possible in your food choices and eating times. Some foods raise blood sugar quickly; others have a more gradual effect. By testing your blood sugar after eating, you can learn how particular foods affect your blood sugar levels.

Timing of meals and coordinating them according to your insulin injections is important. Regular insulin, for example, has its peak glucose-lowering effect approximately 2 hours after injection and acts for 4 to 6 hours. It is usually given before meals. Other insulin preparations are absorbed more slowly and have a longer duration of action.

Insulin regimens should be designed to fit a person's eating habits and lifestyle and should be as consistent as possible on a day-to-day basis. A dietitian can personalize a meal plan to include foods you like. Your physician and diabetes educator can also help.

The DCCT volunteers on intensive treatment learned about the relationship between food choices and blood sugar levels. "Each individual's insulin needs were adjusted to fit his or her lifestyle and diet, rather than trying to match the diet to fit the insulin," says Ms. Linda Delahanty, a dietitian with the DCCT Center at Massachusetts General Hospital in Boston. By understanding the relationship between food choices and blood sugar levels, she notes, volunteers in the intensive therapy group had more flexibility in their daily lives and could adjust their insulin doses to changes in their food intake and activity levels.

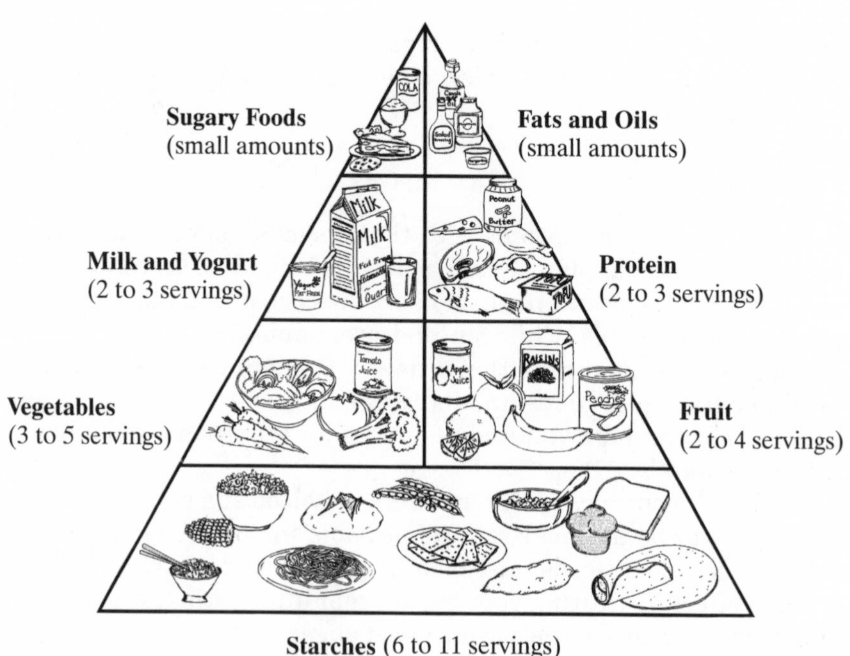


***Figure 10.2.*** *Food Guide Pyramid—a guide to daily food choices.*

*Points to Remember*

- Consult with a dietician to develop a meal plan for you.
- Learn how different foods affect your blood sugar levels.
- Try to keep insulin injections, meals, and activities as consistent as possible on a day-to-day basis.

### *Exercise*

People with IDDM are encouraged to exercise for the same reasons as people without diabetes. Exercise keeps the body in tone and is good for the heart and lungs. Before exercising you should check your blood sugar levels because exercise tends to lower blood sugar. If your blood sugar is too low or if some time has passed since you ate, you should eat a snack before exercising. Sometimes exercise can cause very high blood sugar to rise even higher. If your blood sugar is over 300 mg/dl (before eating), you should give yourself insulin or wait until your blood sugar level falls before beginning to exercise.

"Exercise is an important part of the patient's management plan. Participation in sports and regular exercise helps to improve overall physical fitness," says Dr. Santiago. An exercise program should be planned with the help of a doctor or an experienced physical therapist or trainer.

*Points to Remember*

Exercise can lower blood sugar levels quickly. Before beginning exercise:

- Check your blood sugar levels.
- If your blood sugar is on the low side, eat a snack.
- If your blood sugar is very high, you should bring it under control before beginning to exercise.
- It may also be necessary to lower your insulin dose before planned exercise.

## How Should Diabetic Emergencies Be Handled?

People with diabetes must always balance food, exercise, and insulin to control blood sugar levels. When this balance is disrupted, certain emergency conditions, including low blood sugar (hypoglycemia) or high blood sugar (hyperglycemia) may result. People with IDDM should always wear a medical identification bracelet, necklace, or watch band. These tags state that the wearer has IDDM and list a telephone number to call for help.

## *Hypoglycemia*

Very low blood sugar, called hypoglycemia, is sometimes referred to as an "insulin reaction." This condition can be caused by too much insulin, too little or delayed food, exercise, alcohol, or any combination of these factors. When hypoglycemia occurs, a person can become cranky, tired, sweaty, hungry, confused, and shaky. If blood sugar levels drop too low, a person can lose consciousness or experience a seizure.

Hypoglycemia can usually be treated quickly by eating or drinking something with sugar in it, such as a sweetened drink or orange juice. You should always carry a high-sugar snack that can be used to treat an insulin reaction. Special products to treat insulin reactions, including glucose tablets and gels, are available in drugstores.

If a person loses consciousness or cannot swallow because of hypoglycemia, medical help is necessary. Dial 911 or take the person to a hospital emergency room. An injectable medication called glucagon, available by prescription in drugstores, raises blood sugar quickly. A family member or friend should learn when and how to inject glucagon in an emergency. Your doctor, diabetes educator, or dietitian can give advice about treating hypoglycemia.

In the DCCT, volunteers on intensive treatment had three times as many episodes of hypoglycemia severe enough to require help from another person as the volunteers on standard therapy. Because of this potential danger, intensive management is not recommended for everyone, particularly older adults, children under age 13, or people with heart problems or advanced complications. People who do not experience the usual symptoms of low blood sugar, a condition known as hypoglycemia unawareness, need to take extra care to avoid hypoglycemia. They should measure their blood glucose more often, particularly before driving or operating dangerous machinery.

*Points to Remember*

- Hypoglycemia is low blood sugar.
- Hypoglycemia can develop quickly, especially with exercise.
- Always carry a high-sugar snack to treat low blood sugar.
- Hypogycemia, if not treated in time, can lead to unconsciousness.
- Test blood sugar levels to avoid hypoglycemia, particularly before driving or exercising.

### *Hyperglycemia*

Hyperglycemia is the opposite of hypoglycemia. Hyperglycemia occurs when the body has too much sugar in the blood. This condition may be caused by insufficient insulin, overeating, inactivity, illness, stress, or a combination of these factors. The symptoms of hyperglycemia include extreme thirst, frequent urination, fatigue, blurred vision, vomiting, and weight loss.

If your blood sugar levels are above 250 mg/dl before meals, you should test your urine for ketones. Ketones are chemicals that the body makes when insulin levels are very low and excessive amounts of fat are being burned. Ketone buildup over several hours can lead to serious illness and coma, a condition called ketoacidosis. Ketone testing kits are available in drugstores or at doctors' offices. They should be available for you to use at home when you are ill or when your blood sugar is very high. Signs of ketoacidosis include vomiting, weakness, rapid breathing, and a sweet breath odor.

*Points to Remember*

- Hyperglycemia is high blood sugar.
- Hyperglycemia develops more slowly than hypoglycemia.
- Hyperglycemia can indicate that ketoacidosis may be present.
- If blood sugar is high, test urine for ketones.

## How Does Diabetes Affect Your Body?

Diabetes can cause damage to both large and small blood vessels, resulting in complications affecting the kidneys, eyes, nerves, heart, and gums. The DCCT showed that maintaining blood sugar levels as close to normal as possible prevents or slows the development of many of these complications.

### *Kidney Disease*

Diabetic kidney disease, called diabetic nephropathy, can be a life-threatening complication of IDDM in about 40 percent of people who have had diabetes for 20 or more years. The kidneys are vital to good health because they serve as a filtering system to clean waste products from the blood. Diabetic nephropathy develops when the small blood vessels that filter these wastes are damaged. Sometimes this damage causes the kidneys to stop working. This condition is called kidney failure or end-stage renal disease. People with kidney failure must either have their blood cleaned by a dialysis machine or have a kidney transplant.

High blood pressure (hypertension) also increases a person's chance of developing kidney disease. People with diabetes are more likely to develop high blood pressure than people without diabetes. Therefore, keeping blood pressure under control is especially important for someone with IDDM. Your doctor should check your blood pressure at every visit.

Blood pressure tests measure how hard your heart is working to pump blood to the organs and vessels in your body. If blood pressure is too high, it can be treated with a doctor's help. Left untreated, bladder and kidney infections can also harm the kidneys. Consult your doctor if symptoms such as painful urination occur.

An early sign of kidney disease is albumin or protein in the urine. A doctor should test your urine for protein or albumin once a year. The doctor should also do an annual blood test to evaluate kidney function. More frequent tests may be necessary if findings are not normal.

The DCCT proved that intensive therapy can prevent the development and slow the progression of early diabetic kidney disease. Another recent study has shown that a type of medication called an ACE inhibitor can help protect the kidneys from damage.

### *Eye Disease*

Diabetes can affect the small blood vessels in the back of the eye, a condition called diabetic retinopathy. Retinopathy means disease of the retina, the tissue at the back of the eye that is sensitive to light. Diabetes eventually causes changes in the tiny vessels that supply the retina with blood. These small changes are called background retinopathy. Most people who have had diabetes for a number of years have background retinopathy, which usually does not affect sight. Over time, the blood vessels may rupture or leak fluid. In a minority of patients, most often those with higher blood sugar, retinopathy becomes more severe and new blood vessels may grow on the retina. These vessels may bleed into the clear gel, or vitreous, that fills the eye or detach the retina from its normal position because of bleeding or scar formation.

Laser treatment can help restore vision impaired by diabetic retinopathy. If you have had IDDM for 5 years or more, you should see an eye doctor at least once a year for an examination through dilated pupils. An annual exam is the best way to detect and treat eye damage before the condition becomes severe. Laser treatment, as well as surgical procedures performed by eye doctors who specialize in diabetic problems, can often help preserve useful vision even in cases of advanced retinopathy.

In the DCCT, intensive management reduced the risk of diabetic eye disease by 76 percent in participants with no eye damage at the beginning of the study. In those with early retinopathy, intensive therapy slowed the progression of eye damage by 50 percent.

### *Nerve Disease*

Nerve disease caused by diabetes is called diabetic neuropathy. There are three types of nerve disease: peripheral, autonomic, and mononeuropathy. Peripheral neuropathy affects the hands, feet, legs, toes, or fingers. A person's feet, legs, and fingertips may lose feeling, burn, or become painful. To relieve the pain, doctors prescribe pain-killing drugs and sometimes antidepressant drugs. Scientists are studying other substances to help relieve pain associated with diabetic peripheral neuropathy.

Because of the loss of feeling associated with peripheral neuropathy, feet are especially vulnerable. You should check your feet carefully each day for cuts, bruises, and sores. If you notice anything unusual, see a doctor as soon as possible because foot infections and open sores can be difficult to treat in people with diabetes. Your doctor should check your feet at every visit. At least once a year, the doctor should check your neurological function by testing how well you sense temperature, pinprick, and vibration in your feet and changes of position in your toes. Your doctor may recommend that you see a foot care specialist, called a podiatrist.

Another type of nerve disease that may occur after several years of diabetes is called autonomic neuropathy. Autonomic neuropathy affects the internal organs such as the heart, stomach, sexual organs, and urinary tract. It can cause digestive problems and lead to incontinence (a loss of ability to control urine or bowel movements), and sexual impotence. A doctor can help diagnose problems associated with internal organs and may prescribe medication to help relieve pain and other problems associated with autonomic neuropathy.

Mononeuropathy is a form of nerve disease that affects specific nerves, most often in the torso, leg, or head. Mononeuropathy may cause pain in the lower back, chest, abdomen, or in the front of one thigh. Sometimes, this nerve disease can cause aching in the eye, an inability to focus the eye, or double vision. Mononeuropathy may also cause facial paralysis, a condition called Bell's palsy, or problems with hearing. Mononeuropathies occur most often in older people and can be quite painful. Usually the symptoms improve in weeks or months without causing long-term damage.

Lowering blood sugar levels may help prevent or reduce early neuropathy. DCCT study results showed the risk of significant nerve damage was reduced by 60 percent in persons on intensive treatment.

### Cardiovascular Disease

As with high blood pressure, heart disease is more common in people with diabetes than in people without diabetes. People with diabetes tend to have more fat and cholesterol in their arteries. The arteries are the large blood vessels that keep the heart beating and the blood flowing. When too much fat and cholesterol build up in the arteries, the arteries and heart must work harder. Over time, this extra work can lead to a heart attack. To help avoid heart problems, you should have your blood cholesterol and triglyceride levels checked once a year. Other risk factors that may cause the heart to become overworked include high blood pressure, smoking, age, extra weight, and lack of exercise.

People with diabetes are also at greater risk for stroke and other forms of large blood vessel disease. A stroke is the result of damage to the blood vessels that circulate blood in the brain. Blockage of major blood vessels in the feet, legs, or arms is called peripheral vascular disease. Peripheral vascular disease causes poor circulation and can contribute to foot and leg ulcers.

DCCT participants were checked regularly for heart disease and related problems, although they were not expected to have many heart-related problems because of their young age. Volunteers in the intensive treatment group had fewer heart attacks and significantly lower risks of developing high blood cholesterol, which causes heart disease. The risk was 35 percent lower in these volunteers, suggesting that intensive treatment can help prevent heart disease. The DCCT volunteers on intensive therapy are being followed closely for the next 10 years to see if their risk of heart disease is reduced.

#### *Points to Remember*

To reduce the risk of heart disease:

- Do not smoke.
- Eat a diet low in fat and high in fruits and vegetables.

- Have your blood pressure checked regularly.
- Have your cholesterol checked regularly.

### *Periodontal (Gum) Disease*

People with diabetes, especially those with poor control of their blood sugar, are at risk for developing infections of the gum and bone that hold the teeth in place. Like all infections, gum infections can cause blood sugar to rise and make diabetes harder to control.

Periodontal disease starts as gingivitis, which causes sore, bleeding gums. If not stopped, gingivitis can lead to serious periodontal disease that can damage the bone that holds the tooth in its socket. Without treatment, teeth may loosen and fall out.

Good blood sugar control lowers the risk of gum disease. People with good control have no more gum disease than people without diabetes. Good blood sugar control, daily brushing and flossing, and regular dental checkups are the best defense against gum problems.

*Points to Remember*

Take special care of your teeth and gums.

- Visit your dentist every 6 months.
- Brush and floss teeth at least twice daily.
- Practice other dental care guidelines recommended by the dentist or dental hygienist.

## How Should Special Situations Be Handled?

### *Illness, Stress, and Surgery*

Illness and stress can affect blood sugar levels in people with diabetes. Therefore, during times of illness and stress, you need to be extra careful about keeping blood sugar levels in control. If you develop an illness such as the flu or strep throat, keep in touch with your doctor, test your blood sugar levels often, and check your urine for ketones. Even if you are feeling too sick to eat or have trouble keeping food down, you should continue giving yourself some insulin. In such situations, your doctor will tell you how much insulin to take as well as liquid diets to follow.

A doctor or diabetes nurse educator can also provide guidelines on how to handle stress. If you need hospitalization for an illness or require surgery, doctors and hospital personnel should know that you have diabetes. Your diabetes doctor should also be informed about the hospitalization and should be part of the team that monitors your care. Your doctor will give you advice regarding who to call in case of illness, vomiting, or very high blood sugar levels. In many cases, an early telephone call can prevent lengthy hospitalization.

## *Pregnancy*

Before the 1950s, most pregnant women with diabetes had little chance of having a normal baby. Since the 1960s major advances in diabetes treatment have taken place in Europe and North America. Today, with careful planning, most women with diabetes can become pregnant and deliver a healthy baby with the help of their doctors. Women with diabetes need to discuss their plans with their physicians before they become pregnant. Several studies show that excellent blood glucose control is important at the time a women becomes pregnant. Careful control during the first 2 months of pregnancy can reduce the risk of major birth defects. Later, during the third to ninth months of pregnancy, excellent blood glucose control is essential to protect the health of the baby and reduce complications related to premature delivery.

If you are a pregnant woman with IDDM, you should be treated by a team of doctors or at a center that specializes in the treatment of diabetic pregnancies. The center can provide guidelines for handling such pregnancy-related problems as morning sickness as well as closely monitor your baby before, during, and after delivery.

Because pregnancy sometimes can affect the eyes, kidneys, and blood pressure, your doctors will need to check your eyes, kidneys, and blood pressure before and throughout the pregnancy.

### *Points to Remember*

- Most women with IDDM can have successful pregnancies.
- Blood sugar levels should be in good control before a woman becomes pregnant.
- Women with IDDM must be under the close care of specialists experienced in diabetic pregnancies.

## *School Activities*

Children with IDDM can attend school, do homework, play with friends, and participate in clubs or sports. However, special attention should be paid to diabetes care while the child is in school and involved in daily activities. If old enough, children may keep a blood glucose meter at school or with the school nurse. To safeguard against hypoglycemia, the child can carry extra snacks, or snacks can be given to the teacher for use in case the child's blood sugar level drops. Teachers, friends, club leaders, school nurses, or coaches should be aware that a child has diabetes and should know the signs of low blood sugar and how to treat it in case of emergency.

*Points to Remember*

- Inform teachers and school staff that your child has diabetes and how to treat hypoglycemia.
- Always bring extra snacks in case hypoglycemia occurs with exercise.

### *Social Activities*

Just like people without diabetes, people with diabetes can go to parties and participate in social activities. Some helpful tips are:

- Call ahead to see what foods the host or hostess will serve and at approximately what time. This will help you keep track of how much food you should eat or how much insulin you will need.
- If there does not seem to be food you should eat, offer to bring a snack that everyone, including you, can enjoy.
- Make sure you bring your blood glucose meter to the party to check blood sugar levels before participating in any physical activities, such as strenuous dancing.

Adults with diabetes, even those with IDDM, can drink alcohol safely in moderation. Moderation usually means one or two occasional drinks taken with food. Drinking on an empty stomach and at bedtime can cause blood sugar levels to drop quickly, causing hypoglycemia, with symptoms of shakiness, dizziness, and confusion. People who do not know that someone has diabetes may mistake these symptoms for drunkenness. A dietitian can give guidelines about using alcohol and how to include it in a meal plan. People with nerve damage due to diabetes should avoid frequent alcohol use.

*Points to Remember*

- Alcohol can lower blood glucose.

- Always eat when drinking alcohol.
- Drink in moderation.
- If you have nerve damage due to diabetes, avoid regular alcohol use.

## What Is Happening in Diabetes Research?

The DCCT was one of many recent research programs supported by the Federal Government and by nongovernment organizations to improve the health and well-being of people with diabetes and to find ways to prevent and cure the disorder. A 10-year follow-up to the DCCT, the Epidemiology of Diabetes Intervention and Complications Study, is focusing on the development of macrovascular and renal complications in DCCT volunteers.

The National Institute of Diabetes and Digestive and Kidney Diseases (NIDDK) conducts basic and clinical research in its own laboratories and supports research at centers and hospitals throughout the United States. Other institutes of the National Institutes of Health support studies on diabetic eye, heart, vascular, and nerve disease; pregnancy and diabetes; dental complications; and the immunological aspects of diabetes. This research has led to improved treatments for the complications of diabetes and ways to prevent complications from occurring.

### Preventing Diabetes

Researchers are searching diligently for the causes of all forms of diabetes and ways to delay or prevent the disorder. Much progress has been made. Scientists have identified antibodies in the blood that make a person susceptible to IDDM, making it possible to screen relatives of people with diabetes and determine their risk for developing the disease.

A new NIDDK clinical trial, the Diabetes Prevention Trial—Type 1 (DPT-1), began in 1994. It is identifying relatives at risk for developing IDDM and treating them with low doses of insulin or with oral insulin-like agents in the hope of preventing IDDM. Similar research is being conducted at other medical centers throughout the world. These studies are based on encouraging results in laboratory animals with IDDM and on pilot studies in relatives of people with IDDM.

### Advances in Managing Diabetes

In the past 15 years, many advances have improved treatment for people with diabetes:

- **Genetically engineered insulin.** Because it is identical to insulin produced by the human body, genetically engineered insulin is less apt to cause skin and other allergic reactions. Supplies of genetically engineered insulin are readily available.

- **Self-monitoring of blood glucose.** By testing your own blood sugar, you enable your doctor to offer you much better treatment than was available before 1980 when testing urine for glucose was the only way of estimating diabetes control.

- **Hemoglobin A1c testing.** Using one blood test, doctors can now monitor your average blood sugar control over a period of 2 to 3 months. This test tells you how well you are doing and whether any changes are needed in your management routine.

- **Insulin pumps, insulin pens, and other aids for administering insulin.** Insulin pumps, including implantable pumps now under development, can supply insulin in a more natural pattern, similar to the way the pancreas in a person without diabetes makes insulin. Other injection aids make giving insulin easier and more convenient than in the past, even in young children and people who are visually impaired.

Other improvements in diabetes management being developed include insulin in the form of nasal sprays, patches, or pills and devices to test blood sugar levels without having to prick a finger to get a blood sample. Perhaps one of the most important advances has been the development of an entirely new approach to diabetes management in which IDDM patients take responsibility for much of their own care.

### *Curing Diabetes*

Transplantation of the pancreas or of the insulin-producing islets of the pancreas offer a hope for a cure for IDDM. Many people with IDDM have had successful pancreas transplants, and a few have had islet transplants. Unfortunately, pancreas and islet transplants cannot be offered to everyone with diabetes as yet. The body's immune system rejects "foreign" or transplanted tissue, and people who have transplants must take powerful drugs to prevent rejection. These drugs are costly and may cause serious health problems. Therefore, pancreas or islet transplants are usually given only to people who have had or require a kidney transplant because of advanced complications and are already taking drugs to prevent rejection.

Researchers are working to develop less harmful drugs and better methods of transplanting pancreatic tissue to prevent rejection by the body, such as encapsulating the islet cells in a semi-permeable membrane that offers protection from immune attack, implanting the cells in the thymus gland to induce tolerance by the immune system, and using bioengineering techniques to create artificial islet cells that secrete insulin in response to increased sugar levels in the blood.

### Clinical Trials

Clinical trials are one way to test new treatments that emerge from basic research. NIDDK plans and supports clinical trials related to diabetes, such as the DCCT and DPT-Type 1. For information about NIDDK-supported clinical trials, contact the National Diabetes Information Clearinghouse (NDIC), at 1 Information Way, Bethesda, MD 20892-3560; (301) 654-3327.

Other medical centers also conduct clinical studies. The best way to find out about studies in progress is to contact a nearby university-affiliated hospital or large medical center. Additional information can also be obtained from a local chapter of the American Diabetes Association or Juvenile Diabetes Foundation.

## Acknowledgments

Our thanks to: Julio Santiago, M.D., of Washington University for his careful review of this text.

We also wish to acknowledge the contributions of: Patricia Callahan, R.N., B.S., C.D.E., Linda Delahanty, M.S., R.D., and Alan Jacobson, M.D.

Chapter 11

# Type 2 Diabetes: Noninsulin-Dependent Diabetes

## Introduction

This chapter is about *noninsulin-dependent diabetes*. The word "diabetes" in the text of this chapter refers to noninsulin-dependent diabetes unless otherwise specified.

Of the estimated 13 to 14 million people in the United States with diabetes, between 90 and 95 percent have **noninsulin-dependent or type II diabetes.** Formerly called adult-onset, this form of diabetes usually begins in adults over age 40, and is most common after age 55. Nearly half of people with diabetes don't know it because the symptoms often develop gradually and are hard to identify at first. The person may feel tired or ill without knowing why. Diabetes can cause problems that damage the heart, blood vessels, eyes, kidneys, and nerves.

Although there is no cure for diabetes yet, daily treatment helps control blood sugar, and may reduce the risk of complications. Under a doctor's supervision, treatment usually involves a combination of weight loss, exercise and medication.

This chapter isn't a guide to treatment and it doesn't replace the advice of a doctor. It's one of many sources of extra information about diabetes. Local diabetes groups and clinics sponsor meetings and educational programs about diabetes that also can be helpful. At the end

---

NIH Pub. No. 97-241, September 1992.

of this book is a chapter listing groups that have information on diabetes programs.

## What is Diabetes?

The two types of diabetes, insulin-dependent and noninsulin-dependent, are different disorders. While the causes, short-term effects, and treatments for the two types differ, both can cause the same long-term health problems. Both types also affect the body's ability to use digested food for energy. Diabetes doesn't interfere with digestion, but it does prevent the body from using an important product of digestion, glucose (commonly known as sugar), for energy.

After a meal the digestive system breaks some food down into glucose. The blood carries the glucose or sugar throughout the body, causing blood glucose levels to rise. In response to this rise the hormone insulin is released into the bloodstream to signal the body tissues to metabolize or burn the glucose for fuel, causing blood glucose levels to return to normal. A gland called the pancreas, found just behind the stomach, makes insulin. Glucose the body doesn't use right away goes to the liver, muscle or fat for storage.

In someone with diabetes, this process doesn't work correctly. In people with insulin-dependent diabetes, the pancreas doesn't produce insulin. This condition usually begins in childhood and is also known as type I (formerly called juvenile-onset) diabetes. People with this kind of diabetes must have daily insulin injections to survive.

In people with noninsulin-dependent diabetes the pancreas usually produces some insulin, but the body's tissue don't respond very well to the insulin signal and, therefore, don't metabolize the glucose properly, a condition called insulin resistance. Insulin resistance is an important factor in noninsulin-dependent diabetes.

## Symptoms

The symptoms of diabetes may begin gradually and can be hard to identify at first. They may include fatigue, a sick feeling, frequent urination, especially at night, and excessive thirst. When there is extra glucose in blood, one way the body gets rid of it is through frequent urination. This loss of fluids causes extreme thirst. Other symptoms may include sudden weight loss, blurred vision, and slow healing of skin, gum and urinary tract infections. Women may notice genital itching.

A doctor also may suspect a patient has diabetes if the person has health problems related to diabetes. For instance, heart disease, changes in vision, numbness in the feet and legs or sores that are slow to heal, may prompt a doctor to check for diabetes. These symptoms do not mean a person has diabetes, but anyone who has these problems should see a doctor.

## What Causes Noninsulin-Dependent Diabetes?

There is no simple answer to what causes noninsulin-dependent diabetes. While eating sugar, for example, doesn't cause diabetes, eating large amounts of sugar and other rich, fatty foods, can cause weight gain. Most people who develop diabetes are overweight. Scientists do not fully understand why obesity increases someone's chances of developing diabetes, but they believe obesity is a major factor leading to noninsulin-dependent diabetes. Current research should help explain why the disorder occurs and why obesity is such an important risk factor.

A major cause of diabetes is insulin resistance. Scientists are still searching for the causes of insulin resistance, but they have identified two possibilities. The first could be a defect in insulin receptors on cells. Like an appliance that needs to be plugged into an electrical outlet, insulin has to bind to a receptor to function. Several things can go wrong with receptors. There may not be enough receptors for insulin to bind to, or a defect in the receptors may prevent insulin from binding.

A second possible cause involves the process that occurs after insulin plugs into the receptor. Insulin may bind to the receptor, but the cells don't read the signal to metabolize the glucose. Scientists are studying cells to see why this might happen.

## Who Develops Noninsulin-Dependent Diabetes?

Age, sex, weight, physical activity, diet, lifestyle, and family health history all affect someone's chances of developing diabetes. The chances that someone will develop diabetes increase if the person's parents or siblings have the disease. Experts now know that diabetes is more common in African Americans, Hispanics, Native Americans and Native Hawaiians than whites. They believe this is the result of both heredity and environmental factors, such as diet and lifestyle. The highest rate of diabetes in the world is in an Arizona community of American Indians called the Pimas. While the chances of developing diabetes increase with age, gender isn't a risk factor, although African American women are more likely to develop diabetes than African American men.

While people can't change family history, age, or race, it is possible to control weight and physical fitness. A doctor can decide if someone is at risk for developing diabetes and offer advice on reducing that risk.

## Diagnosing Diabetes

A doctor can diagnose diabetes by checking for symptoms such as excessive thirst and frequent urination and by testing for glucose in blood or urine. When blood glucose rises above a certain point, the kidneys pass the extra glucose in the urine. However, a urine test alone is not sufficient to diagnose diabetes.

A second method for testing glucose is a blood test usually done in the morning before breakfast (fasting glucose test) or after a meal (postprandial glucose test).

The oral glucose tolerance test is a second type of blood test used to check for diabetes. Sometimes it can detect diabetes when a simple blood test does not. In this test, blood glucose is measured before and after a person has consumed a thick, sweet drink of glucose and other sugars. Normally, the glucose in a person's blood rises quickly after the drink and then falls gradually again as insulin signals the body to metabolize the glucose. In someone with diabetes, blood glucose rises and remains high after consumption of the liquid.

A doctor can decide, based on these tests and a physical exam, whether someone has diabetes. If a blood test is borderline abnormal, the doctor may want to monitor the person's blood glucose regularly. If a person is overweight, he or she probably will be advised to lose weight. The doctor also may monitor the patient's heart, since diabetes increases the risk of heart disease.

## Treating Diabetes

The goals of diabetes treatment are to keep blood glucose within normal range and to prevent long-term complications. Why control blood glucose? In the first place, diabetes can cause short-term effects: some are unpleasant and some are dangerous. These include thirst, frequent urination, weakness, lack of ability to concentrate, loss of coordination, and blurred vision. Loss of consciousness is possible with very high or low blood sugar levels, but is more of a danger in insulin-dependent than in noninsulin-dependent diabetes.

In the second place, the long-term complications of diabetes may result from many years of high blood glucose. Research is under way to find out if this is true and to learn if careful control can help prevent complications. Meanwhile, most doctors feel that if people with diabetes keep their blood glucose levels under control, they will reduce the risk of complications.

In 1986, a National Institutes of Health panel of experts recommended that the best treatment for noninsulin-dependent diabetes is a diet that helps the person maintain normal weight. In people who are overweight, losing weight is the one treatment that is clearly effective in controlling diabetes.

In some people, exercise can help keep weight and diabetes under control. However, when diet and exercise alone can't control diabetes, two other kinds of treatment are available: oral diabetes medications and insulin. The treatment a doctor suggests depends on the person's age, lifestyle, and the severity of the diabetes.

## Diabetes Diet

The proper diet is critical to diabetes treatment. It can help someone with diabetes:

- Achieve and maintain desirable weight. Many people with diabetes can control their blood glucose by losing weight and keeping it off.
- Maintain normal blood glucose levels.
- Prevent heart and blood vessel diseases, conditions that tend to occur in people with diabetes.

A doctor will usually prescribe diet as part of diabetes treatment. A dietitian or nutritionist can recommend a diet that is healthy, but also interesting and easy to follow. No one has to be limited to a preprinted, standard diet. Someone with diabetes can get assistance in the following ways:

- A doctor can recommend a local nutritionist or dietitian.
- The local American Diabetes Association, American Heart Association, and American Dietetic Association can provide names of qualified dietitians or nutritionists and information about diet planning.
- Local diabetes centers at large medical clinics, hospitals, or medical universities usually have dietitians and nutritionists on staff.

The guidelines for diabetes diet planning include the following:

- Many experts, including the American Diabetes Association, recommend that 50 to 60 percent of daily calories come from carbohydrates, 12 to 20 percent from protein, and no more than 30 percent from fat.

- Spacing meals throughout the day, instead of eating heavy meals once or twice a day, can help a person avoid extremely high or low blood glucose levels.

- With few exceptions, the best way to lose weight is gradually: one or two pounds a week. Strict diets **must never** be undertaken without the supervision of a doctor.

- People with diabetes have twice the risk of developing heart disease as those without diabetes, and high blood cholesterol levels raise the risk of heart disease. Losing weight and reducing intake of saturated fats and cholesterol, in favor of unsaturated and monounsaturated fats, can help lower blood cholesterol.

  For example, meats and dairy products are major sources of saturated fats, which should be avoided; most vegetable oils are high in unsaturated fats, which are fine in limited amounts; and olive oil is a good source of monounsaturated fat, the healthiest type of fat. Liver and other organ meats and egg yolks are particularly high in cholesterol. A doctor or nutritionist can advise someone on this aspect of diet.

- Studies show that foods with fiber, such as fruits, vegetables, peas, beans, and whole-grain breads and cereals may help lower blood glucose. However, it seems that a person must eat much more fiber than the average American now consumes to get this benefit. A doctor or nutritionist can advise someone about adding fiber to a diet.

- Exchange lists are useful in planning a diabetes diet. They place foods with similar nutrients and calories into groups. With the help of a nutritionist, the person plans the number of servings from each exchange list that he or she should eat throughout the day. Diets that use exchange lists offer more choices than preprinted diets. More information on exchange lists is available from nutritionists and from the American Diabetes Association.

Continuing research may lead to new approaches to diabetes diets. Because one goal of a diabetes diet is to maintain normal blood glucose levels, it would be helpful to have reliable information on the effects of foods on blood glucose. For example, foods that are rich in carbohydrates, like breads, cereals, fruits, and vegetables break down into glucose during digestion, causing blood glucose to rise. However, scientists don't know how each of these carbohydrates affect blood glucose levels. Research is also under way to learn whether foods with sugar raise blood glucose higher than foods with starch. Experts do know that cooked foods raise blood glucose higher than raw, unpeeled foods. A person with diabetes can ask a doctor or nutritionist about using this kind of information in diet planning.

## Alcoholic Beverages

Most people with diabetes can drink alcohol safely if they drink in moderation (one or two drinks occasionally), because in higher quantities alcohol can cause health problems:

- Alcohol has calories without the vitamins, minerals, and other nutrients that are essential for maintaining good health. A doctor can discuss whether it's safe for an individual with diabetes to drink. People who are trying to lose weight need to account for the calories in alcohol in diet planning. A dietitian also can provide information about the sugar and alcohol content of various alcoholic drinks.

- Alcohol on an empty stomach can cause low blood glucose or hypoglycemia. Hypoglycemia is a particular risk in people who use oral medications or insulin for diabetes. It can cause shaking, dizziness, and collapse. People who don't know someone has diabetes may mistake these symptoms for drunkenness and neglect to seek medical help.

- Oral diabetes medications—tolbutamide and chlorpropamide—can cause dizziness, flushing, and nausea when combined with alcohol. A doctor can advise patients on the safety of drinking when taking these and other diabetes medications.

- Frequent, heavy drinking can cause liver damage over time. Because the liver stores and releases glucose, blood glucose levels may be more difficult to control in a person with liver damage from alcohol.

- Frequent heavy drinking also can raise the levels of fats in blood, increasing the risk of heart disease.

## Exercise

Exercise has many benefits, and for someone with diabetes regular exercise combined with a good diet can help control diabetes. Exercise not only burns calories, which can help with weight reduction, but it also can improve the body's response to the hormone insulin. As a result, following a regular exercise program can make oral diabetes medications and insulin more effective and can help control blood glucose levels.

Exercise also reduces some risk factors for heart disease. For example, exercise can lower fat and cholesterol levels in blood, which increase heart disease risk. It also can lower blood pressure and increase production of a cholesterol, called HDL, that protects against heart disease.

However, infrequent, strenuous exercise can strain muscles and the circulatory system and can increase the risk of a heart attack during exercise. A doctor can decide how much exercise is safe for an individual. The doctor will consider how well controlled a person's diabetes is, the condition of the heart and circulatory system, and whether complications require that the person avoid certain types of activity.

Walking is great exercise, especially for an inactive person, and it's easy to do. A person can start off walking for 15 or 20 minutes, three or four times a week, and gradually increase the speed or distance of the walks. The purpose of a good exercise program is to find an enjoyable activity and do it regularly. Doing strenuous exercise for six months and then stopping isn't as effective. People taking oral drugs or insulin need to remember that strenuous exercise can cause dangerously low blood glucose and they should carry a food or drink high in sugar for medical emergencies. Signs of hypoglycemia include hunger, nervousness, shakiness, weakness, sweating, headache, and blurred vision. As a precaution, a person with diabetes should wear an identification bracelet or necklace to alert a stranger that the wearer has diabetes and may need special medical help in an emergency.

A doctor may advise someone with high blood pressure or other complications to avoid exercises that raise blood pressure. For example, lifting heavy objects and exercises that strain the upper body raise blood pressure.

People with diabetes who have lost sensitivity in their feet also can enjoy exercise. They should choose shoes carefully and check their feet regularly for breaks in skin that could lead to infection. Swimming or bicycling can be easier on the feet than running.

## *Oral Medications*

Oral diabetes medicines, or oral hypoglycemics, can lower blood glucose in people who have diabetes, but are able to make some insulin. They are an option if diet and exercise don't work. Oral diabetes medications are not insulin and are not a substitute for diet and exercise. Although experts don't understand exactly how each oral medicine works, they know that they increase insulin production and affect how insulin lowers blood glucose. These medications are most effective in people who developed diabetes after age 40, have had diabetes less than 5 years, are normal weight, and have never received insulin or have taken only 40 units or less of insulin a day. Pregnant and nursing women shouldn't take oral medications because their effect on the fetus and newborn is unknown, and because insulin provides better control of diabetes during pregnancy.

There is also some question about whether oral diabetes medications increase the risk of a heart attack. Experts disagree on this point and many people with noninsulin-dependent diabetes use oral medicines safely and effectively. The Food and Drug Administration (FDA), the agency of the Federal Government that approves medications for use in this country, requires that oral diabetes medicines carry a warning concerning the increased risk of heart attack. Whether someone uses a medication depends on its benefits and risks, something a doctor can help the patient decide.

Six FDA-approved oral diabetes medications are now on the market. Their generic names are tolbutamide, chlorpropamide, tolazamide, acetohexamide, glyburide, and glipizide. The generic name refers to the chemical that gives each medicine its particular effect. Some of these medications are made by more than one pharmaceutical company and have more than one brand name. All six are different types of one class of medication, called sulfonylureas, but each affects metabolism differently. A doctor will choose a patient's medication based on the person's general health, the amount his or her blood glucose needs to be lowered, the person's eating habits, and the medicine's side effects.

The purpose of oral medications is to lower blood glucose.

Therefore, the person taking them must eat regular meals and engage in only light to moderate exercise, to prevent blood glucose from dipping too low. Medications taken for other health problems, including illness, also can lower blood sugar and may react with the diabetes medicine. Therefore, a doctor needs to know all the medications a person is taking to prevent a harmful interaction. Lowering blood sugar too much can cause hypoglycemia with symptoms such as headache, weakness, shakiness, and if the condition is severe enough, collapse.

Oral diabetes medications usually don't cause side effects. However, a few people do experience nausea, skin rashes, headache, either water retention or diuresis (increased urination), and sensitivity to direct sunlight. These effects should gradually subside, but a person should see a doctor if they persist. For reasons that aren't always clear, sometimes oral diabetes medications don't help the person for whom they're prescribed. Investigations are under way to learn why this happens.

## *Insulin*

This chapter is about *noninsulin-dependent diabetes.* The word "diabetes" in the text of this chapter refers to noninsulin-dependent diabetes unless otherwise specified.

Like oral diabetes medications, insulin is an alternative for some people with noninsulin-dependent diabetes who can't control their blood glucose levels with diet and exercise. In special situations, such as surgery and pregnancy, insulin is a temporary but important means of controlling blood glucose. A section of this chapter called "special situations" discusses insulin use during pregnancy and surgery.

Sometimes it's unclear whether insulin or oral medications are more effective in controlling blood glucose; therefore, a doctor will consider a person's weight, age, and the severity of the diabetes before prescribing a medicine. Experts do know that weight control is essential for insulin to be effective. A doctor is likely to prescribe insulin if diet, exercise, or oral medications don't work, or if someone has a bad reaction to oral medicines. A person also may have to take insulin if his or her blood glucose fluctuates a great deal and is difficult to control. A doctor will instruct a person with diabetes on how to purchase, mix, and inject insulin. Various types of insulin are available that differ in purity, concentration, and how quickly they work. They also are made differently. In the past, all commercially available insulin came from the pancreas glands of cows and pigs. Today, human insulin is available in two forms: one uses genetic engineering and the other involves chemically changing pork insulin into human insulin. The best sources of information on insulin are the company that makes it and a doctor.

## Checking Blood Glucose Levels

When a person's body is operating normally, it automatically checks the level of glucose in blood. If the level is too high or too low, the body will adjust the sugar level to return it to normal. This system operates in much the same way that cruise control adjusts the speed of a car. With diabetes, the body doesn't do the job of controlling blood glucose automatically. To make up for this, someone with diabetes has to check blood sugar regularly and adjust treatment accordingly.

A doctor can measure blood glucose during an office visit. However, levels change from hour to hour and someone who visits the doctor only every few weeks won't know what his or her blood glucose is daily. Do-it-yourself tests enable people with diabetes to check their blood sugar daily.

The easiest test someone can do at home is a urine test. When the level of glucose in blood rises above normal, the kidneys eliminate the excess glucose in urine. Glucose in urine, therefore, reflects an excess of glucose in blood.

Urine testing is easy. Tablets or paper strips are dipped in urine. The color change that occurs indicates whether blood glucose is too high. However, urine testing is not completely accurate because the reading reflects the level of blood glucose a few hours earlier. In addition, not everyone's kidneys are the same. Even when the amount of glucose in two people's urine is the same, their sugar levels may be different. Certain drugs and vitamin C also can affect the accuracy of urine tests.

It's more accurate to measure blood glucose directly. Kits are available that allow people with diabetes to test their blood glucose at home. The test involves pricking a finger to draw a drop of blood. A spring-operated "lancet" does this automatically. The drop of blood is placed on a strip of specially coated plastic or into a small machine that "reads" how much glucose is in the blood. A doctor may suggest that someone test his or her blood glucose several times a day. Self blood glucose monitoring can show how the body responds to meals, exercise, stress, and diabetes treatment.

Another test that measures the effectiveness of treatment is a "glycosylated hemoglobin" test. It measures the glucose that has become attached to hemoglobin, the molecule in red blood cells that gives blood its red color. Over time, hemoglobin absorbs glucose, according to its concentration in blood. Once glucose is absorbed by hemoglobin it remains there until the blood cells die and new ones replace them. With the "glycosylated hemoglobin" test, a doctor can tell whether blood glucose has been very high over the last few months.

## Diabetes Complications

A key goal of diabetes treatment is to prevent complications because, over time, diabetes can damage the heart, blood vessels, eyes, kidneys, and nerves, although the person may not know damage is taking place. It's important to diagnose and treat diabetes early, because it can cause damage even before it makes someone feel ill.

How diabetes causes long-term problems is unclear. However, changes in the small blood vessels and nerves are common. These changes may be the first step toward many problems that diabetes causes. Scientists can't predict who among people with diabetes will develop complications, but complications are most likely to occur in someone who has had diabetes for many years. However, because a person can have diabetes without knowing it, a complication may be the first sign.

### *Heart Disease*

Heart disease is the most common life-threatening disease linked to diabetes, and experts say diabetes doubles a person's risk of developing heart disease. In heart disease, deposits of fat and cholesterol build-up in the arteries that supply the heart with blood. If this build-up blocks blood from getting to the heart, a potentially fatal heart attack can occur.

Other risk factors include hypertension or high blood pressure, obesity, high amounts of fats and cholesterol in blood, and cigarette smoking. Eliminating these risk factors, along with treating diabetes, can reduce the risk of heart disease. The American Heart Association has literature that explains what heart disease is and how to prevent it. The association's address is in the resources section of this book.

### *Kidney Disease*

People with diabetes are also more likely to develop kidney disease than other people. The kidneys filter waste products from the blood and excrete them in the form of urine, maintaining proper fluid balance in the body. While people can live without one kidney, those without both must have special treatment, called dialysis. Most people with diabetes will never develop kidney disease, but proper diabetes treatment can further reduce the risk. High blood pressure also can add to the risk of kidney disease. Therefore, regular blood pressure checks and early treatment of the disorder can help prevent kidney disease.

Urinary tract infections are also a cause of kidney problems. Diabetes can affect the nerves that control the bladder, making it difficult for a person to empty his or her bladder completely. Bacteria can form in the unemptied bladder and the tubes leading from it, eventually causing infection. The symptoms of a urinary tract infection include frequent, painful urination, blood in the urine, and pain in the lower abdomen and back. Without prompt examination and treatment by a doctor, the infection can reach the kidneys, causing pain, fever, and possibly kidney damage. A doctor may prescribe antibiotics to treat the infection and may suggest that the person drink large amounts of water.

Kidney problems are one cause of water retention, or edema, a condition in which fluid collects in the body, causing swelling, often in the legs and hands. A doctor can decide if swelling or water retention relates to kidney function.

A nephrologist, a doctor specially trained to diagnose and treat kidney problems, can identify the cause of problems and recommend ways to reduce the risk of kidney disease.

### *Eye Problems*

Diabetes can affect the eyes in several ways. Frequently, the effects are temporary and can be corrected with better diabetes control. However, long-term diabetes can cause changes in the eyes that threaten vision. Stable blood glucose levels and yearly eye examinations can help reduce the risk of serious eye damage.

Blurred vision is one effect diabetes can have on the eyes. The reason may be that changing levels of glucose in blood also can affect the balance of fluid in the lens of the eye, which works like a flexible camera lens to focus images. If the lens absorbs more water than normal and swells, its focusing power changes. Diabetes also may affect the function of nerves that control eyesight, causing blurred vision.

Cataract and glaucoma are eye diseases that occur more frequently in people with diabetes. Cataract is a clouding of the normally clear lens of the eye. Glaucoma is a condition in which pressure within the eye can damage the optic nerve that transmits visual images to the brain. Early diagnosis and treatment of cataract and glaucoma can reduce the severity of these disorders.

### *Diabetic Retinopathy*

Retinopathy, a disease of the retina, the light sensing tissue at the back of the eye, is a common concern among people with diabetes. Diabetic retinopathy damages the tiny vessels that supply the retina with blood. The blood vessels may swell and leak fluid. When retinopathy is more severe, new blood vessels may grow from the back of the eye and bleed into the clear gel that fills the eye, the vitreous.

While most people with diabetes may never develop serious eye problems, people who have had diabetes for 25 years are more likely to develop retinopathy. Experts think high blood pressure may contribute to diabetic retinopathy, and that smoking can cause the condition to worsen. If someone experiences blurred vision that lasts longer than a day or so, sudden loss of vision in either eye, or black spots, lines, or flashing lights in the field of vision, a doctor should be alerted right away.

Treatment for diabetic retinopathy can help prevent loss of vision and can sometimes restore vision lost because of the disease. A yearly eye examination with dilated pupils makes it possible for an ophthalmologist, an eye doctor, to notice changes before the illness becomes harder to treat. Scientists are testing new means of treating diabetic retinopathy. For more information on eye complications of diabetes and the treatment of these conditions, see the resource list at the end of this book.

### *Legs and Feet*

Leg and foot problems can arise in people with diabetes due to changes in blood vessels and nerves in these areas. Peripheral vascular disease is a condition in which blood vessels become narrowed by fatty deposits, reducing blood supply to the legs and feet. Diabetes also can dull the sensitivity of nerves. Someone with this condition, called peripheral neuropathy, might not notice a sore spot caused by tight shoes or pressure from walking. If ignored, the sore can become infected and because blood circulation is poor, the area may take longer to heal.

Proper foot care and regular visits to a doctor can prevent foot and leg sores and ensure that any that do appear don't become infected and painful. Helpful measures include inspecting the feet daily for cuts or sore spots. Blisters and sore spots are not as likely when shoes fit well and socks or stockings aren't tight. A doctor also may suggest washing feet daily, with warm, not hot water; filing thick calluses; and using lotions that keep the feet from getting too dry. Shoe inserts or special shoes can be used to prevent pressure on the foot.

Diabetic neuropathy, or nerve disease, dulls the nerves and can be extremely painful. A person with neuropathy also may be depressed. Scientists aren't sure whether the depression is an effect of neuropathy, or if it's simply a response to pain. Treatment, aimed at relieving pain and depression, may include aspirin and other pain-killing drugs.

Any sore on the foot or leg, whether or not it's painful, requires a doctor's immediate attention. Treatment can help sores heal and prevent new ones from developing. Problems with the feet and legs can cause life-threatening problems that require amputation—surgical removal of limbs—if not treated early.

### *Other Effects of Diabetic Neuropathy*

Nerves provide muscle tone and feeling and help control functions like digestion and blood pressure. Diabetes can cause changes in these nerves and the functions they control. These changes are most frequent in people who have had other complications of diabetes, like problems with their feet. Someone who has had diabetes for some years and has other complications, may find that spells of indigestion or diarrhea are common. A doctor may prescribe drugs to relieve these symptoms. Diabetes also can affect the nerves that control penile erection in men, which can cause impotence that shows up gradually, without any loss of desire for sex. A doctor can find out whether impotence is the result of physical changes, such as diabetes, or emotional changes, and suggest treatment or counseling.

### *Skin and Oral Infections*

People with diabetes are more likely to develop infections, like boils and ulcers, than the average person. Women with diabetes may develop vaginal infections more often than other women. Checking for infections, treating them early, and following a doctor's advice can help ensure that infections are mild and infrequent.

Infections also can affect the teeth and gums, making people with diabetes more susceptible to periodontal disease, an inflammation of tissue surrounding and supporting the teeth. An important cause of periodontal disease is bacterial growth on the teeth and gums. Treating diabetes and following a dentist's advice on dental care can help prevent periodontal disease.

### *Emergencies*

Very high blood glucose levels cause symptoms that are hard to ignore: frequent urination and excessive thirst. However, in someone who is elderly or in poor health these symptoms may go unnoticed. Without treatment, a person with high blood glucose or hyperglycemia can lose fluids, become weak, confused, and even unconscious. Breathing will be shallow and the pulse rapid. The person's lips and tongue will be dry, and his or her hands and feet will be cool. A doctor should be called immediately.

The opposite of high blood glucose, very low blood glucose or hypoglycemia, is also dangerous. Hypoglycemia can occur when someone hasn't eaten enough to balance the effects of insulin or oral medicine. Prolonged, strenuous exercise in someone taking oral diabetes drugs or insulin also can cause hypoglycemia, as can alcohol.

Someone whose blood glucose has become too low may feel nervous, shaky, and weak. The person may sweat, feel hungry, and have a headache. Severe hypoglycemia can cause loss of consciousness. A person with hypoglycemia who begins to feel weak and shaky should eat or drink something with sugar in it immediately, like orange juice. If the person is unconscious, he or she should be taken to a hospital emergency room right away. An identification bracelet or necklace that states that the wearer has diabetes will let friends know that these symptoms are a warning of illness that requires urgent medical help.

## Special Situations

### *Surgery*

Surgery is stressful, both physically and mentally. It can raise blood glucose levels even in someone who is careful about control. To make sure that surgery and recovery are successful for someone with diabetes, a doctor will test blood glucose and keep it under careful control, usually with insulin. Careful control makes it possible for someone with diabetes to have surgery with little or no more risk than someone without diabetes.

To plan a safe and successful surgery, the surgeon and attending physicians must know that the person they're treating has diabetes.

While tests done before surgery can detect diabetes, the patient should inform the doctor of his or her condition. A surgical team also will evaluate the possible effect of complications of diabetes, such as heart or kidney problems.

## *Pregnancy*

Bearing a child places extra demands on a woman's body. Diabetes makes it more difficult for her body to adjust to these demands and it can cause problems for both mother and baby. Some woman may develop a form of diabetes during pregnancy called gestational diabetes. Gestational diabetes develops most frequently in the middle and later months of pregnancy, after the time of greatest risk for birth defects. Although this kind of diabetes often disappears after the baby's birth, treatment is necessary during pregnancy to make sure the diabetes doesn't harm the mother or fetus.

A woman who knows she has diabetes should keep her condition under control before she becomes pregnant, so that her diabetes won't increase the risk of birth defects. A woman whose diabetes isn't well controlled may have an unusually large baby. Diabetes also increases the risk of premature birth and problems in the baby, such as breathing difficulties, low blood sugar and occasionally, death.

Blood glucose monitoring and treatment with insulin can ensure that a baby born to a mother with diabetes will be healthy. Oral diabetes drugs aren't given during pregnancy because the effects of these drugs on the unborn baby aren't known. By following the advice of a doctor trained to treat gestational diabetes, the mother can make sure her blood glucose is normal and her baby is well nourished.

Approximately half of women with gestational diabetes will no longer have abnormal blood glucose tests shortly after giving birth. However, many women with gestational diabetes will develop noninsulin-dependent diabetes later in their lives. Regular check-ups can ensure that if a woman does develop diabetes later, it will be diagnosed and treated early.

## *Is Diabetes Hereditary?*

Scientists estimate that the child of a parent with noninsulin-dependent diabetes has approximately a 10 to 15 percent chance of developing noninsulin-dependent diabetes. If both parents have diabetes, the child's risk of having the disease increases. The child's health habits throughout his or her life will affect the risk of developing diabetes. Obesity, for example, may increase the risk of diabetes or cause it to occur earlier in life.

Noninsulin-dependent diabetes in a parent has no effect on the chances that his or her child will have insulin-dependent diabetes, the more severe form of diabetes.

### Stress and Illness

One way the body responds to stress is to increase the level of blood glucose. In a person with diabetes, stress may increase the need for treatment to lower blood glucose levels. Illnesses such as colds and flu are forms of physical stress that a doctor can treat. The doctor will advise the person to drink plenty of fluids. When blood glucose is high, the body gets rid of glucose through urine, and this fluid needs to be replaced.

If nausea makes eating or taking oral diabetes drugs a problem, a doctor should be consulted. Not eating can increase the risk of low blood glucose, while stopping oral medications or insulin during illness can lead to very high blood glucose. A doctor may prescribe insulin temporarily for someone with diabetes who can't take medicine by mouth.

Great thirst, rapid weight loss, high fever, or very high urine or blood glucose are signs that blood sugar is out of control. If a person has these symptoms, a doctor should be called immediately.

Like illness, stress that results from losses or conflicts at home or on the job can affect diabetes control. Urine and blood glucose checks can be clues to the effects of stress. If someone finds that stress is making diabetes control difficult, a doctor can advise treatment and suggest sources of help.

## Dealing with Diabetes

Good diabetes care requires a daily effort to follow a diet, stay active, and take medicine when necessary. Talking to people who have diabetes or who treat diabetes may be helpful for someone who needs emotional support. The list of organizations at the end of this book can help patients find discussion groups or counselors familiar with diabetes. It's very important for people with diabetes to understand how to stay healthy, follow a proper diet, exercise, and be aware of changes in their bodies. People with diabetes can live long, healthy lives if they take care of themselves.

## Finding Help

A person with diabetes is responsible for his or her daily care and a doctor is the best source of information on that care. A doctor in family practice or internal medicine can diagnose and treat diabetes, and may refer the patient to a doctor who specializes in treating diabetes. "Endocrinologists" and "diabetologists" are doctors with advanced training and experience in diabetes treatment. The local chapters of the American Diabetes Association or the Juvenile Diabetes Foundation have lists of doctors who specialize in diabetes. Another alternative is to contact a university-based medical center. These centers may have special diabetes clinics or may be able to suggest diabetes doctors who practice in the community.

## Printed Information

While information in books and magazines can't replace a doctor's personal advice, it can provide a clear explanation of diabetes and describe advancements in diabetes treatment. The American Diabetes Association and Juvenile Diabetes Foundation have brochures about diabetes and diabetes treatment. These publications are for people without a medical background. The addresses of these organizations are in the resources section at the end of this book.

Brochures and books about diabetes also are available from public libraries and bookstores. Local chapters of the American Diabetes Association, hospitals, and medical centers frequently sponsor educational programs on diabetes and diabetes treatment. Information about diabetes programs is also available from a doctor's office, a local hospital or health department, or a local diabetes organization.

Chapter 12

# Gestational Diabetes

For the purpose of this chapter the words *sugar* and *glucose* are used synonymously.

Approximately 3 to 5 percent of all pregnant women in the United States are diagnosed as having gestational diabetes. These women and their families have many questions about this disorder. Some of the most frequently asked questions are:

- What is gestational diabetes and how did I get it?
- How does it differ from other kinds of diabetes?
- Will it hurt my baby?
- Will my baby have diabetes?
- What can I do to control gestational diabetes?
- Will I need a special diet?
- Will gestational diabetes change the way or the time my baby is delivered?
- Will I have diabetes in the future?

This chapter will address these and many other questions about diet, exercise, measurement of blood sugar levels, and general medical and obstetric care of women with gestational diabetes. It must be emphasized that these are general guidelines and only your health care professional(s) can tailor a program specific to your needs. You should feel free to discuss any concerns you have with your doctor or

NIH Pub. No. 93-2788, February 1993.

other health care provider, as no one knows more about you and the condition of your pregnancy.

### *What is gestational diabetes and what causes it?*

Diabetes (actual name is diabetes mellitus) of any kind is a disorder that prevents the body from using food properly. Normally, the body gets its major source of energy from glucose, a simple sugar that comes from foods high in simple carbohydrates (e.g., table sugar or other sweeteners such as honey, molasses, jams, and jellies, soft drinks, and cookies), or from the breakdown of complex carbohydrates such as starches (e.g., bread, potatoes, and pasta). After sugars and starches are digested in the stomach, they enter the blood stream in the form of glucose. The glucose in the blood stream becomes a potential source of energy for the entire body, similar to the way in which gasoline in a service station pump is a potential source of energy for your car. But, just as someone must pump the gas into the car, the body requires some assistance to get glucose from the blood stream to the muscles and other tissues of the body. In the body, that assistance comes from a hormone called insulin. Insulin is manufactured by the pancreas, a gland that lies behind the stomach. Without insulin, glucose cannot get into the cells of the body where it is used as fuel. Instead, glucose accumulates in the blood to high levels and is excreted or "spilled" into the urine through the kidneys.

When the pancreas of a child or young adult produces little or no insulin we call this condition juvenile-onset diabetes or Type I diabetes (insulin-dependent). This is not the type of diabetes you have. Unlike women with Type I diabetes, women with gestational diabetes have plenty of insulin. In fact, they usually have more insulin in their blood than women who are not pregnant. However, the effect of their insulin is partially blocked by a variety of other hormones made in the placenta, a condition often called insulin resistance.

The placenta performs the task of supplying the growing fetus with nutrients and water from the mother's circulation. It also produces a variety of hormones vital to the preservation of the pregnancy. Ironically, several of these hormones such as estrogen, cortisol, and human placental lactogen (HPL) have a blocking effect on insulin, a "contra-insulin" effect. This contra-insulin effect usually begins about midway (20 to 24 weeks) through pregnancy. The larger the placenta grows, the more these hormones are produced, and the greater the insulin resistance becomes. In most women the pancreas is able to make additional insulin to overcome the insulin resistance. When the pancreas makes all the insulin it can and there still isn't enough to overcome the effect of the placenta's hormones, gestational diabetes results. If we could somehow remove all the placenta's hormones from the mother's blood, the condition would be remedied. This, in fact, usually happens following delivery.

### *How does gestational diabetes differ from other types of diabetes?*

There are several different types of diabetes. Gestational diabetes begins during pregnancy and disappears following delivery. Another type is referred to as juvenile-onset diabetes (in children) or Type I (in young adults). These individuals usually develop their disease before age 20. People with Type I diabetes must take insulin by injection every day. Approximately 10 percent of all people with diabetes have Type I (also called insulin-dependent diabetes).

Type II diabetes or noninsulin-dependent diabetes (formerly called adult-onset diabetes) is also characterized by high blood sugar levels, but these patients are often obese and usually lack the classic symptoms (fatigue, thirst, frequent urination, and sudden weight loss) associated with Type I diabetes. Many of these individuals can control their blood sugar levels by following a careful diet and exercise program, by losing excess weight, or by taking oral medication. Some, but not all, need insulin. People with Type II diabetes account for roughly 90 percent of all diabetics.

### *Who is at risk for developing gestational diabetes and how is it detected?*

Any woman might develop gestational diabetes during pregnancy. Some of the factors associated with women who have an increased risk are obesity; a family history of diabetes; having given birth previously to a very large infant, a stillbirth, or a child with a birth defect; or having too much amniotic fluid (polyhydramnios). Also, women who are older than 25 are at greater risk than younger individuals. Although a history of sugar in the urine is often included in the list of risk factors, this is not a reliable indicator of who will develop diabetes during pregnancy. Some pregnant women with perfectly normal blood sugar levels will occasionally have sugar detected in their urine.

The Council on Diabetes in Pregnancy of the American Diabetes Association strongly recommends that all pregnant women be screened for gestational diabetes. Several methods of screening exist. The most common is the 50-gram glucose screening test. No special preparation is necessary for this test, and there is no need to fast before the test. The test is performed by giving 50 grams of a glucose drink and then measuring the blood sugar level 1-hour later. A woman with a blood sugar level of less than 140 milligrams per deciliter (mg/dl) at 1-hour is presumed not to have gestational diabetes and requires no further testing. If the blood sugar level is greater than 140 mg/dl the test is considered abnormal or “positive.” Not all women with a positive screening test have diabetes. Consequently, a 3-hour glucose tolerance test must be performed to establish the diagnosis of gestational diabetes.

If your physician determines that you should take the complete 3-hour glucose tolerance test, you will be asked to follow some special instructions in preparation for the test. For 3 days before the test, eat a diet that contains at least 150 grams of carbohydrates each day. This can be accomplished by including one cup of pasta, two servings of fruit, four slices of bread, and three glasses of milk every day. For 10 to 14 hours before the test you should not eat and not drink anything but water. The test is usually done in the morning in your physician’s office or in a laboratory. First, a blood sample will be drawn to measure your fasting blood sugar level. Then you will be asked to drink a full bottle of a glucose drink (100 grams). This glucose drink is extremely sweet and occasionally makes some people feel nauseated. Finally, blood samples will be drawn every hour for 3 hours after the glucose drink has been consumed. The normal values for this test are shown in Table 12.1.

**Table 12.1.** 3-Hour Glucose Tolerance Test for Gestational Diabetes

| | **Diagnostic Criteria** Blood Glucose Level | **Normal Mean Values** Blood Glucose Level |
|---|---|---|
| Fasting | 105 mg/dl | 80 mg/dl |
| 1 hour | 190 mg/dl | 120 mg/dl |
| 2 hour | 165 mg/dl | 105 mg/dl |
| 3 hour | 145 mg/dl | 90 mg/dl |

*From 752 Unselected Pregnancies*

If two or more of your blood sugar levels are higher than the diagnostic criteria, you have gestational diabetes. This testing is usually performed at the end of the second trimester or the beginning of the third trimester (between the 24th and 28th weeks of pregnancy) when insulin resistance usually begins. If you had gestational diabetes in a previous pregnancy or there is some reason why your physician is unusually concerned about your risk of developing gestational diabetes, you may be asked to take the 50-gram glucose screening test as early as the first trimester (before the 13th week). Remember, merely having sugar in your urine or even having an abnormal blood sugar on the 50-gram glucose screening test does not necessarily mean you have gestational diabetes. The 3-hour glucose tolerance test must be abnormal before the diagnosis is made.

### *How does gestational diabetes affect pregnancy and will it hurt my baby?*

The complications of gestational diabetes are manageable and preventable. The key to prevention is careful control of blood sugar levels just as soon as the diagnosis of gestational diabetes is made.

You should be reassured that there are certain things gestational diabetes does not usually cause. Unlike Type I diabetes, gestational diabetes generally does not cause birth defects. For the most part, birth defects originate sometime during the first trimester (before the 13th week) of pregnancy. The insulin resistance from the contra-insulin hormones produced by the placenta does not usually occur until approximately the 24th week. Therefore, women with gestational diabetes generally have normal blood sugar levels during the critical first trimester.

One of the major problems a woman with gestational diabetes faces is a condition the baby may develop called "macrosomia." Macrosomia means "large body" and refers to a baby that is considerably larger than normal. All of the nutrients the fetus receives come directly from the mother's blood. If the maternal blood has too much glucose, the pancreas of the fetus senses the high glucose levels and produces more insulin in an attempt to use the glucose. The fetus converts the extra glucose to fat. Even when the mother has gestational diabetes, the fetus is able to produce all the insulin it needs. The combination of high blood glucose levels from the mother and high insulin levels in the fetus results in large deposits of fat which causes the fetus to grow excessively large, a condition known as macrosomia. Occasionally, the baby grows too large to be delivered through the vagina and a cesarean delivery becomes necessary. The obstetrician can often determine if the fetus is macrosomic by doing a physical examination. However, in many cases a special test called an ultrasound is used to measure the size of the fetus. This and other special tests will be discussed later.

In addition to macrosomia, gestational diabetes increases the risk of hypoglycemia (low blood sugar) in the baby immediately after delivery. This problem occurs if the mother's blood sugar levels have been consistently high causing the fetus to have a high level of insulin in its circulation. After delivery the baby continues to have a high insulin level, but it no longer has the high level of sugar from its mother, resulting in the newborn's blood sugar level becoming very low. Your baby's blood sugar level will be checked in the newborn nursery and if the level is too low, it may be necessary to give the baby glucose intravenously. Infants of mothers with gestational diabetes are also vulnerable to several other chemical imbalances such as low serum calcium and low serum magnesium levels.

All of these are manageable and preventable problems. The key to prevention is careful control of blood sugar levels in the mother just as soon as the diagnosis of gestational diabetes is made. By maintaining normal blood sugar levels, it is less likely that a fetus will develop macrosomia, hypoglycemia, or other chemical abnormalities.

### *What can be done to reduce problems associated with gestational diabetes?*

In addition to your obstetrician, there are other health professionals who specialize in the management of diabetes during pregnancy including internists or diabetologists, registered dietitians, qualified nutritionists, and diabetes educators. Your doctor may recommend that you see one or more of these specialists during your pregnancy. In addition, a neonatologist (a doctor who specializes in the care of newborn infants) should also be called in to manage any complications the baby might develop after delivery.

One of the essential components in the care of a woman with gestational diabetes is a diet specifically tailored to provide adequate nutrition to meet the needs of the mother and the growing fetus. At the same time the diet has to be planned in such a way as to keep blood glucose levels in the normal range (60 to 120 mg/dl). Specific details about diet during pregnancy are discussed later.

An obstetrician, diabetes educator, or other health care practitioner can teach you how to measure your own blood glucose levels at home to see if levels remain in an acceptable range on the prescribed diet. The ability of patients to determine their own blood sugar levels with easy-to-use equipment represents a major milestone in the management of diabetes, especially during pregnancy. The technique called "self blood glucose monitoring" (discussed in detail later) allows you to check your blood sugar levels at home or at work without costly and time-consuming visits to your doctor. The values of your blood sugar levels also determine if you need to begin insulin therapy sometime during pregnancy. Short of frequent trips to a laboratory, this is the only way to see if blood glucose levels remain under good control.

### *What is self blood glucose monitoring?*

Once you are diagnosed as having gestational diabetes, you and your health care providers will want to know more about your day-to-day blood sugar levels. It is important to know how your exercise habits and eating patterns affect your blood sugars. Also, as your pregnancy progresses, the placenta will release more of the hormones that work against insulin. Testing your blood sugar level at important times during the day will help determine if proper diet and weight gain have kept blood sugar levels normal or if extra insulin is needed to help keep the fetus protected.

Self blood glucose monitoring is done by using a special device to obtain a drop of your blood and test it for your blood sugar level. Your doctor or other health care provider will explain the procedure to you. Make sure that you are shown how to do the testing before attempting it on your own. Some items you may use to monitor your blood sugar levels are:

- **Lancet**—a disposable, sharp needle-like sticker for pricking the finger to obtain a drop of blood.
- **Lancet device**—a spring-loaded finger sticking device.
- **Test strip**—a chemically treated strip to which a drop of blood is applied.
- **Color chart**—a chart used to compare against the color on the test strip for blood sugar level.
- **Glucose meter**—a device which "reads" the test strip and gives you a digital number value.

Your health care provider can advise you where to obtain the self-monitoring equipment in your area. You may want to inquire if any places rent or loan glucose meters, since it is likely you won't be needing it after your baby is born.

### How often and when should I test?

You may need to test your blood several times a day. Generally, these times are fasting (first thing in the morning before you eat) and 2 hours after each meal. Occasionally, you may be asked to test more frequently during the day or at night. As each person is an individual, your health care provider can advise the schedule best for you.

### How should I record my test results?

Most manufacturers of glucose testing products provide a record diary, although some health care providers may have their own version. A Self Blood Glucose Monitoring Diary example is included (Figure 12.8.) at the end of this chapter.

You should record any test result immediately because it's easy to forget what the reading was during the course of a busy day. You should always have this diary with you when you visit your doctor or other health care provider or when you contact them by phone. These results are very important in making decisions about your health care.

### Are there any other tests I should know about?

In addition to blood testing, you may be asked to check your urine for ketones. Ketones are by-products of the breakdown of fat and may be found in the blood and urine as a result of inadequate insulin or from inadequate calories in your diet. Although it is not known whether or not small amounts of ketones can harm the fetus, when large amounts of ketones are present they are accompanied by a blood condition, acidosis, which is known to harm the fetus. To be on the safe side, you should watch for them in your urine and report any positive results to your doctor.

### How do I test for ketones?

To test the urine for ketones, you can use a test strip similar to the one used for testing your blood. This test strip has a special chemically treated pad to detect ketones in the urine. Testing is done by passing the test strip through the stream of urine or dipping the strip in and out of urine in a container. As your pregnancy progresses, you might find it easier to use the container method. All test strips are disposable and can be used only once. This applies to blood sugar test strips also. You cannot use your blood sugar test strips for urine testing, and you cannot use your urine ketone test strips for blood sugar testing.

### When do I test for ketones?

Overnight is the longest fasting period, so you should test your urine first thing in the morning every day and any time your blood sugar level goes over 240 mg/dl on the blood glucose test. It is also important to test if you become ill and are eating less food than normal. Your health care provider can advise what's best for you.

### Is it ever necessary to take insulin?

Yes, despite careful attention to diet some women's blood sugars do not stay within an acceptable range. A pregnant woman free of gestational diabetes rarely has a blood glucose level that exceeds 100 mg/dl in the morning before breakfast (fasting) or 2 hours after a meal. The optimum goal for a gestational diabetic is blood sugar levels that are the same as those of a woman without diabetes.

There is no absolute blood sugar level that necessitates beginning insulin injections. However, many physicians begin insulin if the fasting sugar exceeds 105 mg/dl or if the level 2 hours after a meal exceeds 120 mg/dl on two separate occasions. Blood sugar levels measured by you at home will help your doctor know when it is necessary to begin insulin. The ability to perform self blood glucose monitoring has made it possible to begin insulin therapy at the earliest sign of high sugar levels, thereby preventing the fetus from being exposed to high levels of glucose from the mother's blood.

### Will my baby be healthy?

The ultimate concern of any expectant mother is, "Will my baby be all right?" There is an array of simple, safe tests used to assess the condition of the fetus before birth and these can be particularly valuable during a pregnancy complicated by gestational diabetes. Tests that may be given during your pregnancy include:

***Ultrasound.*** Ultrasound uses short pulses of high-frequency, low-intensity sound waves to create images. Unlike x rays, there is no radiation exposure to the fetus. First used during World War II to detect enemy submarines below the surface of the water, ultrasound has since been used safely in obstetrics. Occasionally, the date of your last menstrual period is not sufficient to determine a due date. Ultrasound can provide an accurate gestational age and due date that may be very important if it is necessary to induce labor early or perform a cesarean delivery. Ultrasound can also be used to determine the position of the placenta if it is necessary to perform an amniocentesis (another test discussed later).

***Fetal movement records.*** Recording fetal movement is a test you can do by yourself to help determine the condition of the baby. Fetal activity is generally a reassuring sign of well-being. Women are often asked to count fetal movements regularly during the last trimester of pregnancy. You may be asked to set aside specific times to lie down on your back or side and count the number of times the baby moves or kicks. Three or more movements in a 2-hour period is considered normal. Contact your obstetrician if you feel fewer than three movements to determine if other tests are needed.

***Fetal monitoring.*** Modern instruments make it possible to monitor the baby's heart rate before delivery. Currently, there are two types of fetal monitors—internal and external. The internal monitor consists of a small wire electrode attached directly to the scalp of the fetus after the membranes have ruptured. The external monitor uses transducers secured to the mother's abdomen by an elastic belt. One transducer records the baby's heart rate by a sensitive microphone called a doppler. The other transducer measures the firmness of the abdomen during a contraction of the uterus. It is a crude measure of the strength and frequency of contractions. Fetal monitoring is the basis for the non-stress test and the oxytocin challenge test described below.

***Non-stress test.*** The "non-stress" test refers to the fact that no medication is given to the mother to cause movement of the fetus or contraction of the uterus. It is often used to confirm the well-being of the fetus based on the principle that a healthy fetus will demonstrate an acceleration in its heart rate following movement. Fetal activity may be spontaneous or induced by external manipulation such as rubbing the mother's abdomen or making a loud noise above the abdomen with a special device. When movement of the fetus is noted, a recording of the fetal heart rate is made. If the heart rate goes up, the test is normal. If the heart rate does not accelerate, the fetus may merely be "sleeping"; if, after stimulation, the fetus still does not react, it may be necessary to perform a "stress test" (oxytocin challenge test).

***Stress test (oxytocin challenge test).*** Labor represents a stress to the fetus. Every time the uterus contracts, the fetus is momentarily deprived of its usual blood supply and oxygen. This is not a problem for most babies. However, some babies are not healthy enough to handle the stress and demonstrate an abnormal heart rate pattern. This test is often done if the non-stress test is abnormal. It involves giving the hormone oxytocin (secreted by every mother when normal labor begins) to the mother to stimulate uterine contractions. The contractions are a challenge to the baby, similar to the challenge of normal labor. If the baby's heart rate slows down rather than speeds up after a contraction, the baby may be in jeopardy. The stress test is considered more accurate than the non-stress test. Nevertheless, it is not 100 percent fool-proof and your obstetrician may want to repeat it on another occasion to ensure its accuracy. Most women describe this test as mildly uncomfortable but not painful.

***Amniocentesis.*** Amniocentesis is a method of removing a small amount of fluid from the amniotic sac for analysis. Either the fluid itself or the cells shed by the fetus into the fluid can be studied. In mid-pregnancy the cells in amniotic fluid can be analyzed for genetic abnormalities such as Down syndrome. Many women over the age of 35 have amniocentesis for just this reason. Another important use for amniocentesis late in pregnancy is to study the fluid itself to determine if the lungs of the fetus are mature and able to withstand early delivery. This information can be very important in deciding the best time for a woman with Type I diabetes to deliver. It is not done as frequently to women with gestational diabetes.

Amniocentesis can be performed in an obstetrician's office or on an outpatient basis in a hospital. For genetic testing, amniocentesis is usually performed around the 16th week when the placenta and fetus can be located easily with ultrasound and a needle can be inserted safely into the amniotic sac. The overall complication rate for amniocentesis is less than 1 percent. The risk is even lower during the third trimester when the amniotic sac is larger and easily identifiable.

### *Does gestational diabetes affect labor and delivery?*

Most women with gestational diabetes can complete pregnancy and begin labor naturally. Any pregnant woman has a slight chance (about 5 percent) of developing preeclampsia (toxemia), a sudden onset of high blood pressure associated with protein in the urine, occurring late in pregnancy. If preeclampsia develops, your obstetrician may recommend an early delivery. When an early delivery is anticipated, an amniocentesis is usually performed to assess the maturity of the baby's lungs.

Gestational diabetes, by itself, is not an indication to perform a cesarean delivery, but sometimes there are other reasons your doctor may elect to do a cesarean. For example, the baby may be too large (macrosomic) to deliver vaginally, or the baby may be in distress and unable to withstand vaginal delivery. You should discuss the various possibilities for delivery with your obstetrician so there are no surprises.

Careful control of blood sugar levels remains important even during labor. If a mother's blood sugar level becomes elevated during labor, the baby's blood sugar level will also become elevated. High blood sugars in the mother produce high insulin levels in the baby. Immediately after delivery high insulin levels in the baby can drive its blood sugar level very low since it will no longer have the high sugar concentration from its mother's blood.

Women whose gestational diabetes does not require that they take insulin during their pregnancy, will not need to take insulin during their labor or delivery. On the other hand, a woman who does require insulin during pregnancy may be given insulin by injection on the morning labor begins, or in some instances, it may be given intravenously throughout labor. For most women with gestational diabetes there is no need for insulin after the baby is born and blood sugar level returns to normal immediately. The reason for this sudden return to normal lies in the fact that when the placenta is removed the hormones it was producing (which caused the insulin resistance) are also removed. Thus, the mother's insulin is permitted to work normally without resistance. Your doctor may want to check your blood sugar level the next morning, but it will most likely be normal.

### *Should I expect my baby to have any problems?*

One of the most frequently asked questions is, "Will my baby have diabetes?" Almost universally the answer is no. However, the baby is at risk for developing Type II diabetes later in life, and of having other problems related to gestational diabetes, such as hypoglycemia (low blood sugar) mentioned earlier. If your blood sugars were not elevated during the 24 hours before delivery, there is a good chance that hypoglycemia will not be a problem for your baby. Nevertheless, a neonatologist (a doctor who specializes in the care of newborn infants) or other doctor should check your baby's blood sugar level and give extra glucose if necessary.

Another problem that may develop in the infant of a mother with gestational diabetes is jaundice. Jaundice occurs when extra red blood cells in the baby's circulation are destroyed, releasing a substance called bilirubin. Bilirubin is a pigment that causes a yellow discoloration of the skin (jaundice). A minor degree of jaundice is common in many newborns. However, the presence of large amounts of bilirubin in the baby's system can be harmful and requires placing the baby under special lights which help get rid of the pigment. In extreme cases, blood transfusions may be necessary.

### *Will I develop diabetes in the future?*

For most women gestational diabetes disappears immediately after delivery. However, you should have your blood sugars checked after your baby is born to make sure your levels have returned to normal. Women who had gestational diabetes during one pregnancy are at greater risk of developing it in a subsequent pregnancy. It is important that you have appropriate screening tests for gestational diabetes during future pregnancies as early as the first trimester.

Pregnancy is a kind of "stress test" that often predicts future diabetic problems. In one large study more than one-half of all women who had gestational diabetes developed overt Type II diabetes within 15 years of pregnancy. Because of the risk of developing Type II diabetes in the future, you should have your blood sugar level checked when you see your doctor for your routine check-ups. There is a good chance you will be able to reduce the risk of developing diabetes later in life by maintaining an ideal body weight and exercising regularly.

### *Why is a special diet recommended?*

A nutritionally balanced diet is always essential to maintaining a healthy mother and successful pregnancy. The foods you choose become the nutrient building blocks for the growth of the fetus. For a woman with gestational diabetes, proper diet alone often keeps blood sugar levels in the normal range and is generally the first step to follow before resorting to insulin injections. Careful attention should be paid to the total calories eaten daily, to avoid foods which increase blood sugar levels, and to emphasize the use of foods which help the body maintain a normal blood sugar. A registered dietitian is the best person to help you with meal planning to meet your individual needs.

Your physician can help you find a dietitian if this service is not a part of his or her office or clinic. Your local chapter of the American Dietetic Association or the American Diabetes Association can also help you locate a registered dietitian.

### How much weight should I gain?

Of all questions asked by pregnant women, this is the most common. The answer is particularly important for women with gestational diabetes. The weight that you gain is a rough indication of how much nutrition is available to the fetus for growth. An inadequate weight gain may result in a small baby who lacks protective calorie reserves at birth. This baby may have more illness during the first year of life. An excessive weight gain during pregnancy, however, has an insulin-resistant effect, just like the hormones produced by the placenta, and will make your blood sugar level higher.

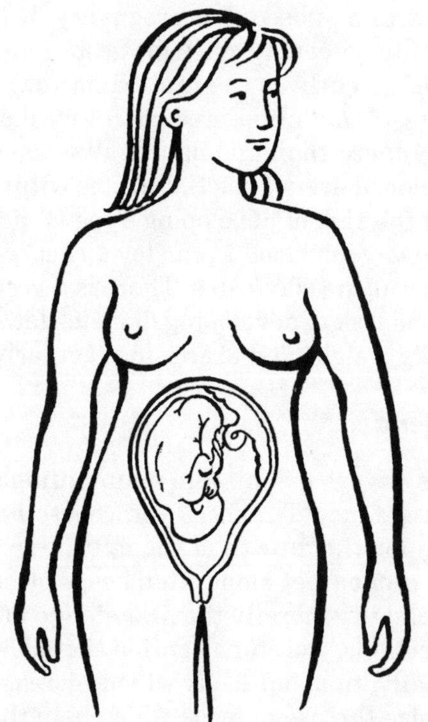

**Weight in Pounds**

7.5 - 8.5 Fetus

7.5 Stores of Fat & Protein

4.0 Blood

2.7 Tissue Fluids

2.0 Uterus

1.8 Amniotic Fluic

1.5 Placenta & Umbilical Cord

1.0 Breasts

**28 - 29.0 Pounds**

***Figure 12.2.*** *Distribution of weight gain during pregnancy.*

The "optimal" weight to gain depends on the weight that you are before becoming pregnant. Your pre-pregnancy weight is also a rough indication of how well-nourished you are before becoming pregnant. If you are at a desirable weight for your body size before you become pregnant, a weight gain of 24 to 27 pounds is recommended. If you are approximately 20 pounds or more above your desirable weight before pregnancy, a weight gain of 24 pounds is recommended. Many overweight women, however, have healthy babies and gain only 20 pounds. If you become pregnant when you are underweight, you need to gain more weight during the pregnancy to give your baby the extra nutrition he or she needs for the first year. You should gain 28 to 36 pounds, depending on how underweight you are before becoming pregnant. Your nutrition advisor or health care provider can recommend an appropriate weight gain. How your weight gain is distributed is illustrated in Figure 12.2.

Total recommended weight gain is often not as helpful as a weekly rate of gain. Most women gain 3 to 5 pounds during the first trimester (first 3 months) of pregnancy. During the second and third trimesters, a good rate of weight gain is about three-quarters of a pound to one pound per week. Gaining too much weight (2 or more pounds per week) results in putting on too much body fat. This extra body fat produces an insulin-resistant effect which requires the body to produce more insulin to keep blood sugar levels normal. An inability to produce more insulin, as in gestational diabetes, causes your blood sugar levels to rise above acceptable levels. If weight gain has been excessive, often limiting weight gain to approximately three-quarters of a pound per week (3 pounds per month) can return blood sugar levels to normal. Fetal growth and development depend on proper nourishment and will be placed at risk by drastically reducing calories. However, you can limit weight gain by cutting back on excessive calories and by eating a nutritionally-sound diet that meets your needs and the needs of your baby. Remember that dieting and severely cutting back on weight gain may increase the risk of delivering prematurely. If blood sugar levels continue to go up and you are not gaining excessive weight or eating improperly, the safest therapy for the well-being of the fetus is insulin.

Occasionally, your weight may go up rapidly in the last trimester (after 28 weeks) and you may notice an increase in water retention, such as swelling in the feet, fingers, and face. If there is any question as to whether the rapid weight gain is due to eating too many calories or too much water retention, keeping records of how much food you eat and your exercise patterns at this time will be very helpful.

A Food and Exercise Record Sheet example is included at the end of this chapter (Figure 12.9.) By examining your Food and Exercise Record Sheet, your nutrition advisor can help you determine which is causing the rapid weight gain. In addition, by examining your legs and body for signs of fluid retention, your physician can help you to determine the cause of your weight gain. If your weight gain is due to water retention, cutting back drastically on calories may actually cause more fluid retention. Bed rest and resting on your side will help you to lose the build-up of fluid. Limit your intake of salt (sodium chloride) and very salty foods, as they tend to contribute to water retention.

Marked fluid retention when combined with an increase in blood pressure and possibly protein in the urine are the symptoms of preeclampsia. This is a disorder of pregnancy that can be harmful to both the mother and baby. Inform your obstetrician of any rapid weight gain, especially if you are eating moderately and gaining more than 2 pounds per week. Should you develop preeclampsia, be especially careful to eat a well-balanced diet with adequate calories.

After being diagnosed as having gestational diabetes, many women notice a slower weight gain as they start cutting the various sources of sugar out of their diet. This seems to be harmless and lasts only 1 or 2 weeks. It may be that sweets were contributing a substantial amount of calories to the diet.

### *How should I eat during my pregnancy?*

As with any pregnancy, it is important to eat the proper foods to meet the nutritional needs of the mother and fetus. An additional goal for women with gestational diabetes is to maintain a proper diet to keep blood sugars as normal as possible.

The daily need for calories increases by 300 calories during the second and third trimesters of pregnancy. If non-pregnant calorie intake was 1800 calories per day and weight gain was maintained, a calorie intake of 2100 calories per day is usual from 14 weeks until delivery. This is the equivalent of an additional 8 ounce glass of 2% milk and one-half of a sandwich (1 slice of bread, approximately 1 ounce of meat, and 1 teaspoon of margarine, mayonnaise, etc.) per day. The need for protein also increases during pregnancy. Make sure your diet includes foods high in protein, but not high in fat. See Table 12.3 for some examples. Most vitamins and minerals are also needed in larger amounts during pregnancy. This can be attained by increasing dairy products, especially those low in fat, and making sure you include whole grain cereals and breads, as well as fruits and vegetables in your diet each day. To make sure you get enough folate (a B vitamin critical during pregnancy) and iron, your obstetrician will probably recommend a prenatal vitamin. Prenatal vitamins do not replace a good diet; they merely help you to get the nutrients you need. To absorb the most iron from your prenatal vitamin, take it at night before going to bed, or in the morning on an empty stomach.

The Daily Food Guide (Table 12.4.) serves as a guideline for food sources that provide important vitamins and minerals, as well as carbohydrates, protein, and fiber during pregnancy. The recommended minimal servings per day appear in parentheses after each food group listed. This guide emphasizes foods that are low in fat and in sugar (discussed later).

The food guide is divided into six groups: milk and milk products; meat, poultry, fish, and meat substitutes; breads, cereals, and other starches; fruits; vegetables; and fats. Each group provides its own combination of vitamins, minerals, and other nutrients which play an important part in nutrition during pregnancy. Omitting the foods from one group will leave your diet inadequate in other nutrients. Plan your meals using a variety of foods within each food group, in the amounts recommended, and you'll be most likely to get all the vitamins, minerals, and other nutrients the fetus needs for growth and development.

**Table 12.3.** Protein Equivalents

| Food | Grams of Protein |
|---|---|
| 1 cup 2% milk | 8 |
| 1 cup plain nonfat yogurt | 8 |
| 1 ounce American processed cheese | 7 |
| 1 ounce low-fat cheese | 7 |
| 1 tbsp. peanut butter | 7 |
| 1/4 cup cottage cheese | 7 |
| 1/2 cup cooked dried beans | 7 |
| 1 slice whole wheat bread | 3 |
| 1/2 cup flaked cereal, bran or corn | 3 |

**Table 12.4a.** Daily Food Guide (Each item equals one serving)

| | | |
|---|---|---|
| **Milk and Milk Products**<br>*(4 Servings Per Day)* | 1 cup milk, skim or low-fat<br>1/3 cup powdered non-fat milk<br>1 cup reconstituted powdered non-fat milk<br>1½ oz. low-fat cheese* (no more than 6 grams of fat per ounce)<br>1 cup low-fat yogurt** | (high protein calcium, vitamin D) |
| **Meat, Poultry, Fish, and Meat Substitutes**<br>*(5-6 Servings Per Day)* | 1 oz. cooked poultry, fish, or lean meat (beef, lamb, pork)<br>1 tbsp. peanut butter<br>1 egg<br>1/4 cup low-fat cottage cheese<br>1/2 cup cooked dried beans or lentils | (high protein, B vitamins, iron) |
| **Breads, Cereals, and Other Starches**<br>*(5-6 Servings Per Day)* | 1 slice whole grain bread<br>5 crackers<br>1 muffin, biscuit, pancake, or waffle<br>3/4 cup dry cereal, unsweetened<br>1/2 cup pasta (macaroni, spaghetti), rice, mashed potatoes, or cooked cereal<br>1/3 cup sweet potatoes or yams<br>1/2 cup cooked dried beans or lentils<br>1/2 bagel, 1/2 english muffin, or 1/2 flour tortilla<br>1 small baked potato<br>2 taco shells | (high complex carbohydrates)<br>(emphasize whole grains, or use fortified or enriched)<br>(a good source of protein, B-vitamins, fiber and minerals) |

**Table 12.4b.** Daily Food Guide (Each item equals one serving)

| | | |
|---|---|---|
| **Fruit**<br>*(2 servings per day)* | 1/2 cup fresh fruit, 1/2 banana, or 1 medium-sized fruit (apple, orange)<br><br>1/2 cup, orange, grapefruit, or other juice fortified with vitamin C<br><br>1/2 medium-sized grapefruit<br><br>1 cup strawberries<br><br>1/2 cup fresh apricots, nectarines, purple plums, cantaloup, or 4 halves dried apricots (vitamin A source) | (fresh fruit provides fiber)<br><br>(include one vitamin C source daily) |
| **Vegetables*****<br>*(2 servings per day)* | 1/2 cup cooked or 1 cup raw: broccoli, spinach, carrots, (vitamin A source)<br><br>1/3 cup mixed vegetables | (include good vitamin A sources at least every other day) |
| **Fats** | 1 tsp. butter or margarine<br><br>1 tsp. oil or mayonnaise<br><br>1 tbsp. regular salad dressing<br><br>2 tbsp. low-calorie salad dressing<br><br>1/4 cup nuts or seeds | |

**1 oz. low-fat cheese can also be used as 1 serving from the Meat, Poultry, Fish, and Meat Substitutes group if sufficient calcium is already being provided from 4 servings.*

***This refers to plain yogurt. Commercially fruited yogurt contains a lot of added sugar.*

****Starchy vegetables such as corn, peas, and potatoes are included in Breads, Cereals, and Other Starches list.*

### *Other Nutritional and Non-Nutritional Considerations*

**Alcohol.** There is no known safe level of alcohol to allow during pregnancy. Daily heavy alcohol intake causes severe defects in development of the body and brain of the fetus, called Fetal Alcohol Syndrome. Even moderate drinking is associated with delayed fetal growth, spontaneous abortions, and lowered birth weight in babies. The Surgeon General's office warns: "Women who are pregnant or even considering pregnancy should avoid alcohol completely and should be aware of the alcohol content of food and drugs."

**Salt.** Salt restriction is no longer routinely advised during pregnancy. Recent research shows that during pregnancy the body needs salt to help provide the proper fluid balance. Your health care provider may recommend that you use salt in moderation.

**Caffeine.** Studies conflict on the potential danger of caffeine to the fetus. Caffeine is found primarily in coffee, tea, and some sodas (Table 12.5). Moderation is recommended. Talk to your doctor or other health professional about the maximum amount of caffeine recommended.

**Table 12.5.** Caffeine Comparisons

| Food | Serving | Amount of Caffeine |
|---|---|---|
| Regular coffee | 8 oz. | 80-200 mg. |
| Instant coffee | 8 oz. | 60-100 mg. |
| Decaffeinated coffee | 8 oz. | 3-5 mg. |
| Tea | 8 oz. | 60-65 mg. |
| Carbonated drinks, e.g., colas | 12 oz. | 30-65 mg. |
| Hot chocolate | 8 oz. | 13 mg. |

**Megavitamins.** Megavitamins are defined as 10 times the Recommended Dietary Allowance (dietary allowances established by the National Academy of Sciences—National Research Council) of vitamins and minerals and are not recommended for pregnant women. Although it is possible to get all of the necessary nutrients from food alone, your doctor may prescribe some prenatal vitamins and minerals. If taken regularly, along with a balanced diet, you will be getting all the vitamins and minerals needed during your pregnancy.

**Smoking.** Research has shown without question that smoking during pregnancy increases the risk of fetal death and preterm delivery, impairs fetal growth, and can lead to low birth weight. It is best to stop smoking entirely and permanently, or at the very least, to cut back drastically on the number of cigarettes you smoke.

### *What foods patterns help keep blood sugar levels normal?*

The following outlines food patterns which help to keep blood sugar levels within an acceptable range.

**Avoid sugar and foods high in sugar.** Most women with gestational diabetes, just like those without diabetes, have a desire for something sweet in their diet. In pregnant women, sugar is rapidly absorbed into the blood and requires a larger release of insulin to maintain normal blood sugar levels. Without the larger release of insulin, blood sugar levels will increase excessively when you eat sugar-containing foods.

There are many forms of sugar such as table sugar, honey, brown sugar, corn syrup, maple syrup, turbinado sugar, high fructose corn syrup, and molasses. Generally, food that ends in "ose" is a sugar (e.g., sucrose, dextrose, and glucose).

Foods that usually contain high amounts of sugar include pies, cakes, cookies, ice cream, candy, soft drinks, fruit drinks, fruit packed in syrup, commercially fruited yogurt, jams, jelly, doughnuts, and sweet rolls. Many of these foods are high in fat as well.

Be sure to check the list of ingredients on food products. Ingredients are listed in order of amount. If an ingredient is first on the list, it is present in the highest amount. If some type of sugar is listed first, second, or third on the list of ingredients, the product should be avoided. If sugar is further down, fourth, fifth, or sixth, it probably will not cause your blood sugar levels to go up excessively.

Fruit juices should only be taken with a meal and limited to 6 ounces. Tomato juice is a good choice because it is low in sugar. Six ounces of most other juice (apple, grapefruit, orange) with no sugar added still contain approximately 4 to 5 teaspoons of sugar. However, these do not contain much of the fiber of a piece of fruit which normally would act to slow the absorption of sugar into the blood. If you drink juice frequently to quench your thirst during the day, a high blood sugar level may result. Use only whole fruit for snacks.

To help with the occasional sweet tooth that we all have, artificial sweeteners may be used in foods. Aspartame has been extensively tested for safety. Use during pregnancy has been approved by the Food and Drug Administration and by the American Medical Association's Review Board. However, aspartame has not been tested for long-term safety and has not been on the market very long. It may be best to avoid its use until more tests have been done.

Saccharin is not advised during pregnancy. Likewise, use of mannitol, xylitol, sorbitol, or other artificial sweeteners is not recommended until further research is done.

Fructose is a special type of sugar that is slowly absorbed into the system. A small amount of fructose can be used if your blood sugar levels are within normal range. However, fructose still has 4 calories per gram, as much as table sugar. High fructose corn syrup is part fructose and part corn syrup, making it very similar to table sugar in composition. It will raise blood sugar levels and should definitely be avoided.

**Emphasize the use of complex carbohydrates.** These include vegetables, cereal, grains, beans, peas, and other starchy foods. A well-balanced diet with plenty of fiber provided by vegetables, dried beans, cereals, and other starchy foods decreases the amount of insulin your body needs to keep blood sugars within a normal range. Anything that decreases the need for insulin is beneficial. The American Diabetes Association recommends that at least one-half of your calories come from complex carbohydrates. Starchy foods include pasta, rice, grains, cereals, crackers, bread, potatoes, dried beans, peas, and legumes. Also, contrary to popular belief, carbohydrates are not highly fattening when eaten in moderate amounts and without the rich sauces and toppings often added.

**Emphasize foods high in dietary fiber.** Fiber is the edible portion of foods of plant origin that is not digested (e.g., skins, membranes, seeds, bran). Foods with a high fiber content include whole grain cereals and breads, fruits, vegetables, and legumes (dried peas and beans). Fiber aids digestion and helps prevent constipation. The fiber found in fruits, vegetables, and legumes also helps keep your blood sugar level from becoming too high without requiring extra insulin.

**Keep your diet low in fat.** Some fat is needed to help with the absorption of certain vitamins and to provide the essential fatty acids necessary for fetal growth. A diet which is high in fat causes the insulin to react in a less efficient manner, necessitating more insulin to keep blood sugar levels within normal range. Foods high in saturated fats such as fatty meats, butter, bacon, cream (light, coffee, sour cream, etc.), and whole milk cheeses are likely to be high in total fat. Most foods with saturated fat are also high in cholesterol because they are fats from animal origin. However, foods such as crackers made with coconut, palm, or palm kernel oil can be high in saturated fats as well. Read labels carefully. Unsaturated fats are found in foods such as fish, margarine and vegetable oils. Keep your use of salad dressings to a minimum and whenever possible use those prepared with olive oil. To help keep the diet lower in fat, avoid adding extra fats such as rich sauces and creamy desserts, and bake or broil foods instead of frying them. Replacing fatty foods with those high in complex carbohydrates is also helpful.

**Include a bedtime snack that is a good source of protein and complex carbohydrates.** Women with gestational diabetes have a tendency toward lower than normal blood sugar levels during the night. This causes the body to increase its utilization of fats as a fuel source. As fat is used, ketones (discussed later) are produced as a by-product of the breakdown of fats, and in large amounts, may be harmful to the fetus. This can be prevented by having a bedtime snack that provides protein and complex carbohydrates such as starchy foods. Starch will stabilize your blood sugar level in the early night, while protein acts as a long-acting stabilizer. Examples of a bedtime snack are:

- 1 oz. American-processed cheese + 5 crackers
- 1/2 chicken sandwich on whole wheat bread
- 3 cups unbuttered popcorn + 1/4 cup nuts

If you need to take insulin, a bedtime snack is critical and you should not omit it. When taken by injection, insulin acts to lower blood sugar level, even during the night when meals are not eaten. A bedtime snack is protective against low blood sugars while sleeping or upon arising. If a bedtime snack causes heartburn, sleep with your head raised on pillows, and be careful that you are not eating too large a bedtime snack.

### *How do I plan meals?*

A registered dietitian or qualified nutritionist can help you plan a meal pattern that is right for you. Most women with gestational diabetes need three meals and a bedtime snack each day. It is unwise for anyone who is pregnant to go long periods of time (greater than 5 hours) without eating, as this will produce ketones. Extra snacks are necessary if your schedule results in a long time between meals. Blood sugars will be easier to keep in the normal range if meal times and amounts (total calories) are evenly spaced. It's more likely that a higher blood sugar will result if the majority of calories are eaten at dinner, than if they are distributed more evenly throughout the day. If insulin injections prove necessary, the time at which meals are eaten and the amounts eaten should be approximately the same from day to day. Do not skip meals and snacks, as this often results in hypoglycemia (low blood sugar), which may be harmful to the fetus and makes you feel irritable, shaky, or may result in a headache.

**Table 12.6.** Sample menu—2,000 calories

This diet is planned for women whose normal non-pregnant weight should be 130-135 lbs. For women who weigh less than 130 before pregnancy, the diet should contain fewer calories. Women who are overweight are at higher risk for gestational diabetes. Your health care provider can discuss this and help you make necessary changes.

**BREAKFAST**

1/2 grapefruit
3/4 cup oatmeal, cooked
1 tsp. raisins
1 cup 2% milk
1 whole wheat English muffin
1 tsp. margarine

**LUNCH**

Salad with:
- 1 cup romaine lettuce
- 1/2 cup kidney beans, cooked
- 1/2 fresh tomato

1 oz. part skim mozzarella cheese
2 tbsp. low-calorie Italian dressing
1 bran muffin
1/2 cup cantaloupe chunks

**AFTERNOON SNACK**

2 rice cakes
6 oz. low-fat yogurt, plain
1/2 cup blueberries

**DINNER**

3/4 cup vegetable soup with
- 1/4 cup cooked barley

3 oz. chicken, without skin
1 baked potato
1/2 cup cooked broccoli
1 piece whole wheat bread
1 tbsp. margarine
1 fresh peach

**BEDTIME SNACK**

1 apple
2 cups popcorn, plain
1/4 cup peanuts

## *What can be done to slow weight gain during pregnancy?*

Gaining too much weight during pregnancy will make blood sugar levels higher than normal for women with gestational diabetes. Yet, for many pregnant women it is very difficult to gain weight slowly and still get all of the recommended nutrients. Luckily, fat, which is high in calories (9 calories per gram), is needed in only small amounts during pregnancy. Carbohydrates and protein, in contrast to fat, provide only 4 calories per gram. To cut calories without depriving the fetus of any necessary nutritional factors, it is best to avoid fats and fatty foods.

- Avoid high-fat meats. Choose lean cuts of beef, pork, and lamb. Emphasize more fish and poultry (without the skin).
- Avoid frying meat, fish, or poultry in added oil, shortening, or lard. Bake, broil, or roast instead.
- Avoid foods fried in oil such as chips, french fries, and doughnuts. Substitute pretzels, unbuttered popcorn, or breadsticks instead.
- Avoid using cream sauces and butter sauces, as well as salt pork for seasoning on vegetables. Season with herbs instead.
- Avoid using the fat drippings from meat or poultry for gravy. Use broth or bouillon instead and thicken with cornstarch.
- Avoid using mayonnaise or oil for salads. Use vinegar, lemon juice, or low-calorie salad dressings instead.

To help reduce calories choose low-fat dairy products. During pregnancy you need 1200 mg calcium daily to build the fetal skeleton without drawing from maternal calcium stores. Table 12.7 points out foods in which the calcium content is almost the same, yet the calories are not due to the difference in fat content.

The difference between 600 calories and 340 calories is only 260 calories and may seem insignificant. Yet, if your diet is cut by 260 calories daily for 1 week, your weight gain slows down by approximately ½ pound per week. In other words, instead of gaining 1½ pounds per week you will only gain 1 pound per week.

If cheese is a part of your daily diet, use low-fat cheeses such as low-fat cottage cheese, Neufchatel, mozzarella, farmers, and pot cheese. Avoid using cream cheese, as it has little protein and most of its calories come from fat.

Even though pregnancy can be a very hectic time, with little time for meal preparation, eat less and less often at "fast food" restaurants. Studies have shown that some foods from fast food restaurants average 40 to 60 percent of their calories from fat, and are quite high in calories (*Fast Food Facts: Nutritive and Exchange Values for Fast Food Restaurants,* Marion J. Franz, International Diabetes Center, Minneapolis, Minnesota, 1987. 54 pp.). For example, chicken and fish that are coated with batter and deep-fried in fat may contain more fat and calories than a hamburger or roast beef sandwich.

Go lightly when using butter and margarine. Adding only an extra three pats of butter or margarine (same calories) daily could add an extra pound of weight gain next month. It may be better to emphasize the use of foods rich in complex carbohydrates that don't use butter, margarine, or cream sauce to make them palatable. Many people find rice, noodles, and spaghetti tasty without a lot of butter. Use a variety of spices and herbs (such as curry, garlic, and parsley) to flavor rice and tomato sauce to flavor pasta without additional fats.

It is also a good idea to eat small amounts frequently, thereby keeping the edge off your appetite. This will assist your "self-control" in avoiding large portions of food that you should not have. Avoid skipping meals or trying to cut back drastically on breakfast or lunch. It will leave you too hungry for the next meal to exercise any control. Your doctor or dietitian can help you determine how you can cut extra calories.

You may find it helpful to keep food records of what you eat, as most of us tend to forget or not realize the extent of our snacking.

**Table 12.7.** Calorie Comparisons

| Food | Calories |
|---|---|
| 4-8 oz. glasses whole milk | 600 |
| 4-8 oz. glasses 2% milk | 480 |
| 4-8 oz. glasses skim milk | 340 |
| 2-8 oz. glasses whole milk plus 3 oz. American processed cheese | 600 |
| 2-8 oz. glasses 2% milk plus 3 oz. American processed cheese | 540 |
| 2-8 oz. glasses skim milk plus 3 oz. American processed cheese | 470 |

Recording everything you eat or drink tends to be a sobering and instructive experience. A Food and Exercise Record Sheet example is included at the end of this chapter (Figure 12.9).

Be careful to maintain a weight gain of at least ½ pound per week, over several weeks, if you are in the second trimester (14 weeks or more of gestation). Cutting back more than this may increase the risk of having a low-birth-weight infant.

### *Is breast-feeding recommended?*

Breast-feeding is strongly encouraged. For most women this represents the easiest way back to pre-pregnancy weight after delivery. The body draws on the calories stored during the first part of pregnancy to use in milk production. Approximately 800 calories per day are used during the first 3 months of milk production, and even more during the next 3 months. By 6 weeks after delivery, women who breast-feed usually have lost 4 pounds more than women who bottle-feed. This can be a very important factor, as it is strongly recommended that women with gestational diabetes return to their desirable body weight 4 to 5 months postpartum. As previously mentioned, maintaining a weight appropriate for your height and frame may reduce the risk of developing diabetes later in life.

In addition, breast-feeding has many advantages for your baby. Protection from infection and allergies are transferred to the baby through breast milk. This milk is also easier to digest than formula, and its minerals are better absorbed than those in formula.

### *Should I exercise?*

A daily exercise program is an important part of a healthy pregnancy. Daily exercise helps you feel better and reduces stress. In addition, being physically fit protects against back pain, and maintains muscle tone, strength, and endurance. For women with gestational diabetes, exercise is especially important.

- Regular exercise increases the efficiency or potency of your body's own insulin. This may allow you to keep your blood sugar levels in the normal range while using less insulin.
- Moderate exercise also helps blunt your appetite, helping you to keep your weight gain down to normal levels. Maintaining the correct weight gain is very important in preventing high blood sugar levels.

Talk with your doctor about what exercise program is right for you. Your doctor can advise you about limitations, warning signs, and any special considerations. Generally, you can continue any exercise program or sport you participated in prior to pregnancy. Use caution, however, and avoid sports or exercises where you might fall, or that involve jolting. Pre-pregnancy bicycling, jogging, and cross-country skiing are good exercises to continue during pregnancy. If you plan to start an exercise program during pregnancy, talk to your doctor before beginning and start slowly. Vigorous walking is good for women who need to start exercising and have not been active before pregnancy.

Exercising frequently, 4 to 5 days per week, is necessary to get the "blood sugar lowering" advantages of an exercise program. Don't omit a warm-up period of 5 to 10 minutes and a cool-down period of 5 to 10 minutes. Always stop exercising if you feel pain, dizziness, shortness of breath, faintness, palpitations, back or pelvic pain, or experience vaginal bleeding. Also, avoid vigorous exercise in hot, humid weather or if you have a fever. It is important to prevent dehydration during exercise, especially during pregnancy. The American College of Obstetricians and Gynecologists (ACOG) recommends drinking fluids prior to and after exercise, and if necessary, during the activity to prevent dehydration.

An ACOG report (*Home Exercise Program: Exercise During Pregnancy and the Postnatal Period*. American College of Obstetricians and Gynecologists. May 1985. 6 pp.) issued in 1985, warned that target heart rates for pregnant and postpartum women should be set approximately 25 to 30 percent lower than rates for non-pregnant women. It may be that exercising too vigorously will direct blood flow away from the uterus and fetus. ACOG recommends that pregnant women measure their heart rate during activity and that maternal heart rate not exceed 140 beats per minute.

If you need to be on insulin during your pregnancy, take a few precautions. Because both insulin and exercise lower blood sugar levels, the combination can result in hypoglycemia or low blood sugar. You need to be aware that this is a potential problem, and you should be familiar with the symptoms of hypoglycemia (confusion, extreme hunger, blurry vision, shakiness, sweating). When exercising, take along sugar in the form of hard, sugar-sweetened candies just in case your blood sugar becomes too low. When on insulin, you should always carry some form of sugar for potential episodes of hypoglycemia.

It may be necessary for you to eat small snacks between meals if the exercise results in low blood sugar levels.

- One serving of fruit will keep blood sugars normal for most short-term activities (approximately 30 minutes).
- One serving of fruit plus a serving of starch will be enough for activities that last longer (60 minutes or more).

If you exercise right after a meal, eat the snack after the exercise. If the exercise is 2 hours or more after a meal, eat the snack before the exercise.

## *What happens if diet and exercise fail to control my blood sugars?*

If your blood sugars tend to go over the acceptable levels (105 mg/dl or below for fasting, 120 mg/dl or below 2 hours after a meal) you may need to take insulin injections. Insulin is a protein and would be digested like any other protein in food if it were given orally. The needles used to inject insulin are extremely fine, so there is little discomfort. If insulin injections are necessary, you will be taught how to fill the syringe and how to do the injections yourself.

Your physician will calculate the amount of insulin needed to keep blood sugar levels within the normal range. It is very likely that the amount or dosage of insulin needed to keep your levels of blood sugar normal will increase as your pregnancy advances. This does not mean your gestational diabetes is getting worse. As any healthy pregnancy progresses, the placenta will grow and produce progressively higher levels of contra-insulin hormones. As a result you will likely need to inject more insulin to overcome their effect. Some women may even require two injections each day. This does not imply anything about the severity of the problem or the outcome of the pregnancy. The goal is to maintain normal blood sugar levels with whatever dosage of insulin is needed.

## *Can my blood sugar level go too low, and if so, what do I do?*

Occasionally, your blood sugar level may get too low if you are taking insulin. This can happen if you delay a meal or exercise more than usual, especially at the time your insulin is working at its peak. This low blood sugar is called "hypoglycemia" or an "insulin reaction." This is a medical emergency and should be promptly treated, never ignored.

The symptoms of insulin reaction vary from sweating, shakiness, or dizziness to feeling faint, disoriented, or a tingling sensation. Remember, if you take insulin injections, you need to keep some form of sugar-sweetened candy in your purse, at home, at work, and in your car. In case of an episode of hypoglycemia, you will be prepared to treat it immediately. Be sure to eat something more substantial afterward. Also, report any insulin reactions or high blood sugar levels to your doctor right away in case an adjustment in your treatment needs to be made.

As you can see, extra care, work, and commitment on the part of you and your spouse or partner are required to provide the special medical care necessary. Don't worry if you occasionally go off your diet or miss a planned exercise program. Your doctor and other health care professionals will work along with you to make sure you receive the specialized care that has resulted in dramatically improved pregnancy outcome.

An ounce of prevention is worth a pound of cure! Eat as directed. Exercise as directed. Monitor as directed. Do these things and you are doing your part toward a happy, healthy pregnancy.

**Self Blood Glucose Monitoring Diary**

| DATE | Before eating **am** | 2 hr. after **breakfast** | 2 hr. after **lunch** | 2 hr. after **dinner** | Amount of **insulin** | NOTES |
|---|---|---|---|---|---|---|
| | | | | | | |
| | | | | | | |
| | | | | | | |
| | | | | | | |
| | | | | | | |
| | | | | | | |
| | | | | | | |
| | | | | | | |
| | | | | | | |
| | | | | | | |
| | | | | | | |
| | | | | | | |
| | | | | | | |
| | | | | | | |
| | | | | | | |
| | | | | | | |
| | | | | | | |
| | | | | | | |
| | | | | | | |
| | | | | | | |
| | | | | | | |
| | | | | | | |
| | | | | | | |
| | | | | | | |
| | | | | | | |
| | | | | | | |
| | | | | | | |
| | | | | | | |
| | | | | | | |
| | | | | | | |

***Figure 12.8.*** *Example of a self blood glucose monitoring diary.*

**Food and Exercise Record Sheet**

The following chart is intended to help you and your health care providers keep track of your food and exercise habits and enable you to plan a regimen tailored to your particular needs.

1) Write down everything you eat or drink.

2) Write down items added to foods (e.g., sugar, butter).

3) Write down how your food was prepared (e.g., broiled, fried, baked).

4) Write down the amount you eat in household measures (e.g., 1/2 cup or 2 tbsp.).

5) Write down any exercising you have done, type of exercise, and time spent.

| DAY | TIME | FOOD AND TYPE OF PREPARATION | AMOUNT | EXERCISE |
|---|---|---|---|---|
| | | | | |
| | | | | |
| | | | | |
| | | | | |
| | | | | |
| | | | | |
| | | | | |
| | | | | |
| | | | | |
| | | | | |
| | | | | |
| | | | | |
| | | | | |
| | | | | |

***Figure 12.9.*** *Example of a food and exercise record.*

# Chapter 13

# *Maternal Diabetes*

Pregnancy is a time of wonder and excitement. But if you have diabetes, you may worry whether you'll have a healthy baby. As recently as 20 years ago, women with diabetes were often advised to avoid having children. Those who did become pregnant were hospitalized for most of the pregnancy.

The good news is that now, with prenatal planning, careful management of your diabetes, and close monitoring of your baby with advanced technology, you can have a healthy pregnancy and a healthy baby. But it takes planning and a lot of work to make your success story come true.

## *Planning for Pregnancy*

Preparing for a healthy pregnancy begins with excellent care of your diabetes even before you conceive. This is true whether you have type 1or type 2 diabetes. In fact, all women with diabetes need to plan carefully for pregnancy from their teenage years to menopause. Even if you aren't considering a pregnancy in the near future, you still need to realize the importance of good control before conception. If you are of child-bearing age and don't wish to become pregnant, discuss birth control options with your doctor to prevent an unintended pregnancy.

---

Bartholomew, Sallie P., "Make Way for Baby." Vol. 50, *Diabetes Forecast*, 12-01-1997, pp 20(9). 

It's crucial for your blood glucose levels to be well controlled during early pregnancy to help prevent birth defects. A baby's organs, including the heart and the neural tube (the foundation for the brain, spinal column, muscles, and nerves), are formed by six to eight weeks of pregnancy.

However, you may not realize you're pregnant until after you've missed a period. This means you won't even know you're pregnant until six weeks or more have passed. Unless you've cared for your diabetes well before conceiving, you've missed the opportunity to decrease the risk of birth defects. In fact, studies show that when the diabetes is well controlled, the risk of birth defects drops from 17 percent to 3 to 5 percent, which is the same as that of women who don't have diabetes.

Poorly controlled diabetes also leads to a higher risk for miscarriage in the early weeks. The rate of miscarriage is about twice as high for women with uncontrolled diabetes as for those without diabetes. Keeping blood glucose levels in the near-normal range also lowers this risk.

## Three to Six Months Before Becoming Pregnant

If you are considering a pregnancy soon, see your diabetes team and discuss your plans for pregnancy. If you don't have a team, this is the time to assemble one. Team members should include:

- an endocrinologist or physician who specializes in diabetes and is skilled in treating pregnant women
- a diabetes nurse educator
- a dietitian
- an ophthalmologist (eye doctor)
- an obstetrician (OB)

A complete assessment of your diabetes should be done, including length of time you've had diabetes, overall patterns of blood glucose control, your history of diabetic ketoacidosis, and any problems with severe hypoglycemia. Your weight and blood pressure should be checked. Urinalysis will be done to check for protein, ketones, and signs of infection.

### Blood Glucose Control

A glycohemoglobin test (one type is HbA1c) should be done to measure your average blood glucose level over the previous two to three months.

During your pregnancy, you'll be monitoring your blood glucose levels before and after eating. This means you may be testing anywhere from six to ten times every day. It's a good idea to begin testing at least four times a day now. This gets you into the habit of doing what will be required while you're pregnant. Bring your meter to a health care visit to compare its results with the lab's for accuracy. Your diabetes educator can instruct you on how best to use your meter and will assess your technique.

The acceptable range for blood glucose during pregnancy is lower than when you are not pregnant (see Table 13.1). These goals may need to be modified, especially if you have trouble detecting hypoglycemia. Discuss with your doctor the appropriate range for you.

Because you'll be going for tighter control during pregnancy, your insulin regimen should be evaluated. If you plan to switch to intensive therapy using multiple daily injections or an insulin pump, it's best to do so at least three to six months before you become pregnant.

**Table 13.1.** Acceptable Range for Blood Glucose during Pregnancy

| Time of Test | Blood Glucose Range |
|---|---|
| Fasting or before meals | 70 to 100 mg/dl |
| One hour after eating | under 140 mg/dl |
| Two hours after eating | under 120 mg/dl |
| Glycohemoglobin | within normal range* |

*Normal range depends on which glycohemoglobin test is done. A common normal range is 4 to 6 percent.

### *Meal Planning*

Paying close attention to what you eat is important for both your blood glucose control and for the health of your baby, and this is the time to see your dietitian to review your current meal plan, weight, and calorie needs. Your dietitian will give you guidelines for healthy eating during pregnancy. In addition, he or she can help with your diabetes management by teaching you how to detect the effects of certain foods on your blood glucose levels, match your food with insulin, and space meals appropriately. Your dietitian can also provide tips for handling pregnancy challenges such as morning sickness and heartburn.

### *Diabetic Complications*

If you have diabetic complications, pregnancy may worsen them. Therefore, you should be evaluated for complications. Then, in light of the results, discuss with your doctor the risks of pregnancy to you and your baby.

Retinopathy may worsen during pregnancy because of the increase in the mother's blood volume and blood pressure. If tests show you have serious retinopathy, you'll need laser treatments before becoming pregnant or as soon as problems are detected.

You'll be screened for nephropathy (kidney disease) with a 24-hour urine collection. If you have mild kidney disease, it may still be safe for you to get pregnant. However, if you have advanced kidney disease, you'll be advised not to get pregnant. Kidney disease may result in fetal growth restriction, and for the mother, excess fluid retention and toxemia (also called preeclampsia or pregnancy-induced hypertension).

Gastroparesis affects how well the stomach empties and how quickly food is absorbed. This will have an impact on your after-meal blood glucose levels and may affect your appetite and make morning sickness worse. Although you can still become pregnant, you will need to be advised how best to handle this situation.

Although cardiovascular disease is very rare at this stage of life, you may need to be screened if you have had diabetes for more than 10 years and have other risk factors, such as high blood pressure or an abnormal EKG. This is a special situation and needs careful attention from specialists. Advanced cardiovascular disease is dangerous for the mother and baby, so if it's present, you will be advised not to become pregnant.

### *Other Concerns*

Cigarette smoking and drinking alcohol affect your developing baby. Quit now!

If you're on blood pressure medication, make sure it's one that's safe to use during pregnancy. If you're on an ACE inhibitor, you'll need to switch to another type of medication. If you're on a beta blocker or diuretic, you may need to switch.

Finally, as you're considering pregnancy, realize that managing diabetes during pregnancy is time-consuming and expensive. There will be more doctor visits, special tests, more frequent blood glucose testing, and more insulin injections each day. There will also be more time away from work. Depending on your condition, your OB may ask you to reduce your hours or stop work by the late weeks of pregnancy. You and your partner need to be aware of these factors and discuss their impact on your finances and lifestyle.

### *If You Have Type 2 Diabetes*

Unfortunately, type 2 diabetes is often considered more "mild" or "not as bad" as type 1 diabetes. Nothing is farther from the truth, especially when planning a pregnancy. You need to be as careful about blood glucose control as a woman with type 1. But you may have different medication needs.

If you're on diet therapy alone, you may need no insulin until later in your pregnancy. However, if you're on oral agents, you'll need to switch to insulin before becoming pregnant.

Being overweight makes diabetes control more difficult, so your prepregnancy planning should include a visit with the dietitian to help you with weight control and to design a meal plan to fit you. It's very important to discuss your plans for starting a family with your doctor before becoming pregnant so that these issues can be addressed.

## *First Trimester: 1 to 13 Weeks (Counting from the First Day of Your Last Period)*

### *The Baby*

During the first trimester your baby develops from a one-celled organism to a tiny, miniature human being. By the 6th week the heart is prominent, and the buds for arms and legs can be seen. Fingers, toes, nails, and the beginnings of the baby's eyes, ears, mouth, and nose are present by the 8th week. The heartbeat is detectable by ultrasound (sound waves) by about 5 to 6 weeks and can be heard with a Doppler (sound detection) instrument by 8 to 10 weeks. By the 12th week, the baby is about 7 cm (3 inches) long and begins to move spontaneously.

In addition, the placenta develops during the first trimester. This incredible organ connects to the baby through the umbilical cord. Glucose is one of the many nutrients that cross the placenta, so your glucose does reach your baby. Insulin, however, does not. By the 13th week, your baby is producing its own insulin.

### *The Mother*

Again, you may not even realize you're pregnant until you are about 6 to 8 weeks along. Early signs of pregnancy include a missed period, fatigue, morning sickness, increased urination, and breast tingling. All of these are side effects of the hormonal changes of pregnancy.

*Insulin Needs*

Your sensitivity to insulin may be much greater during these early weeks, and you may find you need less insulin than you did before you became pregnant.

*Watch Out For Lows!*

The risk for sudden, unexplained hypoglycemia (low blood sugar) is highest from the 10th to the 16th week. Monitor frequently, especially if you have trouble recognizing the symptoms of hypoglycemia. Observe yourself carefully for even the most subtle symptoms. It's easy to think you feel "funny," "not quite right," "emotional," or "tired" because you're pregnant when, in fact, these feelings may be due to low blood glucose.

*Don't Guess. Test!*

Carry glucose tablets or other food with you to treat low blood glucose promptly. Check your blood glucose before you drive—even if you have no symptoms of a "low"—to prevent a car accident caused by hypoglycemia.

Although the risk for hypoglycemia may diminish after 16 to 18 weeks, it doesn't disappear completely, so stay vigilant.

*Things to Do during the First Trimester*

Inform your diabetes team and obstetrician as soon as you think you're pregnant. A home pregnancy test may be helpful but only a blood test can positively confirm a pregnancy.

You'll be seen by your team right away and every one to four weeks after that, depending on your control. If you have not recently had a meter assessment and nutrition counseling, these should be done now. Discuss strategies for adjusting insulin doses to deal with any morning sickness.

If you have not done so already, start testing your blood glucose before and one to two hours after each meal.

Laboratory tests include a blood glucose level measurement and urinalysis, and a glycohemoglobin now and about every six weeks.

Inform your ophthalmologist that you're pregnant. If you have not had a recent eye exam, schedule one now.

Your obstetrician may do a pelvic exam to confirm the pregnancy. An ultrasound should be done to determine the due date.

### *DKA: Medical Emergency for Type 1 Mom and Baby*

Insulin controls the flow of fuels in the body. Without it, the body can no longer use its main fuel, glucose. Instead, it switches to burning fats and proteins. This produces ketones and acids, hence the name, diabetic ketoacidosis (DKA). DKA occurs in people with type 1 diabetes when they don't get enough insulin. It's a medical emergency for you and your baby.

DKA is more likely to occur when you're sick because your body needs more insulin than usual during an illness. Be sure to discuss sick-day guidelines with your diabetes team, including ketone testing, and preventing and treating DKA. An illness, especially nausea and vomiting, should alert you to call your diabetes doctor and your OB immediately.

## *Second Trimester: 14 to 27 Weeks*

### *The Baby*

Your baby is structurally formed by 14 to 15 weeks. It is now growing steadily as its organs mature. You can feel the baby's movements by 18 to 20 weeks. At 22 weeks, the baby weighs about 350 grams (3/4 pound) and begins to lay down some body fat. By 26 weeks the baby is covered with a thin layer of red skin and weighs about 1,000 grams (2 pounds). Your baby can hear sounds and even moves in rhythm to your voice.

### *The Mother*

Many women find that this is the most enjoyable time of pregnancy. The discomforts of the early weeks subside, and you may feel more energetic.

#### *Insulin Needs*

Around 22 to 23 weeks, the pregnancy hormones begin to increase and your insulin requirements may start to rise. However, it's usually a small change at this point.

At 26 to 28 weeks, the pregnancy hormones increase even more and so does their interference with insulin's ability to work. You may notice blood glucose levels beginning to rise more now, along with your need for larger doses of insulin. Careful, frequent monitoring before and after meals will help you and your diabetes team make appropriate insulin adjustments at the right time.

*Things to Do during the Second Trimester*

Continue to see your diabetes team every one to four weeks, depending on your control. Have your eyes checked by your ophthalmologist. You should be seen by your OB every three to four weeks.

You may be advised to have a blood test called alpha-fetoprotein (AFP) at around 16 weeks. This is a screening test for neural tube defects (which includes spina bifida) and Down syndrome. This is not a diagnostic test. It can't say whether the fetus does or does not have one of these conditions. It's a screening test, identifying fetuses that are at high risk.

It's been reported that women with diabetes have more falsely high results than nondiabetic women. That's because a different normal range is used to interpret the results for diabetic women. So don't be surprised if your test comes back abnormal. You'll be advised to get other tests, such as ultrasound and amniocentesis, to more accurately assess whether there is a problem.

An ultrasound at 18 to 20 weeks should be done to determine the size of your baby and screen for defects. Babies of mothers with diabetes—especially poorly controlled diabetes—have an increased risk of heart defects. By 20 weeks the baby's heart is well developed and large enough that a detailed ultrasound or fetal echocardiogram can show most problems.

## Third Trimester: 28 to 40 Weeks

### The Baby

Your baby grows rapidly during this time. The lungs and liver are the last two organs to reach full maturity.

Poorly controlled diabetes during the late weeks can lead to problems for the baby:

*Large Birth Weight and Low Blood Glucose*

Blood glucose crosses the placenta, so if your blood glucose is high, your baby's is, too. The high glucose level stimulates the baby to produce more of its own insulin, which causes the baby to form extra layers of fat. This causes a large birth weight, which makes delivery difficult for the mother and the baby. It may also lead to weight problems for the child later in life.

The mother's high blood glucose levels can also cause hypoglycemia in the newborn at birth. The baby has been producing extra insulin to deal with the extra glucose. At birth, when the baby is cut off from its mother's high glucose supply, its blood glucose may drop too low.

*A Delay in Lung Development*

Delayed lung development may cause the baby to have difficulty breathing when it's born. Controlling your diabetes decreases this risk greatly. Also, the baby's lungs can be checked for their maturity and ability to function with amniocentesis before delivery. This helps your OB make a decision about the safest timing of delivery.

*Stillbirth*

A frightening risk in the late weeks is that of stillbirth. It's thought to be due to deterioration of the placenta. This risk gets higher the closer to the actual due date you get. For this reason, many OB' s will decide to deliver the baby a week or two early. Fortunately, the risk of stillbirth is very small. Excellent diabetes control and frequent, close assessment of the baby lowers the risk to that of women without diabetes.

*Jaundice*

Keeping your blood glucose under good control during these late weeks greatly reduces this risk.

### ***The Mother***

*Insulin Needs*

Pregnancy hormones reach their peak during the third trimester. They cause your body's cells to be resistant to insulin, which means you'll need higher doses of insulin to keep your blood glucose under control.

Your need for insulin will increase dramatically from about 28 weeks to 36 weeks. You may need to make adjustments frequently, sometimes as often as every three to seven days. This varies for each mother, so self-monitoring of blood glucose is essential to make the appropriate adjustments at the right time.

After 36 weeks, your need for insulin may plateau or even decrease. In fact, frequent hypoglycemia after 36 weeks means that the pregnancy hormone levels are changing and delivery may be soon. Notify your diabetes doctor and your OB if you begin having more frequent episodes of low blood glucose.

*Complications*

Women with diabetes are more likely to develop a condition of pregnancy known as preeclampsia. This is characterized by high blood pressure, a lot of swelling of the hands and face, and leakage of protein into the urine. Preeclampsia affects the kidneys, liver, and placenta, and so may affect the health of the mother and child.

If you develop preeclampsia, your OB will probably recommend that you reduce your activities, limit your work hours, or be on bedrest. Preeclampsia could lead to a more serious condition called toxemia of pregnancy, which usually requires hospitalization.

If you have a history of retinopathy, kidney disease, or high blood pressure, you should be monitored carefully for changes, as they will be greatest now because of the greater volume of circulating blood and the hormonal effects on the blood vessels. The tests done in early pregnancy for these complications are used as a baseline and compared to your condition now, so appropriate decisions are made about your care.

*Things to Do in the Third Trimester*

Visits to your diabetes team and OB will be more frequent now. Although it may seem inconvenient and difficult to keep all these appointments, they are extremely important for both you and your baby. Your diabetes team will see you every one to two weeks. Your blood glucose control will be evaluated and insulin adjustments made. Towards the end of your pregnancy you'll receive instructions for handling your insulin at delivery. Be sure to see your ophthalmologist one more time.

The following OB tests may begin as early as 28 weeks if there are complications, or at about 32 to 34 weeks if things are going well. All of these tests help the OB monitor the health and development of your baby and decide when best to deliver.

- An ultrasound is done to check your baby's size, the placenta, and the amount of fluid surrounding the baby.
- Non-stress tests will be done to measure your baby's movements in correlation with its heart rate. These may be done weekly and then twice a week by the end of the pregnancy.
- You may be asked to do kick counts at home to assess the baby's movements each day.
- A biophysical profile may be done, which includes an ultrasound, measurement of your baby's breathing, movements, fetal tone, and fluid volume.

## Labor and Delivery

After months of hard work, it's now time for your little one to arrive. Delivery should take place in a center where skilled doctors and nurses are available to care for you and your newborn. The type of delivery you have will depend on how early the delivery is and the size of the baby. Your blood pressure, the amount of swelling, protein in the urine, the presence of any complications of diabetes., and your baby's condition will also be considered.

If your diabetes has been well controlled, you are doing well, and the baby's size is healthy, you may go to term and have a vaginal delivery.

If the baby is large or if you are experiencing eye problems, kidney problems, or high blood pressure, you may need to deliver early, possibly by cesarean section.

If you need to deliver earlier than 38 weeks, your OB will most likely perform an amniocentesis to test the baby's lungs for development. This helps with decisions about timing of the delivery and allows doctors to anticipate what the baby's condition will be when it is born.

### Insulin Needs

Your need for insulin will change dramatically at delivery. The hormones of pregnancy are no longer present, and you will need much less insulin. Before delivery, discuss the plan for handling your insulin with your diabetes doctor, who will write orders for the hospital. You may want to do your own monitoring at least part of the time, and the hospital needs to be aware of that, also. Bring your own meter and supplies, and treatments for hypoglycemia, to the hospital.

During delivery you will get fluids containing glucose through an IV to prevent hypoglycemia. If you have type 1 diabetes you will still need some insulin, but the dose is usually even less than what you were on before pregnancy. If you have type 2 diabetes, you may go off of insulin altogether at delivery. You might remain off medication for a while and then resume it later.

For either type of diabetes, over the next few days and weeks, continue to monitor your blood glucose levels closely and follow up with your doctor to re-evaluate your need for medication.

## The Baby

Your newborn will be checked for development, weight, ability to breathe, color, movement, hypoglycemia, and jaundice. The closer to term that you deliver, the more likely it is that your baby will go to the regular newborn nursery. A newborn who has a birth injury, birth defect, hypoglycemia, is large or small for gestational age, or has difficulty breathing will be placed in a specialty unit. Remember that these problems also occur in mothers who do not have diabetes. With good newborn care, even babies born with problems can do very well.

### *The Early Days after Delivery*

All your hard work has paid off, and you are now the mother of a beautiful newborn baby. But diabetes care cannot be abandoned after you deliver. Babies need healthy moms to care for them. You will still need to test your blood sugars and adjust your insulin based on the results. However, you can monitor less frequently, and your goals for blood glucose levels are no longer as strict. In fact, it's wise to err on the side of preventing low blood sugar since this is more likely to occur in the early weeks after delivery.

Yes, it takes a lot of work to control your diabetes during pregnancy. But that healthy baby in your arms makes it all worthwhile. Now it's time to enjoy your newborn.

## Breastfeeding

Breastfeeding has many wonderful advantages for both you and your baby. Breast milk provides the complete nutrition your baby needs, including the perfect amount of calories, protein, iron, and vitamins necessary for growth. Breast milk contains antibodies, thus giving your baby immunity to diseases. Your baby's stomach can easily digest breast milk, so problems with constipation and diarrhea are less common. Babies who were breast-fed have fewer problems with allergies as children. Adults who were breast-fed have lower cholesterol levels and fewer problems with obesity.

Another incredible bonus is that breastfeeding has been associated with a lower chance of developing type 1 diabetes.

There's good news for mom, too. Breastfeeding helps use up the fat stored during pregnancy. It also lowers the risk of breast cancer and protects against osteoporosis. It's less expensive than formula and many women find it more convenient than formula and bottles. Best of all, for moms with diabetes, breastfeeding removes glucose from the bloodstream, which leads to a lower need for insulin. This is an enjoyable benefit, as you can eat more food but take less insulin.

Your growing baby stimulates milk production, and your insulin and food needs will change over time. Therefore it's essential to monitor your blood glucose, insulin doses, and need for calories during this time.

### *A Strong Word of Caution*

You are much more sensitive to insulin in the first few weeks after delivery, and the risk of hypoglycemia is high. Combine this with breastfeeding, which lowers blood glucose, and you see that you must take extra care to prevent hypoglycemia. Hypoglycemia is very dangerous, especially while caring for a newborn. To avoid hypoglycemia:

- Don't keep super-tight control. Your blood glucose goals are now higher than they were during pregnancy. Err on the side of preventing hypoglycemia.
- Have a snack while nursing your baby.
- Check your blood glucose level about an hour after nursing.

*—by Sallie P. Bartholomew*

Sallie P. Bartholomew, RN, BSN, CDE, is the diabetes nurse educator at the Endocrine and Diabetes Management Center, in Richmond, VA. She has had type 1 diabetes for 26 years. She has two children: Erik 6½, and Emily Joy, 10 months. Her first pregnancy was planned and she maintained tight control with multiple daily injections. Erik was born at 36 weeks weighing 8 pounds, 14 ounces.

Attempts at a second pregnancy failed. Then Bartholomew developed retinopathy, which required laser treatments to both eyes. Another pregnancy was just too risky. Shortly after giving up on the whole idea, including selling all baby and maternity things, a welcome, but not formally planned second pregnancy occurred.

Fortunately, she was using an insulin pump and was in excellent control. Her second pregnancy was much easier than the first because she didn't experience severe hypoglycemia and excessive fluid retention as she did the first time. The pregnancy went smoothly, and Emily Joy arrived healthy at 39 weeks weighing 7 pounds, 7 ounces.

## Chapter 14

# Hypoglycemia

### What Is Hypoglycemia?

Glucose, a form of sugar, is the body's main fuel. Hypoglycemia, or low blood sugar, occurs when blood levels of glucose drop too low to fuel the body's activity.

Carbohydrates (sugars and starches) are the body's main dietary sources of glucose. During digestion, the glucose is absorbed into the blood stream (hence the term "blood sugar"), which carries it to every cell in the body. Unused glucose is stored in the liver as glycogen.

Hypoglycemia can occur as a complication of diabetes, as a condition in itself, or in association with other disorders.

### How Does the Body Control Glucose?

The amount of glucose in the blood is controlled mainly by the hormones insulin and glucagon. Too much or too little of these hormones can cause blood sugar levels to fall too low (hypoglycemia) or rise too high (hyperglycemia). Other hormones that influence blood sugar levels are cortisol, growth hormone, and catecholamines (epinephrine and norepinephrine).

The pancreas, a gland in the upper abdomen, produces insulin and glucagon. The pancreas is dotted with hormone-producing tissue called the islets of Langerhans, which contain alpha and beta cells.

---

National Institute of Diabetes and Digestive and Kidney Diseases (NIDDK), NIH Pub. No. 95-3926, May 1995.

When blood sugar rises after a meal, the beta cells release insulin. The insulin helps glucose enter body cells, lowering blood levels of glucose to the normal range. When blood sugar drops too low, the alpha cells secrete glucagon. This signals the liver to release stored glycogen and change it back to glucose, raising blood sugar levels to the normal range. Muscles also store glycogen that can be converted to glucose.

## Blood Sugar Range

The normal range for blood sugar is about 60 mg/dl (milligrams of glucose per deciliter of blood) to 120 mg/dl, depending on when a person last ate. In the fasting state, blood sugar can occasionally fall below 60 mg/dl and even to below 50 mg/dl and not indicate a serious abnormality or disease. This can be seen in healthy women, particularly after prolonged fasting. Blood sugar levels below 45 mg/dl are almost always associated with a serious abnormality.

## What Are the Symptoms of Hypoglycemia?

A person with hypoglycemia may feel weak, drowsy, confused, hungry, and dizzy. Paleness, headache, irritability, trembling, sweating, rapid heart beat, and a cold, clammy feeling are also signs of low blood sugar. In severe cases, a person can lose consciousness and even lapse into a coma.

The symptoms associated with hypoglycemia are sometimes mistaken for symptoms caused by conditions not related to blood sugar. For example, unusual stress and anxiety can cause excess production of catecholamines, resulting in symptoms similar to those caused by hypoglycemia but having no relation to blood sugar levels.

## Hypoglycemia in Diabetes

The most common cause of hypoglycemia is as a complication of diabetes. Diabetes occurs when the body cannot use glucose for fuel because either the pancreas is not able to make enough insulin or the insulin that is available is not effective. As a result, glucose builds up in the blood instead of getting into body cells.

The aim of treatment in diabetes is to lower high blood sugar levels. To do this, people with diabetes may use insulin or oral drugs, depending on the type of diabetes they have or the severity of their condition. Hypoglycemia occurs most often in people who use insulin to lower their blood sugar. All people with insulin-dependent diabetes (IDDM or Type I) and some people with noninsulin-dependent diabetes (NIDDM or Type II) use insulin. People with Type II diabetes who take oral drugs called sulfonylureas are also vulnerable to low blood sugar episodes.

Conditions that can lead to hypoglycemia in people with diabetes include taking too much medication, missing or delaying a meal, eating too little food for the amount of insulin taken, exercising too strenuously, drinking too much alcohol, or any combination of these factors. People who have diabetes often refer to hypoglycemia as an "insulin reaction."

### *Managing Hypoglycemia in Diabetes*

People with diabetes should consult their health care providers for individual guidelines on target blood sugar ranges that are best for them. The lowest safe blood sugar level for an individual varies, depending on the person's age, medical condition, and ability to sense hypoglycemic symptoms. A target range that is safe for a young adult with no diabetes complications, for example, may be too low for a young child or an older person who may have other medical problems.

Because they are attuned to the symptoms, people with diabetes can usually recognize when their blood sugar levels are dropping too low. They can treat the condition quickly by eating or drinking something with sugar in it such as candy, juice, or nondiet soda. Taking glucose tablets or gels (available in drug stores) is another convenient and quick way to treat hypoglycemia.

People with IDDM are most vulnerable to severe insulin reactions, which can cause loss of consciousness. A few patients with long-standing insulin-dependent diabetes may develop a condition known as hypoglycemia unawareness, in which they have difficulty recognizing the symptoms of low blood sugar. For emergency use in patients with IDDM, physicians often prescribe an injectable form of the hormone glucagon. A glucagon injection (given by another person) quickly eases the symptoms of low blood sugar, releasing a burst of glucose into the blood.

Emergency medical help may be needed if the person does not recover in a few minutes after treatment for hypoglycemia. A person suffering a severe insulin reaction may be admitted to the hospital so that blood sugar can be stabilized.

People with diabetes can reduce or prevent episodes of hypoglycemia by monitoring their blood sugar levels frequently and learning to recognize the symptoms of low blood sugar and the situations that may trigger it. They should consult their health care providers for advice about the best way to treat low blood sugar. Friends and relatives should know about the symptoms of hypoglycemia and how to treat it in case of emergency.

Episodes of hypoglycemia in people with IDDM may become more common now that research has shown that carefully controlled blood sugar helps prevent the complications of diabetes. Keeping blood sugar in a close-to-normal range requires multiple injections of insulin each day or use of an insulin pump, frequent testing of blood glucose, a diet and exercise plan, and guidance from health care professionals.

## Other Causes of Hypoglycemia

Hypoglycemia in people who do not have diabetes is far less common than once believed. However, it can occur in some people under certain conditions such as early pregnancy, prolonged fasting, and long periods of strenuous exercise. People on beta blocker medications who exercise are at higher risk of hypoglycemia, and aspirin can induce hypoglycemia in some children. Drinking alcohol can cause blood sugar to drop in some sensitive individuals, and hypoglycemia has been well documented in chronic alcoholics and binge drinkers. Eating unripe ackee fruit from Jamaica is a rare cause of low blood sugar.

### Diagnosis

To diagnose hypoglycemia in people who do not have diabetes, the doctor looks for the following three conditions:

- The patient complains of symptoms of hypoglycemia
- Blood glucose levels are measured while the person is experiencing those symptoms and found to be 45 mg/dl or less in a woman or 55 mg/dl or less in a man
- The symptoms are promptly relieved upon ingestion of sugar.

For many years, the oral glucose tolerance test (OGTT) was used to diagnose hypoglycemia. Experts now realize that the OGTT can actually trigger hypoglycemic symptoms in people with no signs of the disorder. For a more accurate diagnosis, experts now recommend that blood sugar be tested at the same time a person is experiencing hypoglycemic symptoms.

The doctor will also check the patient for health conditions such as diabetes, obtain a medication history, and assess the degree and severity of the patient's symptoms. Laboratory tests to measure insulin production and levels of C-peptide (a substance that the pancreas releases into the bloodstream in equal amounts to insulin) may be performed.

### Reactive Hypoglycemia

A diagnosis of reactive hypoglycemia is considered only after other possible causes of low blood sugar have been ruled out. Reactive hypoglycemia with no known cause is a condition in which the symptoms of low blood sugar appear 2 to 5 hours after eating foods high in glucose.

Ten to 20 years ago, hypoglycemia was a popular diagnosis. However, studies now show that this condition is actually quite rare. In these studies, most patients who experienced the symptoms of hypoglycemia after eating glucose-rich foods consistently had normal levels of blood sugar—above 60 mg/dl. Some researchers have suggested that some people may be extra sensitive to the body's normal release of the hormone epinephrine after a meal.

People with symptoms of reactive hypoglycemia unrelated to other medical conditions or problems are usually advised to follow a healthy eating plan. The doctor or dietitian may suggest that such a person avoid foods high in carbohydrates; eat small, frequent meals and snacks throughout the day; exercise regularly; and eat a variety of foods, including whole grains, vegetables, and fruits.

### Rare Causes of Hypoglycemia

Fasting hypoglycemia occurs when the stomach is empty. It usually develops in the early morning when a person awakens. As with other forms of hypoglycemia, the symptoms include headache, lack of energy, and an inability to concentrate. Fasting hypoglycemia may be caused by a variety of conditions such as hereditary enzyme or hormone deficiencies, liver disease, and insulin-producing tumors.

In hereditary fructose intolerance, a disorder usually seen in children, the body is unable to metabolize the natural sugar fructose. Attacks of hypoglycemia, marked by seizures, vomiting, and unconsciousness, are treated by giving glucose and eliminating fructose from the diet.

Galactosemia, a rare genetic disorder, hampers the body's ability to process the sugar galactose. An infant with this disorder may appear normal at birth, but after a few days or weeks of drinking milk (which contains galactose), the child may begin to vomit, lose weight, and develop cataracts. The liver may fail to release stored glycogen into the blood, triggering hypoglycemia. Removing milk from the diet is the usual treatment.

A deficiency of growth hormone causes increased sensitivity to insulin. This sensitivity occurs because growth hormone opposes the action of insulin on muscle and fat cells. For this reason, children with growth hormone deficiency sometimes suffer from hypoglycemia, which goes away after treatment.

People with insulin-producing tumors, which arise in the islet cells of the pancreas, suffer from severe episodes of hypoglycemia.

To diagnose these tumors, called insulinomas, a doctor will put the patient on a 24- to 72-hour fast while measuring blood levels of glucose, insulin, and proinsulin. High levels of insulin and proinsulin in the presence of low levels of glucose strongly suggest an insulin-producing tumor. These tumors are usually benign and can be surgically removed.

In rare cases, some cancers such as breast cancer and adrenal cancer may cause hypoglycemia through secretion of a hormone called insulin-like growth factor II. The treatment is removal of the tumor, if possible.

## Research

The National Institute of Diabetes and Digestive and Kidney Diseases (NIDDK) was established by Congress in 1950 as one of the National Institutes of Health, the research arm of the Public Health Service under the U.S. Department of Health and Human Services.

The NIDDK conducts and supports research in diabetes, glucose metabolism, insulin action, and the hormonal controls of blood sugar. Current studies also focus on fasting hypoglycemia, obesity, and insulin resistance.

## Resources on Hypoglycemia

**American Diabetes Association (ADA)**
**National Service Center**
1660 Duke Street
Alexandria, VA 22314
(800) 232-3472 or (703) 549-1500

The ADA is a private, voluntary organization that fosters public awareness of diabetes and supports and promotes diabetes research and education. The ADA distributes printed information on many aspects of diabetes, and local affiliates sponsor community programs. Local affiliates, located in every state, are listed in telephone directories or can be located by contacting the national office.

**The American Dietetic Association**
**National Center for Nutrition and Dietetics**
216 West Jackson Boulevard
Chicago, IL 60606-6995
(800) 366-1655 or (312) 899-0040

The American Dietetic Association is a professional organization for registered dietitians. It publishes a variety of materials for patient and professional education and supports an information and referral service for the general public.

**Juvenile Diabetes Foundation (JDF) International**
432 Park Avenue, South
New York, NY 10016
(800) 223-1138 or (212) 889-7575

The JDF is a private, voluntary organization that promotes research and public education in diabetes, primarily insulin-dependent diabetes. Local chapters, located across the country, are listed in telephone directories or can be found by contacting the national office.

**National Diabetes Information Clearinghouse (NDIC)**
1 Information Way
Bethesda, MD 20892-3560
(301) 654-3827

The NDIC is a service of NIDDK. The clearinghouse distributes a variety of diabetes-related materials to the public and to health professionals, including a literature search listing publications and articles about hypoglycemia in diabetes.

## Additional Readings

Bennion, Lynn J., "Hypoglycemia: A diagnostic challenge," *Clinical Diabetes*, July/August 1985, pp. 85-90.

DCCT Research Group, "Epidemiology of Severe Hypoglycemia in the Diabetes Control and Complications Trial," *The American Journal of Medicine*, vol. 90, April 1991, pp. 450-459.

Field, James B., "Hypoglycemia: Definition, clinical presentations, classifications and laboratory tests," in *Endocrinology and Metabolism Clinics of North America*, vol. 18, no. 1, March 1989.

Foster, Daniel & Rubenstein, Arthur, "Hypoglycemia, insulinoma, and other hormone-secreting tumors of the pancreas" in *Principles of Internal Medicine*. Ed. E. Braunwald et al. [K. J. Isselbacher, R. G. Petersdorf, J. D. Wilson, J. B. Martin, & A. S. Fauci] McGraw-Hill Book Company, 1987, pp. 1800-1807.

Metz, Robert J., "Is the problem hypoglycemia?," *Patient Care*, Oct. 15, 1983, pp. 61-89.

Nelson, Roger L., "Oral glucose tolerance test: Indications and limitations," *Mayo Clinic Proceedings*, vol. 63, 1988, pp. 263-269.

Palardy, Jean et al., "Blood glucose measurements during symptomatic episodes in patients with suspected postprandial hypoglycemia," *New England Journal of Medicine*, Nov. 23, 1989, pp. 1421-1425.

Service, F. John, "Hypoglycemic Disorders," *New England Journal of Medicine*, April 27, 1995, pp. 1144-1152.

Service, F. John, "Hypoglycemia," in *Cecil's Textbook of Medicine*. James B. Wyngaarden & Lloyd H. Smith, Jr. (Eds). W. B. Saunders Company, 1988, pp. 1381-1387.

Service, F. John, "Hypoglycemia and the postprandial syndrome," *New England Journal of Medicine*, (Editorial), Nov. 23, 1989, pp. 1472-1474.

# Chapter 15

# *Syndrome X*

Ever wonder why so many people with type II diabetes also have high blood pressure and high blood fat levels? Maybe it's all one disease.

What an a-*maz*-ing coincidence. A lot of people who have non-insulin-dependent (type II) diabetes also have high blood pressure. *And* abnormal levels of blood lipids (fats). *And* too much insulin floating around in their blood. A run of bad luck? Bad, yes. People who have high blood pressure, dyslipidemia (abnormal blood-fat levels), and high levels of insulin have a higher risk of coronary artery disease. Culminating in what is known on the street as a plain ol' heart attack, coronary artery disease is the leading cause of death in people with type II diabetes. But luck? Probably not. If a person rolling dice comes up with snake eyes four times in a row, you might get away with calling it a chance event. But if a whole lot of people come up with snake eyes four rolls in a row, you might start thinking that the dice are loaded.

Gerald Reaven, MD, professor of medicine at Stanford University School of Medicine in Palo Alto, Calif., proposes that insulin resistance, a state in which cells don't respond well to insulin, loads the dice: It may lead to type II diabetes, high blood pressure, dyslipidemia, high insulin levels, or any combination of these. Reaven calls this collection of diseases syndrome X. He says the majority of people with type II started out with syndrome X.

---

## Those Stubborn Muscle Cells

Muscle cells take in glucose with the help of insulin. Cells that don't readily accept the help offered are said to be insulin-resistant. If glucose can't get into the muscle cells, it stays in the blood.

Some people who are insulin-resistant produce extra insulin to overcome the resistance of the muscle cells. Their blood levels of glucose are normal; their insulin levels are high.

Others don't produce enough insulin to overcome the resistance. The result is high blood sugar: diabetes.

## Fat Cells Follow Suit

Fat cells store energy for the body. The body prefers to use glucose for fuel, but when glucose levels are low, the body uses fat. When needed, fat cells break down and release two types of molecules, fatty acids and glycerol, into the bloodstream to be used as energy by other cells.

A fat cell doesn't react directly to low blood glucose levels but rather to low insulin levels. Normally, insulin levels rise only when blood sugar levels rise. So if a fat cell sees insulin, it assumes there is also glucose in the blood. All's well, and the fat cell keeps its energy stores to itself. Insulin suppresses the release of fatty acids.

In a person with syndrome X, the theory goes, the fat cells, like the muscle cells, are insulin-resistant. More insulin is required to keep the fat cells from releasing fatty acids.

But a fat cell requires fewer molecules of insulin to keep it from releasing free fatty acids than a muscle cell requires to take in glucose. A person whose muscle cells are insulin-resistant, but whose pancreas obliges by putting out more insulin, often has more than enough insulin in the blood to keep the fat cells from releasing free fatty acids, even though the fat cells are insulin-resistant. A raised level of insulin that is unable to keep blood glucose levels down might still be enough to keep fat cells in check.

But if the pancreas can't even put out enough insulin to keep the relatively easy-to-please fat cells happy, the free fatty acid levels in the blood go up.

Then the liver gets sucked in to this charade. The liver normally releases glucose when the body needs it. High levels of free fatty acids cause the liver to release more glucose into the bloodstream.

So here's a body with muscle cells that don't readily take up glucose because they're resistant to insulin, and now it's suddenly got extra glucose from the liver. If the pancreas couldn't put out more insulin to suppress fatty acid release, it certainly won't be able to put out the amount needed to deal with the extra glucose the liver is dishing out. Result: high blood sugar. Not great, but as Reaven notes, "High sugar doesn't acutely kill people."

Meanwhile, the free fatty acids hook up with glycerol molecules to form dreaded triglycerides. High levels of certain types of triglycerides are part of dyslipidemia (too much of the bad blood fats, too little of the good fats). Dyslipidemia contributes to the development of coronary artery disease. And that does kill.

## Feeling the Pressure

Just because the muscle and fat cells are resistant to insulin, doesn't mean other types of cells are resistant to insulin's other actions. Enter high blood pressure, and another step towards coronary heart disease, according to Reaven.

High insulin may lead to high blood pressure by affecting the kidneys. The kidneys regulate the amount of water and dissolved substances that get excreted from the body by way of the bladder. Insulin may cause the kidneys to reabsorb sodium, and the water that clings to it. This could raise blood pressure.

Insulin may also raise blood pressure by affecting the nervous system, which causes blood vessels to constrict, raising blood pressure.

Although many studies show an apparent link between high insulin levels and high blood pressure, a link doesn't prove cause and effect. Some scientists think insulin is getting a bad rap; others think the theory of syndrome X, and in particular the insulin resistance-high blood pressure link, may not hold true for all ethnic groups, for example, Black Americans.

## Changing Odds

Insulin resistance is very common. About 25 percent of the people who don't have diabetes are insulin-resistant, but they don't all end up with high triglycerides and high blood pressure. How come? A few good genes may soften syndrome X.

"You might have insulin resistance," Reaven says, "but also have the most powerful natural triglyceride disposal system known to man. In that way, you would overcome this one side effect of insulin resistance.

"There are many genetic factors, and many powerful environmental factors, that can modify—either make better or worse—the effects of insulin resistance or hyperinsulinemia (high insulin levels).

"Weight control and activity levels are incredibly important. You can improve all these things—high blood pressure, high triglycerides—by exercising and decreasing weight. And the heavier you are and the less active you are, the more insulin-resistant you will be, no matter what your genetic makeup."

Why did insulin resistance evolve in the first place? Reaven speculates: "It was useful to have insulin resistance in the old days, because we lived under the constant threat of starvation. The brain needs sugar. If we didn't have enough food, we would break down our muscles to get sugar to feed our brains. If you don't have any muscle left, you can't look for food."

"Let's say both of us need 25 grams of sugar for our brains. My muscle cells are insulin resistant, so more sugar is left in the bloodstream for the brain to use. I don't break down muscle. You break down more muscle to feed the brain."

"Eventually, I'll find a deer, and you won't. So back then, being insulin-resistant was terrific."

## *Syndrome X Make-At-Home Kit*

Don't have syndrome X? Feeling left out? Don't despair—there are a few practices that can greatly increase your chances of becoming insulin-resistant.

One: Become a couch potato, and put on the pounds; insulin resistance won't be far behind. You may also be able to create insulin resistance and put yourself at risk for all the related abnormalities with one simple ingredient: cigarettes.

Reaven and his colleagues at Stanford University and the Veterans Affairs Medical Center in Palo Alto, Calif., compared 20 chronic smokers and 20 non-smokers. After the subjects drank glucose, their blood glucose levels were measured. The glucose levels of both groups were about the same, but the smokers' blood samples were found to have significantly higher levels of insulin than the non-smokers. The smokers' pancreases had to crank out more insulin to deal with the same amount of glucose as the nonsmokers. The smokers were insulin-resistant.

Total cholesterol levels were about the same in both groups, but the level of VLDL-cholesterol (very bad) was higher in the smokers; HDL-cholesterol (good) was—yeah, you guessed it—lower in the smokers.

It is widely accepted that cigarette smoking contributes to the development of heart disease. These researchers suggest that, along with all its other effects, cigarette smoking also has an indirect effect: smoking causes insulin resistance and the cascade of events which, in turn, contribute to heart disease.

*—by Marie McCarren*

Marie McCarren is associate editor of *Diabetes Forecast*.

# Part Three

# Diabetes Management

## Chapter 16

# *Diabetes Demands a Triad of Treatments*

Actress Mary Tyler Moore battles it. Country singer Mark Collie has it. Rhythm and blues singer Pattie LaBelle was diagnosed with it recently.

Celebrities like Moore, Collie and LaBelle are just three well-known faces amid the 16 million Americans suffering from diabetes mellitus, a chronic disease in which the pancreas produces too little or no insulin, impairing the body's ability to turn sugar into usable energy.

In recent years, the Food and Drug Administration has approved a fast-acting form of human insulin and several new oral diabetes drugs, including the most recent, Rezulin (troglitazone), the first of a new class of drugs called insulin sensitizers. This drug is designed to help Type II diabetics make better use of the insulin produced by their bodies and could help as many as 1 million Type II diabetics reduce or eliminate their need for insulin injections.

While it is treatable, diabetes is still a killer. The fourth leading cause of death in America, diabetes claims an estimated 178,000 lives each year. So the treatment is aimed at holding the disease in check, reversing it where possible, and preventing complications.

Philip Cryer, M.D., a professor at Washington University School of Medicine in St. Louis and president of the American Diabetes Association, believes that most people simply don't understand the magnitude of the diabetes problem. "Diabetes is an increasingly common,

---

*FDA Consumer*, May-June1997.

potentially devastating, treatable yet incurable, lifelong disease. It's the leading cause of blindness in working-age adults, the most common cause of kidney failure leading to dialysis or transplants, and is a leading cause of amputation," he says. "The most recent estimate we have of diabetes' cost [in terms of] direct medical care is $90 billion dollars annually—more than heart disease, cancer, or AIDS."

At the heart of diabetes control are dietary management and drug treatment. The increasing emphasis on the importance of a healthy diet, the availability of glucose monitoring devices that can help diabetics keep a close watch over blood sugar levels, and the wide range of drug treatments enable most diabetics to live a near-normal life.

Managing the diet is easier now because of food labeling regulations that went into effect in 1994.

### *Two Types of Diabetes*

There are two main types of diabetes, Type I and Type II. Insulin-dependent, or Type I, diabetes affects about 5 percent of all diabetics. It's also known as juvenile diabetes because it often occurs in people under 35 and commonly appears in children or adolescents. For example, Mary Tyler Moore, a Type I diabetic who is international chairman of the Juvenile Diabetes Foundation, was diagnosed in her late 20s, following a miscarriage. A routine test found her blood sugar level was 750 milligrams per deciliter (mg/dl), as compared with the normal level, 70 mg/dl to 105 mg/dl. And Collie has been diabetic since age 17.

In Type I diabetes, the insulin-secreting cells of the pancreas are destroyed, with insulin production almost ceasing. Experts believe that this may be the result of an immune response after a viral infection.

Type I diabetics must inject insulin regularly under the skin. Insulin cannot be taken by mouth because it cannot be absorbed from the gastrointestinal tract into the bloodstream. Doses range from one or two up to five injections a day, adjusted in response to regular blood sugar monitoring.

Insulin regulates both blood sugar and the speed at which sugar moves into cells. Because food intake affects the cells' need for insulin and insulin's ability to lower blood sugar, the diet is the cornerstone of diabetes management: Insulin is not a replacement for proper diet.

Symptoms of untreated insulin-dependent diabetes include:

- continuous need to urinate
- excessive thirst
- increased appetite

- weakness
- tiredness
- urinary tract infections
- recurrent skin infections, such as boils
- vaginal yeast infections in women
- blurred vision
- tingling or numbness in hands or feet.

If Type I diabetes goes untreated, a life-threatening condition called ketoacidosis can quickly develop. If this condition is not treated, coma and death will follow.

Type II, or non-insulin-dependent, diabetes is the most common type. It results when the body produces insufficient insulin to meet the body's needs, or when the cells of the body have become resistant to insulin's effect. While all Type I diabetics develop symptoms, only a third of those who have Type II diabetes develop symptoms. Many people suffer from a mild form of the disease and are unaware of it. Often it's diagnosed only after complications are detected.

When they occur, Type II symptoms usually include frequent urination, excessive thirst, fatigue, an increase in infections, blurred vision, tingling in hands or feet, impotence in men, and absence of menstrual periods in women.

Type II diabetes usually develops in people over 40, and it often runs in families. For instance, Pattie LaBelle was diagnosed with Type II diabetes at age 50, and her mother died of the disease.

Type II diabetes is often linked to obesity and inactivity and can often be controlled with diet and exercise alone. Type II diabetics sometimes use insulin, but usually oral medications are prescribed if diet and exercise alone do not control the disease.

### *Malfunction in Glucose Metabolism*

In a normal body, carbohydrates (sugars and starches) are broken down in the intestines to simple sugars (mostly glucose), which then circulate in the blood, entering cells, where they are used to produce energy. Diabetics respond inappropriately to carbohydrate metabolism, and glucose can't enter the cells normally.

Insulin—a hormone that is made in the pancreas and released into the bloodstream and carried throughout the body—enables the organs to take sugar from the blood and use it for energy. If body cells become resistant to insulin's effect or if there isn't enough insulin, sugar stays in the blood and accumulates, causing high blood sugar. At the same time, cells starve because there's no insulin to help move sugar into the cells.

Diabetes is diagnosed by measuring blood sugar levels. This can begin with a urine test sampled for glucose because excess sugar in the blood spills over into the urine. Further testing involves taking blood samples after an overnight fast. Normal fasting blood glucose levels are between 70 mg/dl and 105 mg/dl; a fasting blood glucose measurement greater than 140 mg/dl on two separate occasions indicates diabetes.

Diabetes can result in many complications, including nerve damage, foot and leg ulcers, and eye problems that can lead to blindness. Diabetics also are at greater risk for heart disease, stroke, narrowing of the arteries, and kidney failure. But evidence shows that the better the patient controls his or her blood sugar levels, the greater the chances that the disease's serious complications can be reduced.

### *Shot of Insulin*

The first insulin for diabetes was derived from the pancreas of cows and pigs. Today, chemically synthesized human insulin is the most often used. It is prepared from bacteria with DNA technology. Human insulin is not necessarily an advantage over animal insulin, and most doctors don't recommend that patients on animal insulin automatically switch to human insulin. But if they do switch, dosages may change. Human insulin is preferred for those patients who take insulin intermittently.

According to Robert Misbin, M.D., medical officer for metabolic and endocrine drug products in FDA's Center for Drug Evaluation and Research and a practicing physician, some diabetics take beef insulin for religious reasons because of dietary restrictions against pork. "But the vast majority of insulin-dependent diabetics take synthesized human insulin," he says. "Those who are taking a beef or pork insulin and doing well—you don't necessarily change the type of insulin they take. But for new patients I see, I would start them on human insulin."

Diabetics on intensified insulin therapy—that is, those needing multiple daily injections or an insulin pump, which is worn 24 hours a day—can have flexibility in when and what they eat. Other diabetics on insulin therapy must eat at consistent times, synchronized with the time-action of the insulin they use.

In 1996, FDA approved Humalog, which Misbin describes as "a modified human insulin." Humalog is absorbed and dissipated more rapidly than regular human insulin. Misbin says that Humalog is of particular benefit to Type I diabetics who are on very strict regimens.

Julio V. Santiago, M.D., director of the Diabetes Research and Training Center at Washington University's School of Medicine in St. Louis, notes that Humalog is most helpful for diabetics monitoring their blood sugar levels and taking three or more injections of insulin a day. He reports switching most of his Type I patients who fit that profile to the new insulin.

### *Oral Drugs*

Four classes of oral diabetes drugs are now available. The oldest class, sulfonylureas (SFUs), act on the pancreatic tissue to produce insulin. The newest one is Glimepiride, approved by FDA in 1996.

Because SFUs can become less effective after 10 or more years of use, other drugs often are needed. Also, there is some controversy regarding SFUs; some of these agents have been shown in studies to contribute to increased risk of death from cardiovascular disease.

A newer class is the biguanides, including Metformin, which was approved by FDA in 1995. This drug acts by lowering cells' resistance to insulin, a common problem in Type II diabetes.

A third class is the alpha-glucosidase inhibitors, which include Precose, approved by FDA in 1995, and Miglitol, approved in 1996. These drugs slow the body's digestion of carbohydrates, delaying absorption of glucose from the intestines.

In January 1997, FDA approved the first in a new class of diabetes drugs, Rezulin. The new medicine helps Type II diabetics make better use of their own insulin by resensitizing body tissues to the insulin. Parke-Davis, a division of Warner-Lambert of Morris Plains, N.J., plans to begin marketing the drug by summer 1997.

"It will be useful in patients who, despite taking large doses of insulin, still are not achieving adequate glucose control," Misbin says.

Some oral drugs may be used in combination to improve blood sugar control. For example, FDA's Misbin says, Metformin, with an SFU, is particularly useful for Type II diabetics who are obese. "Type II patients who would ordinarily use [only] SFUs do not gain weight with Metformin," he explains. "[The combination] also is used for people taking SFUs but are no longer getting the SFUs' full effect. Studies show that when you add Metformin to a regimen of an SFU, you get a treatment that is better than either drug used alone."

Metformin makes users more sensitive to the body's naturally produced insulin and decreases excessive production of sugar by the liver, another characteristic of Type II diabetes.

The drugs are not without side effects. Metformin, for example, can cause serious cramps and diarrhea, and it can't be used in people with kidney problems. "So if you have to go on this drug, you need to have kidney function tests," Santiago says.

Metformin is also contraindicated in patients with liver dysfunction. "It should be used only in healthy patients, and it's not for the elderly," Misbin says.

Precose is less effective but usually safer to use than Metformin, he points out. Precose's one major side effect is flatulence. Precose stops, or delays, absorption of carbohydrates and in doing so delivers glucose and other carbohydrates, which cause gas, Santiago explains. "Flatulence can occur when the drug is used at high doses, but this can be reduced by beginning the drug at a low dose and going up ... a 'start-low, go-slow' approach."

Product labeling recommends that doctors start patients on lower doses to combat the flatulence problem.

"Although the lowest effective dose is 25 milligrams three times a day with meals, some physicians are starting patients on just 25 mg daily to minimize this side effect," Misbin says.

The newest drug, Rezulin, was well-tolerated in clinical studies. The most commonly reported side effects were infection, pain and headache, but these occurred at rates comparable to those in the placebo-treated patients. The drug should be prescribed with caution in patients with advanced heart failure or liver disease.

Some diabetes experts report that when it comes to prescribing initial therapy for Type II diabetics, some doctors tend to follow a "treatment of laziness"—for example, prescribing SFUs if they perceive difficulties in the patient's ability to change dietary habits or lifestyle.

"Sometimes, patients with diabetes are treated with drugs when it's not really necessary," Misbin says. "Oral pills should be used in Type II diabetes only when diet and exercise are not effective. It's very common for overweight patients who lose weight to lower their own blood sugar levels and come off the medicines. The problem is that it's very difficult to get patients to lose weight."

So, the bottom line in diabetes control still hinges on patients' ability to manage the disease themselves. "I don't know of a chronic disease in which the person who suffers from it is so responsible for its management," says ADA president Cryer. "The patient has to become an expert regarding their own diabetes."

Although drug treatment makes a difference to many diabetics and their quality of life, Cryer adds that current diabetes treatments are still "not ideal." He hopes that continuing research will someday find the answer to the diabetes dilemma.

## Blood Glucose Monitoring Devices

For millions of Americans with diabetes, regular home testing of blood glucose levels is critical in controlling their disease.

"The most near-normal glucose patterns you can get will have a terrific long-term impact on how well people with diabetes do," says Steven Gutman, M.D., director of the division of clinical laboratory devices in FDA's Office of Device Evaluation. But he adds, "Tight control isn't easy because it requires multiple glucose measurements."

For many years, diabetics relied on home urine glucose testing to monitor blood sugar levels. But the method was not without drawbacks. Monitoring glucose levels via the urine is problematic for several reasons: First, blood glucose concentrations above which glucose appears in the urine vary widely among individuals, so the tests are not very reliable. Second, factors such as fluid or vitamin C intakes can influence test results. And third, negative tests can't distinguish between normal, low, and moderately high blood sugar levels.

By the late 1960s, manufacturers began introducing home blood glucose monitoring kits. These kits allowed diabetics to detect blood sugar levels by looking at color changes on a chemical test strip using a single drop of blood from a pricked finger. Portable meters that could electronically read the strip and provide immediate results came along in the late 1970s.

Although today's monitors are small, easier to use than early ones, and reasonably priced at between $50 and $100, they all require users to prick their fingers to provide a blood sample for testing. So diabetics were understandably enthusiastic when a noninvasive glucose sensor monitoring device was developed. It doesn't require a finger prick but instead uses infrared technology to measure blood glucose. But after reviewing data from the device's manufacturer, the Clinical Chemistry and Clinical Toxicology Devices Advisory Panel of FDA's Medical Devices Advisory Committee decided more data were needed to ensure the device's safety and effectiveness.

"The idea of being able to test yourself without a painful prick is very attractive. It would probably increase compliance because some patients simply don't want to prick their fingers," Gutman says. "It's a very promising technology. But you have to balance technology against performance."

Gutman said the criteria the company chose to deem the device successful—that 50 percent of readings agree with 20 percent of readings from the patient's finger-prick device—was not an appropriate target. The panel agreed that success should be defined as having 80 to 90 percent of values correlating to values obtained with finger-prick tests. So, the FDA advisory committee also recommended that the sponsor conduct more studies, doing them at multiple sites and involving more women who develop diabetes while pregnant and more children. Also, the committee suggested that the sponsor base the studies on specific study objectives related to performance claims, with the data sufficient to ensure safety and effectiveness.

Julio V. Santiago, M.D., an internist specializing in diabetes and a former member of FDA's Endocrine Advisory Committee, says, "It's an exciting new technology that diabetics could benefit from, so we were rooting for the company. But they failed to demonstrate that the device worked long term for home use."

Santiago says that current invasive finger-prick devices are very reliable, with accuracy within 15 percent of real measurements 80 to 90 percent of the time. Their biggest disadvantage is cost, since each test strip costs 50 cents, and several are often used in one day. A spokesman for Boehringer Mannheim Corp., Rick Naples, says the cost of test strips and lancets needed to perform self blood-glucose monitoring can average between $600 and $1,000 a year.

Gutman says FDA appreciates the need for noninvasive glucose monitors and is anxious to work with companies early in the development of these devices. The Center for Devices and Radiological Health has implemented an expedited review program for devices like noninvasive glucose monitors so items that may be in the interest of public health can be made available in an expedited way without compromising the devices' safety and effectiveness, he says. "Such expedited reviews are given precedence over routine reviews."

Gutman is optimistic about future approval of a noninvasive blood glucose monitoring kit for diabetics. "I'd be very disappointed if we don't eventually see a noninvasive model in the future," he says.

*—by Audrey Hingley*

Audrey Hingley is a writer in Mechanicsville, Va.

Chapter 17

# Take Charge of Your Diabetes

## Introduction

Diabetes touches almost every part of your life. It's a serious, lifelong condition, but there's so much you can do to protect your health. You can take charge of your health—not only for today, but for the coming years.

Diabetes can cause health problems over time. It can hurt your eyes, your kidneys, and your nerves. It can lead to problems with the blood circulation in your body. Even your teeth and gums can be harmed. And diabetes in pregnancy can cause special problems. Many of these problems don't have to happen. You can do a lot to prevent them, and there are people in your community who can help. This chapter can help you find how to get the help you need to prevent problems.

Today and every day, you need to balance your food, physical activity, and medicine. Testing your own blood glucose (also called blood sugar) helps you see how this balance is working out. You can then make choices that help you feel well day-to-day and protect your health.

Feeling healthy can allow you to play a big part in the life of your family and community. You may even want to join a community group to help others deal with their diabetes.

---

Centers for Disease Control and Prevention. *Take Charge of Your Diabetes*. 2nd edition. Atlanta: U.S. Department of Health and Human Services, 1997. This booklet is also available on the Internet at: http://www.cdc.gov/nccdphp/ddt/ddthome.

*Take Charge of Your Diabetes* was written to help you take important steps to prevent problems caused by diabetes. You'll learn many useful things:

- What problems diabetes can cause.
- How to work with a health care team to prevent problems.
- Why it is important to get your blood glucose closer to normal.
- How to find out about resources in your community to help you prevent problems.

It's important to work with a primary care provider, as well as other members of a team that care about your health. To find out about resources in your community, telephone one of the groups listed below:

- Your state medical association, listed in the business section of your phone book.
- Your state department of health's Diabetes Control Program, listed in the blue pages of your phone book.
- Local hospitals, listed in the yellow pages.
- Diabetes organizations (see Part VIII of this book, Additional Help and Information).

Stay in touch with your health care team so you will know the latest news about diabetes care.

*Balance* is the key word in living well with diabetes. Strive for balance in all parts of your life. With the support of your family and friends, your health care team, and your community, you can take charge of your diabetes.

### *Who and What Is This Chapter for?*

This chapter was mainly written for people who found out they had diabetes as an adult. It's meant to be used along with other information your health care providers give you.

If you've just learned you have diabetes, you'll need more details than you'll find in this chapter. Ask your health care provider for help. See (see part eight of this book, Additional Help and Information) for phone numbers and addresses of places where you can get more information. Find out as much as you can about the three most important things for controlling your diabetes: food, physical activity, and diabetes medicine.

## What Is Diabetes?

Most of the food we eat is turned into **glucose** (sugar) for our bodies to use for energy. The **pancreas**, an organ near the stomach, makes a **hormone** called **insulin** to help glucose get into our body cells. When you have **diabetes**, your body either doesn't make enough insulin or can't use its own insulin very well. This problem causes glucose to build up in your blood.

*Signs and Symptoms of Diabetes*

You may recall having some of these signs before you found out you had diabetes:

- Being very thirsty.
- Urinating a lot—often at night.
- Having blurry vision from time to time.
- Feeling very tired much of the time.
- Losing weight without trying.
- Having very dry skin.
- Having sores that are slow to heal.
- Getting more infections than usual.
- Losing feeling or getting a tingling feeling in the feet.
- Vomiting.

*Types of Diabetes*

There are two main types of diabetes:

- **Type 1.**
- **Type 2.**

Another type of diabetes appears during pregnancy in some women. It's called **gestational diabetes**.

One out of ten people with diabetes has Type 1 diabetes. These people usually find out they have diabetes when they are children or young adults. People with Type 1 diabetes must **inject** insulin every day to live. The pancreas of a person with Type 1 makes little or no insulin. Scientists are learning more about what causes the body to attack its own **beta cells** of the pancreas (an **autoimmune process**) to stop making insulin in people with certain sets of genes.

Most people with diabetes—nine out of ten—have Type 2 diabetes. The pancreas of people with Type 2 diabetes keeps making insulin for some time, but the body can't use it very well. Most people with Type 2 find out about their diabetes after age 30 or 40.

# At-Risk Weight Chart

| Women (shows 20% over ideal weights) | | | Men (shows 20% over ideal weights) | | |
|---|---|---|---|---|---|
| **Height** (without shoes) | | **Weight in Pounds** (without clothing) | **Height** (without shoes) | | **Weight in Pounds** (without clothing) |
| ***Feet*** | ***Inches*** | | ***Feet*** | ***Inches*** | |
| 4 | 9 | 134 | 5 | 1 | 157 |
| 4 | 10 | 137 | 5 | 2 | 160 |
| 4 | 11 | 140 | 5 | 3 | 162 |
| 5 | 0 | 143 | 5 | 4 | 165 |
| 5 | 1 | 146 | 5 | 5 | 168 |
| 5 | 2 | 150 | 5 | 6 | 172 |
| 5 | 3 | 154 | 5 | 7 | 175 |
| 5 | 4 | 157 | 5 | 8 | 179 |
| 5 | 5 | 161 | 5 | 9 | 182 |
| 5 | 6 | 164 | 5 | 10 | 186 |
| 5 | 7 | 168 | 5 | 11 | 190 |
| 5 | 8 | 172 | 6 | 0 | 194 |
| 5 | 9 | 175 | 6 | 1 | 199 |
| 5 | 10 | 178 | 6 | 2 | 203 |
| 5 | 11 | 182 | 6 | 3 | 203 |

***Figure 17.1.***

Certain **risk factors** make people more likely to get Type 2 diabetes. Some of these are:

- A family history of diabetes.
- Lack of exercise.
- Weighing too much.
- Being of African American, American Indian, Hispanic/Latino, or Asian/Pacific Islander heritage.

In Figure 17.1, you'll find a weight chart. If you weigh more than the weight that matches your height on the chart, tell your health care provider. You can help manage your diabetes by controlling your weight, making healthy food choices, and getting regular physical activity. Some people with Type 2 diabetes may also need to take **diabetes pills** or insulin shots to help control their diabetes.

## Controlling Your Diabetes

There's good news for people with diabetes. A new study shows that keeping your **blood glucose** (also called **blood sugar**) close to normal helps prevent or delay some diabetes problems.

Scientists in this study learned that through such control, at least half of the expected eye disease, kidney disease, and nerve damage was prevented or slowed. People who were in the study had **Type 1 diabetes**, but many doctors believe that people who have **Type 2 diabetes** can also benefit by keeping their blood glucose closer to normal.

You can get more information about this study by contacting the National Diabetes Information Clearinghouse at 1-800-GET-LEVEL (1-800-438-5383).

### *Keeping a Balance*

As the eagle learns its position and adjusts what it must do to keep its balance in flight, you must also strive for balance that helps you keep your blood glucose in control. To keep your glucose at a healthy level, you need to keep a balance between three important things:

- What you eat and drink.
- How much physical activity you do.
- What diabetes medicine you take (if your doctor has prescribed **diabetes pills** or **insulin**).

This chapter gives you only some of the facts you need. Your health care team can give you more.

*A Few Things about Food*

Here are some tips for making healthy eating choices:

- *Eat regular meals.* Ask your health care team to help you choose a **meal plan**. Your dietitian may suggest you eat three meals and a snack or two every day at about the same times. Don't skip meals.
- *Eat a variety of foods.* Choose a variety of foods to eat so that your body gets the nutrition it needs. Use the Food Pyramid to choose a variety of foods every day. Eat more from the foods at the bottom of the pyramid and eat less from those at the top. Ask your dietitian for help.
- *Eat less fat.* Avoid fried foods. Foods that are baked, broiled, grilled, boiled, or steamed are more healthy to eat. Eat meats that have little fat. When you eat dairy products (cheese, milk, yogurt, and others) choose those that have little or no fat or cream.
- *Eat less sugar.* You may find that eating less sugar helps you control your blood glucose level. Here are some things you can do to eat less sugar:
    - Read the labels on jars, cans, and food packages—before you buy them. If one of the first four ingredients listed is sucrose, dextrose, corn sweeteners, honey, high-fructose corn syrup, molasses, or powdered sugar, try to buy something with less sugar, or else use less of that food item.
    - Drink sugar-free sodas and other liquids that have no added sugar in them.
    - Eat fewer foods that have extra sugar, such as cookies, cakes, pastries, candy, chocolates, brownies, and sugared breakfast cereals.
- *Eat less salt.* Eating less salt may help control your blood pressure. Here are some ways to eat less salt:
    - Use less salt when you prepare foods.

  - Cut down on processed foods, such as foods you buy in cans and jars, pickled foods, lunch meats ("cold cuts"), and snack foods, such as chips.
  - Taste your food first before adding salt. You may not need to add any.
  - Use herbs and spices instead of salt to flavor your food.

- *A word about drinking alcohol*: Alcohol can cause health problems, especially for people with diabetes. It adds calories and it doesn't give your body any nutrition. Drinking alcohol may cause dangerous reactions with medicines you take. Your blood glucose can go down too low if you drink beer, wine, or liquor on an empty stomach. If you want to include a drink in your food plan once in a while, ask your health care team how to do so safely.

*A Few Things about Physical Activity*

- *It's important to be active*. Physical activity has many benefits. It can help you control your blood glucose and your weight. Physical activity can help prevent heart and circulation problems. Many people say they feel better when they get regular exercise.

- *Start with a little*. If you haven't been doing any physical activity, talk to your health care team before you begin. Walking, working in the yard, and dancing are good ways to start. As you become stronger, you can add a few extra minutes to your physical activity. If you feel pain, slow down or stop and wait until it goes away. If the pain comes back, talk to your health care team right away.

- *Do some physical activity every day*. It's better to walk 10 or 20 minutes each day than one hour once a week.

- *Choose an activity you enjoy*. Do an activity you really like. The more fun it is, the more likely you will do it each day. It's also good to exercise with a family member or friend.

If you're already active now, but want to become more active, talk to your health care team about a safe exercise plan.

*A Few Things about Diabetes Medicine*

If you take diabetes pills or insulin injections to control your diabetes, ask your health care provider to explain how these work. It's important to know how and when to take diabetes medicine. If you take other medicines that are sold with or without a prescription, ask your doctor how these can affect your diabetes control. When you take insulin injections or diabetes pills, your blood glucose levels can get too low. If you inject insulin, your health care team should be able to tell you:

- How to give yourself injections.
- When you need to change your insulin dose.
- How to safely dispose of needles.

## Keeping Track of Your Blood Glucose

It's important to your health to control your **blood glucose** (also called **blood sugar**). Keeping your glucose close to normal helps prevent or delay some diabetes problems, such as eye disease, kidney disease, and nerve damage. One thing that can help you control your glucose level is to keep track of it. You can do this by:

- Testing your own glucose a number of times each day (**self-monitoring blood glucose**). Many people with diabetes test their glucose two to four times a day.

- Getting a **hemoglobin A1c** test from your health care provider about every 3 months if you take **insulin** and at least every 6 months if you don't take insulin.

You'll learn more about these tests on the next pages. These tests can help you and the rest of your diabetes health care team—doctor, diabetes educator, and others—work together to help you control your blood glucose.

### *Testing Your Blood Glucose Each Day*

You can do a test to find out what your blood glucose is at any moment. Your health care team can show you how to do the test yourself. Using a finger prick, you place a drop of blood on a special coated strip, which "reads" your blood glucose. Many people use an electronic meter to get this reading.

Blood glucose testing can help you understand how food, physical activity, and diabetes medicine affect your glucose level. Testing can help you make day-to-day choices about how to balance these things. It can also tell you when your glucose is too low or too high so that you can treat these problems.

Ask your health care team to help you set a goal for your glucose range and show you how to record your glucose readings in a logbook or record sheet. If you need a daily logbook, ask your health care provider for one.

Be sure to write down each glucose reading and the date and time you took it. When you review your records, you can see a pattern of your recent glucose control. Keeping track of your glucose on a day-to-day basis is one of the best ways you can take charge of your diabetes.

### *Getting a Summary Lab Test (Hemoglobin A1c)*

A hemoglobin A1c test uses blood drawn from a vein in your arm to sum up your diabetes control for the past few months. Hemoglobin A1c measures how much glucose has been sticking to part of the hemoglobin in your red blood cells. Since each red blood cell is replaced by a new one every four months, this test summarizes how high the glucose levels have been during the life of the cells.

If most of your recent blood glucose readings have been near normal (70 to 140 mg/dL, with the higher reading occurring after meals), the hemoglobin A1c test will be near normal (usually about 6%-7%). If you've had many readings above normal, the extra glucose sticking to your red blood cells will make your hemoglobin A1c test read higher.

You should get a hemoglobin A1c test at least two times a year. People who take insulin need to get this test about four times a year. Ask your health care provider for the results and record them. This test will help you and your diabetes care team keep track of our average blood glucose control.

Ask your team to tell you the normal range of values and help you set a goal for yourself. Write your goal down. If your hemoglobin A1c is high, work with your team to adjust your balance of food, physical activity, and diabetes medicine. When your hemoglobin A1c test result is near your goal, you'll know you've balanced things well.

### *Having Problems with Low Blood Glucose*

In general, a blood glucose reading lower than 70 mg/dL is too low. If you take **insulin** or **diabetes pills**, you can have **low blood glucose** (also called **hypoglycemia**). Low blood glucose is usually caused by eating less or later than usual, being more active than usual, or taking too much diabetes medicine. Drinking beer, wine, or liquor may also cause low blood glucose or make it worse.

Low blood glucose happens more often when you're trying to keep your glucose level near normal. This is no reason to stop trying to control your diabetes. It just means you have to watch more carefully for low levels. Talk this over with your health care team.

*Signs of Low Blood Glucose*

Some possible signs of low blood glucose are feeling nervous, shaky, or sweaty. Sometimes people just feel tired.

The signs may be mild at first. But a low glucose level can quickly drop much lower if you don't treat it. When your glucose level is very low, you may get confused, pass out, or have seizures.

If you have any signs that your glucose may be low, test it right away. If it's less than 60 to 70 mg/dL, you need to treat it right away. See below for ways to treat low blood glucose.

*Treating Low Blood Glucose*

If you feel like your blood glucose is getting too low but you can't test it right then, play it safe—go ahead and treat it. Eat 10 to 15 grams of **carbohydrate** right away. See Figure 17.2 below for examples of foods and liquids with this amount of carbohydrate.

Check your blood glucose again in 15 minutes. Eat another 10 to 15 grams of carbohydrate every 15 minutes until your blood glucose is above 70 mg/dL or your signs have gone away.

Eating an item on the list on this page will keep your glucose up for only about 30 minutes. So if your next planned meal or snack is more than 30 minutes away, you should go ahead and eat something like crackers and a tablespoon of peanut butter or a slice of cheese.

In your glucose logbook or record sheet, write down the numbers and the times when low levels happen. Think about what may be causing them. If you think you know the reason, write it beside the numbers you recorded. You may need to call your health care provider to talk about changing your diet, activity, or diabetes medicine.

Tell family members, close friends, teachers, and people at work that you have diabetes. Tell them how to know when your blood glucose is low. Show them what to do if you can't treat yourself. Someone will need to give you fruit juice, soda pop (not diet), or sugar.

If you can't swallow, someone will need to give you a shot of **glucagon** and call for help. Glucagon is a prescription medicine that raises the blood glucose and is injected like insulin. If you take insulin, you should have a glucagon kit handy. Teach family members, roommates, and friends when and how to use it.

*Waiting to treat low blood glucose is not safe*. You may be in danger of passing out. If you get confused, pass out, or have a seizure, you need emergency help. Don't try to drive yourself to get help. Be prepared for an emergency.

*Preventing Low Blood Glucose*

**Keep a balance.** Try to stay close to your usual schedule of eating, activity, and medicine. If you're late getting a meal or if you're more active than usual, you may need an extra snack.

**Test your blood glucose.** Keeping track of your blood glucose is a good way to know when it tends to run low. Show your logbook or record sheet to your health care providers. Be sure to let them know if you're having a number of low glucose readings a week.

## Foods and Liquids for Low Blood Glucose

(each item equals about 10 to 15 grams of carbohydrate)

| Food Item | Amount |
| --- | --- |
| Sugar packets | 2 to 3 |
| Fruit juice | 1/2 cup (4 ounces) |
| Soda pop (not diet) | 1/2 cup (4 ounces) |
| Hard candy | 3 to 5 pieces |
| Sugar or honey | 3 teaspoons |
| Glucose tablets | 2 to 3 |

***Figure 17.2.***

To be safe, always check your glucose before doing any of these things:

- Driving a vehicle.
- Using heavy equipment.
- Being very physically active.
- Being active for a long time.

Ask your health care team whether you should test your glucose before (or during) any other activities.

**Be prepared.** Always carry some type of carbohydrate with you so you'll be ready at any time to treat a low glucose level. See Figure 17.2. (above) for snacks that have 10-15 grams of carbohydrate.

Always wear something (like an identification bracelet) that says you have diabetes. Carry a card in your wallet that says you have diabetes and tells if you use medicine to treat it.

### *Having Problems with High Blood Glucose*

For most people, blood glucose levels that stay higher than 140 mg/dL (before meals) are too high. Talk with your health care team about the glucose range that is best for you.

Eating too much food, being less active than usual, or taking too little diabetes medicine are some common reasons for **high blood glucose** (or **hyperglycemia**). Your blood glucose can also go up when you're sick or under stress.

Over time, high blood glucose can damage body organs. For this reason, many people with diabetes try to keep their blood glucose in control as much as they can.

Some people with diabetes are in danger of **diabetic ketoacidosis** when their glucose level stays high. You can tell if you're in diabetic ketoacidosis by checking your urine for **ketones**. If you have ketones in your urine, call your doctor or go to the hospital right away. The most common reason for diabetic ketoacidosis is not taking your insulin. If you have Type 1 diabetes, ask your health care team about diabetic ketoacidosis.

Your blood glucose is more likely to go up when you're sick—for example, when you have the flu or an infection. You'll need to take special care of yourself during these times. The section "Taking Care of Yourself When You're Sick" below can help you do this.

*Signs of High Blood Glucose*

Some common signs of high blood glucose are having a dry mouth, being thirsty, and urinating often. Other signs include feeling tired, having blurred vision, and losing weight without trying. If your glucose is very high, you may have stomach pain, feel sick to your stomach, or even throw up.

If you have any signs that your glucose is high, test your blood. In your logbook or on your record sheet, write down your glucose reading and the time you did the test. If your glucose is high, think about what could have caused it to go up. If you think you know of something, write this down beside your glucose reading.

*Preventing High Blood Glucose*

**Keep a balance.** Try to stay with your food and activity plan as much as you can. Take your diabetes medicine about the same time each day. Work with your health care team to set goals for weight, glucose level, and activity.

**Test your blood glucose.** Keep track of your glucose and go over your records often. You'll learn how certain foods or activities affect your glucose.

**Show your records to your health care team.** Ask how you can change your food, activity, and medicine to avoid or treat high blood glucose. Ask when you should call for help.

## *Taking Care of Yourself When You're Sick*

*Keep Taking Medicine*

Be sure to keep taking your diabetes pills or insulin. Don't stop taking them even if you can't eat. Your health care provider may even advise you to take more insulin during sickness.

*Keep Eating*

Try to eat the same amount of fruits and breads as usual. If you can, eat your regular diet. If you are having trouble doing this, use **food exchanges**: eat enough soft foods or drink enough liquids to take the place of the fruits and breads you usually eat. A food exchange is a measured portion of one type of food that can be eaten instead of another type of food. A food exchange will give you similar nutrients. Use Figure 17.3. to make food exchanges for bread or fruit.

## What to Eat or Drink When You're Sick

(each item equals one bread or fruit exchange*)

| Food Item | Amount |
|---|---|
| Fruit juice | 1/3 to 1/2 cup |
| Fruit-flavored drink | 1/2 cup |
| Soda pop (regular, not diet) | 1/2 cup |
| *Jell-O™ ( regular, not sugar-free) | 1/2 cup |
| *Popsicle™ (not sugar-free, regular) | 1/2 twin |
| Sherbet | 1/4 cup |
| Saltine crackers | 6 squares |
| Milk | 1 cup |
| Thin soup (examples: vegetable, chicken noodle) | 1 cup |
| Thick soup (examples: cream of mushroom, tomato) | 1/2 cup |
| Ice cream (vanilla) | 1/2 cup |
| Pudding (sugar-free) | 1/2 cup |
| Pudding (regular) | 1/4 cup |
| Macaroni, noodles, rice, mashed potatoes | 1/2 cup (cooked) |

*Use of trade names is for identification only and does not imply endorsement by the U.S. Department of Health and Human Services.

**Figure 17.3.**

*Drink Liquids*

Drink extra liquids. Try to drink at least 1/2 cup (4 ounces) to 3 /4 cup (6 ounces) every half-hour to hour, even if you have to do this in small sips. These liquids should not have calories. Water, diet soda pop, or tea without sugar are good choices.

*Check for Changes*

- Test your blood glucose at least every 4 hours. If your glucose is 240 mg/dL or higher, test your urine for ketones. Ketones are chemicals the liver makes when there's not enough insulin in the blood. It's easy to test for ketones. Buy urine ketone strips at the drug store. Urinate on the pad part of the strip. Compare the color that the strip becomes to the color example on the package. If the pad turns a purple color, call your health care provider right away.
- Weigh yourself every day. Losing weight without trying is a sign of high blood glucose.
- Check your temperature every morning and evening. A fever may be a sign of infection.
- Every 4 to 6 hours, check how you're breathing and decide how alert you feel. Having trouble breathing, feeling more sleepy than usual, or not thinking clearly can be danger signs.

*Keep Records*

Use Figure 17.4. "Records for Sick Days," Ask a family member or friend to help if you need it.

*Call for Help*

Ask your health care provider when you should call. During your sick times, you may need to call every day for advice.

You should call your health care provider or go to an emergency room if any of the following happens:

- You feel too sick to eat normally and for more than 6 hours can't keep food or liquids down.
- You have severe diarrhea.
- You lose 5 pounds or more without trying to.
- Your temperature is over 101° F.
- Your blood glucose level is lower than 60 mg/dL or stays over 300 mg/dL.
- You have moderate or large amounts of ketones in your urine.
- You're having trouble breathing.
- You feel sleepy or can't think clearly.

## Records for Sick Days

| How often | Question | Answer | |
|---|---|---|---|
| Every day | How much do you weigh today? | ____pounds | |
| Every evening | How much liquid did you drink today? | ____glasses | |
| Every morning and every evening | What is your temperature? | ____ a.m.<br>____ p.m. | |
| Every 4 hours or before every meal | How much diabetes medicine did you take? | Time | Dose |
| | | ____ | ____ |
| | | ____ | ____ |
| | | ____ | ____ |
| | | ____ | ____ |
| | | ____ | ____ |
| | | ____ | ____ |
| Every 4 hours or each time you pass urine | What is your blood glucose level? | Time | Blood glucose |
| | | ____ | ____ |
| | | ____ | ____ |
| | | ____ | ____ |
| | | ____ | ____ |
| | | ____ | ____ |
| | | ____ | ____ |
| Every 4 hours or each time you pass urine | What are your urine ketones? | Time | Ketones |
| | | ____ | ____ |
| | | ____ | ____ |
| | | ____ | ____ |
| | | ____ | ____ |
| | | ____ | ____ |
| | | ____ | ____ |
| Every 4 to 6 hours | How are you breathing? | Time | Condition |
| | | ____ | ____ |
| | | ____ | ____ |
| | | ____ | ____ |
| | | ____ | ____ |
| | | ____ | ____ |
| | | ____ | ____ |

*Figure 17.4.*

## *Managing Your Diabetes at Work, School, and in Travel*

Staying in charge of your diabetes no matter what your day holds—work, school, travel, or special events—takes planning ahead. Many days will go smoothly, but some days will hold surprises, such as extra activity or delays that throw your schedule off.

Plan ahead for these times by always keeping a treatment for low blood glucose with you (see Figure 17.2. for some choices). If you have any signs that your glucose may be low, go ahead and treat it right away.

Stay as close to your eating, activity, and medicine schedule as you can. Keep track of your glucose so you can pick up changes early. Always wear identification that says you have diabetes.

Talk with your health care team about your planned schedule and activities. Ask for help in planning ahead for work, school, travel, and special events. When you read the rest of this section, you may think of more questions to ask.

### *At Work and School*

Talk with your health care team about the type of activity you do at work or at school. From time to time, you and your health care team may need to make changes in your activity, medicine, or eating.

Many people take supplies for testing their glucose to work and to school so they can test at regular break times. Some people choose to show their fellow workers, their teachers, or their classmates how to help if they should ever have a problem. They teach them how to tell when their glucose is low and how to treat it. Some people like to have written steps on file at their place of work or with their teacher.

### *In Travel*

When you plan a trip, think about your day-to-day schedule and try to stay as close to it as you can. For example, if you usually test your blood glucose at noon and then eat lunch, plan to do this on your trip, as well. Trips can hold surprises—delays and changes. Even the types of food and supplies you can buy on your trip may not be the same as those you get at home.

Before you travel, work with your health care provider to plan your timing for medicine, food, and activity. Talk about what to do if you find changes in your glucose readings.

Plan ahead for trips:

- Keep snacks with you that could be used to prevent—or treat—low blood glucose.
- Carry extra food and drink supplies with you, such as cracker packs and small cans of juices or bottled water.
- Carry plenty of glucose testing supplies with you.
- Take along all the diabetes medicine you'll need.

When you travel, be sure to:

- Test your glucose often and keep track of it.
- Wear identification that says you have diabetes.
- Let others know how they can help you.

If you're traveling in a different time zone, you may need to change your timing of food, medicine, and activity. Ask your health care provider to help you with this. Talk about the food and drink choices that would be healthy for you. If you'll be in another country, ask your doctor to write a letter explaining that you have diabetes. It's also a good idea to get your doctor to write a prescription for you to get insulin or supplies if needed.

## Feelings about Having Diabetes

Living with diabetes isn't easy. It's normal to feel troubled about it. Tell your health care team how you feel. Point out any problems you have with your diabetes care plan. Your diabetes educator or other health care provider may be able to help you think of ways to deal with these problems.

Talk about the stresses you feel at home, school, and work. How do you cope with these pressures? If your feelings are getting in the way of taking care of yourself, you need to ask for help.

### *Support Groups*

It helps to talk with other people who have problems like your own. You may want to think about joining a diabetes **support group**. In support groups, people who have just found out they have diabetes can learn from people who have lived with it for a long time. People can talk about and share how they deal with their diabetes. They can also talk about how they take care of their health, how they prepare food, and how they get physical activity. Family members who do not have diabetes may want to join a support group, too. Ask your health care team about support groups for people with diabetes and their families and friends. If there is not a support group in your area, you may want to call a diabetes organization about starting a group.

### *Counseling*

One-on-one and family counseling sessions may also help. Be sure to see a counselor who knows about diabetes and its care. Ask your health care provider to help you find a counselor.

## *Eye Problems*

**Diabetic eye disease** (also called diabetic **retinopathy**) is a serious problem that can lead to loss of sight. There's a lot you can do to take charge and prevent such problems. A recent study shows that keeping your **blood glucose** closer to normal can prevent or delay the onset of diabetic eye disease. Keeping your blood pressure under control is also important. Finding and treating eye problems early can help save sight.

### *Signs of Diabetic Eye Disease*

Since diabetic eye disease may be developing even when your sight is good, regular eye exams are important for finding problems early. Some people may notice signs of vision changes. If you're having trouble reading, if your vision is blurred, or if you are seeing rings around lights, dark spots, or flashing lights, you may have eye problems. Be sure to tell your health care team or eye doctor about any eye problems you may have.

### *Protecting Your Sight*

*Keep Your Blood Glucose Under Control*

**High blood glucose** can damage your eyes as time goes by. Work with your health care team to keep your glucose levels as close to normal as you can.

*Keep Your Blood Pressure Under Control*

**High blood pressure** can damage your eyes. Have your health care provider check your **blood pressure** at least four times a year. If your blood pressure is higher than 140/90, you may want to buy a blood pressure cuff and check your blood pressure at home. Ask your health care provider where you can buy a cuff.

*Get Regular Eye Exams*

Even if you're seeing fine, you need regular, complete eye exams to protect your sight. Ask your health care provider to help you find an eye doctor who cares for people with diabetes. Before the exam, a doctor or nurse will put drops in your eyes to dilate the pupils.

You should have your eyes dilated and examined once a year. Keep track of these exams. Even if you've lost your sight from diabetic eye disease, you still need to have regular eye care. If you haven't already had a complete eye exam, you should have one now if any of these conditions apply to you:

- You've had **Type 1 diabetes** for 5 or more years.
- You have **Type 2 diabetes**.
- You're going through puberty and you have diabetes.
- You're pregnant and you have diabetes.
- You're planning to become pregnant and you have diabetes.

If you can't afford an eye exam, ask about a payment plan or a free exam. If you're 65 or older, Medicare may pay for diabetic eye exams (but not glasses). Ask your eye doctor to accept the Medicare fee as full payment.

*Discuss Your Physical Activity Plan*

If you have diabetic eye disease, talk with your health care provider about the kind of physical activity that is best for you.

### *Treating Diabetic Eye Disease*

Treating eye problems early can help save sight. **Laser surgery** may help people who have advanced diabetic eye disease. An operation called **vitrectomy** may help those who have lost their sight from bleeding in the back of the eye.

If your sight is poor, an eye doctor who is an expert in low vision may be able to give you glasses or other devices that can help you use your limited vision more fully. You may want to ask your health care provider about support groups and job training for people with low vision.

## Kidney Problems

Diabetes can cause **diabetic kidney disease** (also called diabetic **nephropathy**), which can lead to kidney failure. There's a lot you can do to take charge and prevent kidney problems. A recent study shows that controlling your **blood glucose** can prevent or delay the onset of kidney disease. Keeping your blood pressure under control is also important.

The **kidneys** keep the right amount of water in the body and help filter out harmful wastes. These wastes then pass from the body in the urine. Diabetes can cause kidney disease by damaging the parts of the kidneys that filter out wastes. When the kidneys fail, a person has to have his or her blood filtered through a machine (a treatment called dialysis) several times a week or has to get a kidney transplant.

## Testing Your Kidneys

Your health care provider can learn how well your kidneys are working by testing for **albumin** (a protein) in the urine. Albumin in the urine is an early sign of diabetic kidney disease. You should have your urine checked for albumin every year.

Your health care provider can also do a yearly blood test to measure your kidney function. If the tests show albumin in the urine or if your kidney function isn't normal, you'll need to be checked more often.

Write down the dates and the results of these tests. Ask your health care provider to explain what the results mean.

## Protecting Your Kidneys

### *Keep Your Blood Glucose Under Control*

**High blood glucose** can damage your kidneys as time goes by. Work with your health care team to keep your glucose levels as close to normal as you can.

### *Keep Your Blood Pressure Under Control*

**High blood pressure** can damage your kidneys. You may want to check your **blood pressure** at home to be sure it stays lower than 140/90. Have your health care provider check your blood pressure at least four times a year. Your doctor may have you take a blood pressure pill, called an ACE inhibitor, to help protect your kidneys.

### *Choose Healthy Foods*

You may want to talk to your health care team about cutting back on foods that are high in proteins (such as meat, milk, and cheese). A diet high in proteins can cause more damage to your kidneys over time. Eating less salt is also a good idea.

### *Preventing and Treating Infections*

**Bladder** and kidney infections can damage your kidneys. Call your health care provider right away if you have any of these signs of bladder infection:

- Cloudy or bloody urine.
- Pain or burning when you urinate.
- An urgent need to urinate often.

Call your health care provider right away if you have any of these signs of kidney infections:

- Back pain.
- Chills.
- Fever.
- **Ketones** in the urine.

Your health care provider will test your urine. If you have a bladder or kidney infection, you'll be given medicine to stop the infection. After you take all the medicine, have your urine checked again to be sure the infection is gone.

#### *Know the Effects of Some Medicines and X-Ray Dyes*

If you have kidney disease, ask your health care provider about the possible effects that some medicines and X-ray dyes can have on your kidneys.

## Heart and Blood Vessel Problems

Heart and blood vessel problems are the main causes of sickness and death among people with diabetes. These problems can lead to **high blood pressure**, **heart attacks**, and **strokes**. Heart and blood vessel problems can also cause poor blood flow (circulation) in the legs and feet.

You're more likely to have heart and blood vessel problems if you smoke cigarettes, have high blood pressure, or have too much **cholesterol** or other fats in your blood. Talk with your health care team about what you can do to lower your risk for heart and blood vessel problems.

## Signs of Heart and Blood Vessel Problems

If you feel dizzy, have sudden loss of sight, slur your speech, or feel numb or weak in one arm or leg, you may be having serious heart and blood vessel problems. Your blood may not be getting to your brain as well as it should.

Danger signs of circulation problems to the heart include chest pain or pressure, shortness of breath, swollen ankles, or irregular heartbeats. If you have any of these signs, go to an emergency room or call your health care provider right away.

Signs of circulation problems to your legs are pain or cramping in your buttocks, thighs, or calves during physical activity. Even if this pain goes away with rest, report it to your health care provider.

## Preventing and Controlling Heart and Blood Vessel Problems

### *Eat Right and Get Physical Activity*

Choose a healthy diet, low in salt. Work with a dietitian to plan healthy meals. If you're overweight, talk about how to safely lose weight. Ask about a physical activity or exercise program for you.

### *Don't Use Tobacco*

Smoking cigarettes causes hundreds of thousands of deaths each year. When you have diabetes and also use tobacco, the risk of heart and blood vessel problems is even greater. One of the best choices you can make for your health is to never start smoking—or if you smoke, to quit.

At least once a year, your health care provider will ask you about tobacco use. If you smoke, ask your provider about things you can do to help you stop, such as joining a stop-smoking program.

### *Check Your Blood Pressure*

Get your **blood pressure** checked at each visit. Record these numbers. If your blood pressure is higher than 140/90, you may want to buy a blood pressure cuff and check your blood pressure at home. Ask your health care provider where you can buy a cuff.

If your blood pressure is still high after 3 months, you may need medicine to help control it. Many medicines are available to treat high blood pressure. If you have side effects from the medicine, ask your health care provider to change it.

*Check Your Cholesterol*

Get your cholesterol checked once a year. Record the results. Your total cholesterol should be lower than 200 mg/dL. Ask your health care team to explain what your **HDL** and **LDL** levels are.

If your cholesterol is higher than 200 mg/dL on two or more checks, you can do several things to lower it. You can work with your health care team to improve your **blood glucose** control, you can lose weight (if you're overweight), and you can cut down on foods that are high in fat and cholesterol. Ask your health care team about foods that are low in fats. Also ask about a physical activity program.

If your cholesterol is still high after 6 months, you may need a medicine to help control it. Your health care provider will advise you about what medicine to take.

*Ask if You Need an Electrocardiogram (EKG)*

If you're having heart and blood circulation problems, an EKG may help you and your health care provider know if you need to change your treatment.

## Nerve Damage

**Diabetic nerve damage** (also called diabetic **neuropathy**) is a problem for many people with diabetes. Over time, **high blood glucose** levels damage the delicate coating of nerves. This damage can cause a number of problems, such as pain in your feet. There's a lot you can do to take charge and prevent nerve damage. A recent study shows that controlling your **blood glucose** can help prevent or delay these problems. Controlling your blood glucose may also help reduce the pain from some types of nerve damage.

### *Some Signs of Diabetic Nerve Damage*

Some signs of diabetic nerve damage are pain, burning, tingling, or loss of feeling in the feet and hands. It can cause you to sweat abnormally, make it hard for you to tell when your blood glucose is low, and make you feel light-headed when you stand up.

Nerve damage can lead to other problems. Some people develop problems swallowing and keeping food down. Nerve damage can also cause bowel problems, make it hard to urinate, cause dribbling with urination, and lead to bladder and kidney infections. Many people with nerve damage have trouble having sex. For example, men can have trouble keeping their penis erect, a problem called **impotence**. If you have any of these problems, tell your health care provider. There are ways to help in many cases.

### *Protecting Your Nerves from Damage*

*Keep Your Blood Glucose in Control*

High blood glucose can damage your nerves as time goes by. Work with your health care team to keep your glucose levels as close to normal as you can.

*Have a Physical Activity Plan*

Physical activity or exercise may help keep some nerves healthy, such as those in your feet. Ask your health care team about an activity that is healthy for you.

*Get Tests for Nerve Damage*

Nerve damage can happen slowly. You may not even be aware you're losing feeling in your feet. Ask you health care provider to check your feet at each visit. At least once a year, your provider should test how well you can sense temperature, pinprick, vibration, and position in your feet. If you have signs of nerve damage, your provider may want to do more tests. Testing can help your provider know what is wrong and how to treat it. Keep track of your foot exams

*Check Your Feet for Changes*

If you've lost feeling in your feet, you'll need to take special care of them. Check your feet each day. Wear shoes that fit well. You'll read more about foot care in the next section.

## Foot Problems

Nerve damage, circulation problems, and infections can cause serious foot problems for people with diabetes. There's a lot you can do to prevent problems with your feet. Controlling your **blood glucose** and not smoking or using tobacco can help protect your feet. You can also take some simple safeguards each day to care for and protect your feet. Measures like these have prevented many amputations.

It's helpful to understand why foot problems happen. Nerve damage can cause you to lose feeling in your feet. Sometimes nerve damage can deform or misshape your feet, causing pressure points that can turn into blisters, sores, or **ulcers**. Poor circulation can make these injuries slow to heal.

### *Signs of Foot Problems*

Your feet may tingle, burn, or hurt. You may not be able to feel touch, heat, or cold very well. The shape of your feet can change over time. There may even be changes in the color and temperature of your feet. Some people lose hair on their toes, feet, and lower legs. The skin on your feet may be dry and cracked. Toenails may turn thick and yellow. Fungus infections can grow between your toes.

Blisters, sores, ulcers, infected **corns**, and ingrown toenails need to be seen by your health care provider or foot doctor (podiatrist) right away.

### *Protecting Your Feet*

#### *Get Your Health Care Provider to Check Your Feet at Least Four Times a Year*

Ask your health care provider to look at your feet at least four times a year. As a reminder, take off your shoes and socks when you're in the exam room. Have your sense of feeling and your pulses checked at least once a year. If you have nerve damage, deformed or misshaped feet, or a circulation problem, your feet need special care. Ask your health care provider to show you how to care for your feet. Also ask if special shoes would help you.

#### *Check Your Feet Each Day*

You may have serious foot problems yet feel no pain. Look at your feet every day to see if you have scratches, cracks, cuts, or blisters. Always check between your toes and on the bottoms of your feet. If you can't bend over to see the bottoms of your feet, use a mirror that won't break. If you can't see well, ask a family member or friend to help you. Call your health care provider at once if you have a sore on your foot. Sores can get worse quickly.

#### *Wash Your Feet Daily*

Wash your feet every day. Dry them with care, especially between the toes. Don't soak your feet—it can dry out your skin, and dry skin can lead to infections. If you have dry skin, rub a thin coat of oil, lotion, or cream on the tops and bottoms of your feet—but not between your toes. Moisture between the toes will let germs grow that could cause an infection. Ask your health care provider for the name of a good lotion or cream.

*Trim Your Toenails Carefully*

Trim your toenails after you've washed and dried your feet—the nails will be softer and safer to cut. Trim the nails to follow the natural curve of your toes. Don't cut into the corners. Use an emery board to smooth off the edges.

If you can't see well, or if your nails are thick or yellowed, get them trimmed by a foot doctor or another health care provider. Ask your health care provider for the name of a foot doctor. If you see redness around the nails, see your health care provider at once.

*Treat Corns and Calluses Gently*

Don't cut corns and **calluses**. Ask your health care provider how to gently use a pumice stone to rub them. Don't use razor blades, corn plasters, or liquid corn or callus removers—they can damage your skin.

*Protect Your Feet from Heat and Cold*

Hot water or hot surfaces are a danger to your feet. Before bathing, test the water with a bath thermometer (90 to 95° F is safe) or with your elbow. Wear shoes and socks when you walk on hot surfaces, such as beaches or the pavement around swimming pools. In summer, be sure to use a sunscreen on the tops of your feet.

You also need to protect your feet from the cold. In winter, wear socks and footwear such as fleece-lined boots to protect your feet. If your feet are cold at night, wear socks. Don't use hot water bottles, heating pads, or electric blankets—they can burn, your feet. Don't use strong antiseptic solutions or adhesive tape on your feet.

*Wear Shoes and Socks Always*

Wear shoes and socks at all times. Don't walk barefoot—not even indoors.

Wear shoes that fit well and protect your feet. Don't wear shoes that have plastic uppers and don't wear sandals with thongs between the toes. Ask your health care provider what types of shoes are good choices for you.

New shoes should be comfortable at the time you buy them—don't expect them to stretch out. Slowly break in new shoes by wearing them only one or two hours a day.

Always wear socks or stockings with your shoes. Choose socks made of cotton or wool—they help keep your feet dry.

Before you put on your shoes each time, look and feel inside them. Check for any loose objects, nail points, torn linings, and rough areas—these can cause injuries. If your shoe isn't smooth inside, wear other shoes.

*Be Physically Active*

Physical activity can help increase the circulation in your feet. There are many ways you can exercise your feet, even during times you're not able to walk. Ask your health care team about things you can do to exercise your feet and legs.

## Dental Disease

Because of **high blood glucose**, people with diabetes are more likely to have problems with their teeth and gums. There's a lot you can do to take charge and prevent these problems. Caring for your teeth and gums every day can help keep them healthy. Keeping your **blood glucose** under control is also important. Regular, complete dental care helps prevent dental disease.

### Signs of Dental Disease

Sore, swollen, and red gums that bleed when you brush your teeth are a sign of a dental problem called **gingivitis**. Another problem, called **periodontitis**, happens when your gums shrink or pull away from your teeth. Like all infections, dental infections can make your blood glucose go up.

### Preventing Dental Problems

*Keep Your Blood Glucose in Control*

High blood glucose can cause problems with your teeth and gums. Work with your health care team to keep your glucose levels as close to normal as you can.

*Brush Your Teeth Often*

Brush your teeth at least twice a day to prevent gum disease and tooth loss. Be sure to brush before you go to sleep. Use a soft toothbrush and toothpaste with fluoride. To help keep bacteria from growing on your toothbrush, rinse it after each brushing and store it upright with the bristles at the top. Get a new toothbrush at least every 3 months.

*Floss Your Teeth Daily*

Besides brushing, you need to floss between your teeth each day to help remove **plaque**, a film that forms on teeth and can cause tooth problems. Flossing also helps keep your gums healthy. Your dentist or dental hygienist will help you choose a good method to remove plaque, such as dental floss, bridge cleaners, or water spray. If you're not sure of the right way to brush or floss, ask your dentist or dental hygienist for help.

*Get Regular Dental Care*

Get your teeth cleaned and checked at your dentist's office at least every 6 months. If you don't have a dentist, find one or ask your health care provider for the name of a dentist in your community.

See your dentist right away if you have any signs of dental disease, including bad breath, a bad taste in your mouth, bleeding or sore gums, red or swollen gums, sore or loose teeth, or trouble chewing.

Give your dentist the name and telephone number of your diabetes health care provider. Each time you make a visit, remind your dentist that you have diabetes.

Plan dental visits so they don't change the times you take your **insulin** and meals. Don't skip a meal or diabetes medicine before your visit. Right after breakfast may be a good time for your visit.

## Vaccinations

If you have diabetes, take extra care to keep up-to-date on your **vaccinations** (also called **immunizations**). Vaccines can prevent illnesses that can be very serious for people with diabetes. This section talks about some vaccines you need to know about.

***Influenza Vaccine***

**Influenza** (often called the **flu**) is not just a bad cold. It's a serious illness that can lead to pneumonia and even death. The flu spreads when influenza viruses pass from one person to the nose or throat of others. Signs of the flu may include sudden high fever, chills, body aches, sore throat, runny nose, dry cough, and headache.

People with diabetes who come down with the flu may become very sick and may even have to go to a hospital. If you get the flu, you'll need to take special care of yourself (see section "Taking Care of Yourself When You're Sick.")

You can help keep yourself from getting the flu by getting a flu shot every year. Everyone with diabetes—even pregnant women—should get a yearly flu shot. The best time to get one is between October and mid-November, before the flu season begins. This vaccine is fully covered under Medicare Part B.

### Pneumococcal Vaccine

Pneumococcal disease is a major source of illness and death. It can cause serious infections of the lungs (pneumonia), the blood (bacteremia) and the covering of the brain (meningitis). Pneumococcal polysaccharide vaccine (often called PPV) can help prevent this disease.

PPV can be given at the same time as flu vaccine—or at any time of the year. Most people only have to take PPV once in their life. Ask your health care provider whether you are in the small group of people—such as people on dialysis—who might need a second vaccination. This vaccine is fully covered under Medicare Part B.

### Tetanus/Diphtheria (Td) Toxoid

Tetanus (or lockjaw) and diphtheria are serious diseases. Tetanus is caused by a germ that enters the body through a cut or wound. Diphtheria spreads when germs pass from one person to the nose or throat of others.

You can help prevent tetanus and diphtheria with a combined shot called Td toxoid. Most people get Td toxoid as part of their routine childhood vaccinations, but all adults need a Td booster shot every 10 years. Other vaccines may be given at the same time as Td toxoid.

### Other Vaccines

You may need vaccines to protect you against other illnesses. Ask your health care provider if you need any of these:

- Measles/Mumps/Rubella vaccine
- Hepatitis A and B vaccines

- Varicella (chickenpox) vaccine
- Polio vaccine
- Vaccines for travel to other countries

### *How to Get More Information*

Call the immunization program in your state health department to find out where you can get vaccinations in your area. Keep your vaccination records up-to-date so you and your health care provider will know what vaccines you may need.

For more information on vaccination, call the National Immunization Information Hotline at 1-800-232-2533 (English) or 1-800-232-0233 (Spanish). These are toll-free calls.

## *Pregnancy, Diabetes, and Women's Health*

### *Becoming Pregnant When You Have Diabetes*

Women with diabetes can have healthy babies, but it takes planning ahead and effort. Pregnancy can make both **high** and **low blood glucose** levels happen more often. It can make **diabetic eye disease** and **diabetic kidney disease** worse. High glucose levels during pregnancy are dangerous for the baby, too.

If you don't want to become pregnant, talk with your health care provider about birth control.

### *Protecting Your Baby and Yourself*

Keeping your glucose levels near normal before and during pregnancy can help protect you and your baby. That's why it's so important to plan your pregnancies ahead of time.

If you want to have a baby, discuss it with your health care provider. Work with your diabetes care team to get and keep your blood glucose in the normal or near-normal range before you become pregnant. Your glucose records and your **hemoglobin A1c** test results will show when you have maintained a safe range for a period of time.

You may need to change your **meal plan** and your usual physical activity, and you may need to take more frequent **insulin** shots. Testing your glucose several times a day will help you see how well you're balancing things. Record the test results in your logbook or on a log sheet.

Get a complete check of your eyes and kidneys before you try to become pregnant. Don't smoke, drink alcohol, or use drugs—doing these things can harm you and your baby.

### *Having Diabetes During Pregnancy*

Some women have diabetes only when they're pregnant. This condition, which is called **gestational diabetes**, can be controlled just like other kinds of diabetes. Glucose control is the key. Your health care team can help you take charge of gestational diabetes.

### *Controlling Diabetes for Women's Health*

Some women with diabetes may have specials problems, such as **bladder** infections. If you have an infection, it needs to be treated right away. Call your doctor.

Some women get **yeast infections** in their vagina, especially when their blood glucose is high. A sign of a yeast infection may be itching in the vagina. If you notice vaginal itching, tell your health care provider. You may learn about medicines you can buy at the drugstore and about how to prevent yeast infections.

Some women with diabetes may have trouble with sexual function. Discomfort caused by vaginal itching or dryness can be treated.

Ask your doctor how often you should get a Pap smear and a mammogram (breast X-ray). Regular Pap smears and mammograms help detect cervical and breast cancer early. All women—whether or not they have diabetes—need to keep up with these tests.

## Some Words of Thanks

This guide was written by the Centers for Disease Control and Prevention's Division of Diabetes Translation, which is part of the National Center for Chronic Disease Prevention and Health Promotion. We work with partners who share with us a mission to reduce the burden of diabetes in communities.

William H. Herman, M.D., M.P.H., was the general editor of the first book, *Take Charge of Your Diabetes: A Guide for Care*, printed in 1991. We asked people with diabetes who read the first book to help us make this second book even more helpful.

The American Association of Diabetes Educators did a survey among people with diabetes and diabetes educators to learn what people liked and didn't like about the first book. Special thanks for helping conduct this survey go to Betty Brackenridge, Linda Haas, Julie Meyer, Jean Betschart, Kris Ernst, and Robert Anderson. Focus groups made up of persons with diabetes were held by Health Promotion Council of SE Pennsylvania and Casals and Associates of

Washington, D.C. The groups gave us valuable input to help make this book more useful.

Important support for this book's emphasis on glucose control came from the Diabetes Control and Complications Trial. Conducted by the National Institute of Diabetes and Digestive and Kidney Diseases, this important study provided scientific proof that glucose control can help prevent or delay complications of diabetes.

Dawn Satterfield and Patricia Mitchell of the division's Health Communications Section were the lead writers. Claudia Martinez and Hope Woodward also helped with the writing. Rick Hull reviewed and edited the final version of this guide. Most of the drawings were provided by the Public Health Practice Program Office, Centers for Disease Control and Prevention. Chris Rigaux and Ward Nyholm of Cygnus Corporation assisted with design and layout.

## Chapter 18

# Questions to Ask Your Doctor about Blood Sugar Control

The Diabetes Control and Complications Trial (DCCT) showed that people with insulin-dependent diabetes who keep blood sugar levels as close to normal as possible can reduce their risk of eye, kidney and nerve diseases.

Ask your doctor how you can improve blood sugar control. Questions you may want to ask include:

- What is my glycosylated hemoglobin (a test that measures average blood sugar level over the past 2 to 3 months)? What is a normal glycosylated hemoglobin?
- How can I get my glycosylated hemoglobin in the normal range?
- How often and under what conditions should I test my blood sugar? What should I do with the results? What patterns should I try to achieve?
- What changes should we make in my program as a result of the findings of the Diabetes Control and Complications Trial (DCCT)?
- Do I have microalbuminuria (detection of tiny amounts of albumin in urine indicating early diabetic kidney disease)?
- What effect has diabetes had on my eyes and kidneys?
- When should I get together with a dietitian to review what I eat?

---

National Diabetes Information Clearinghouse, February 1998.

- What exercises are best for me? What adjustments to my food or insulin should I make if I plan to exercise?
- What should my family and friends do if my blood sugar goes so low that I need their help?
- (For women) What should I do about taking care of my diabetes if I plan to become pregnant?
- How should I take care of my feet?
- Are there any diabetes groups that I could attend in our area?

## For More Information

For an information kit write:

National Diabetes Outreach Program
One Diabetes Way
Bethesda, Maryland 20892-3600
or
Call 1-800-GET LEVEL
1-800-438-5383

***National Diabetes Information Clearinghouse***
1 Information Way
Bethesda, MD 20892-3560
E-mail: ndic@info.niddk.nih.gov

The National Diabetes Information Clearinghouse (NDIC) is a service of the National Institute of Diabetes and Digestive and Kidney Diseases (NIDDK). The NIDDK is part of the National Institutes of Health under the U.S. Public Health Service. Established in 1978, the clearinghouse provides information about diabetes to people with diabetes and their families, health care professionals, and the public. NDIC answers inquiries; develops, reviews, and distributes publications; and works closely with professional and patient organizations and government agencies to coordinate resources about diabetes.

Publications produced by the clearinghouse are reviewed carefully for scientific accuracy, content, and readability.

# Chapter 19

# *Diabetes on a Shoe-String Budget*

Sarah, an elderly caller, sounded distraught. Through her tears she described the bitter facts of her diabetes to an operator at the National Center of the American Diabetes Association:

Both Sarah and her husband have insulin-dependent diabetes. They are in financial straits, but not poor enough to qualify for government assistance. They are old, but not old enough to qualify for Medicare. They have no medical insurance.

To make ends meet, Sarah has been cutting back on her insulin for some time. That way her husband can get the larger doses he needs. Now, she is beginning to have diabetes complications. Could the operator please help her?

Sad to say, Sarah's story is not unusual. The American Diabetes Association National Center receives half a dozen "help" calls like hers every day. State affiliates and local chapter offices get even more. For example, the Los Angeles chapter of the ADA California Affiliate reports receiving from 8 to 10 such calls every day.

Some organizations have documented the sheer number of people with diabetes in programs for the indigent. Consider the network of federally funded Healthcare for the Homeless clinics that serve indigent people across the nation. In 1992, these clinics offered health care to 11,750 people with diabetes, out of a total of 83,133 patients—just over 14 percent of the clientele.

---

Dawson, Leslie. "Diabetes on a Shoe-String Budget," *Diabetes Forecast* Vol. 47, No. 11 November 1994 © American Diabetes Association; reprinted with permission.

The good news is that a surprising number of government, nonprofit, and voluntary clinics and organizations are helping needy people with diabetes. The clinics, in turn, are subsidized by large pharmaceutical companies that make significant donations of insulin and oral medications.

Indigent and homeless people *can* find primary diabetes health care, although it does take extra effort, time, and extraordinary patience. A good number of nonprofit organizations will help pay for major expenses such as eye surgery, and Medicare covers major kidney disease for people of all ages.

Even very poor people can manage their diabetes successfully. Many can keep their blood sugars at low to moderate levels, despite the stresses of poverty.

Joan Werblun, RN, CDE, works at the medical center of the University of California at Davis as a patient educator for medically indigent and homeless people in Sacramento. She says that some of her patients who are homeless tell her, "It just takes a little common sense." According to Werblun, these patients enjoy reasonably good health.

Beatrice Nordberg, RN, CDE, MA, is the diabetes nurse specialist at the University of Maryland in Baltimore. Most of her patients are indigent, unemployed, or employed on a part-time basis. Most rely upon her clinic for donated supplies of insulin, oral medications, and syringes. Even without their own blood testing supplies, Nordberg's patients maintain glucose levels of 200 milligrams per deciliter (mg/dl). "Far from perfect" she admitted. But she was quick to add, "Their goal is not diabetes management. Their goal is survival." Under those circumstances, she credits them with doing pretty well.

Diabetes is an expensive disease. Insulin, oral medications, and equipment necessary for proper care do not come cheaply. Test strips cost more than 60 cents apiece, and many people use two or three strips daily. When the expense of hospital and outpatient care for the complications associated with the disease are added in, the costs soar to stratospheric levels.

The burden of diabetes on the nation shows up in the burden it places on charitable organizations. "Our diabetics eat up our pharmacy budget," said Randi Abramson, MD, medical coordinator of the Zaccheus Free Clinic in Washington, D.C. She said that her clinic, which primarily serves the working poor, receives most of the District of Columbia's medically indigent diabetic patients. Other clinics reject them; apparently because of the expense.

## Resources for Survival

Elderly people on fixed incomes, unemployed workers, and those with disabilities often rely on government programs such as Medicare, Medicaid, or Medicare and Medicaid combined, to pay their medical expenses. Approximately a quarter of all Americans are covered by these sources, and they are the lucky ones. At least a safety net of government-defined medical services is available to them. In certain cases, those in Medicare programs have better health coverage than people in some inexpensive employer-paid insurance programs, according to Carol Ko, RD, CDE, manager of Nutritional Health Education for CIGNA Health Care of California. She treats people in both groups in a health maintenance organization (HMO).

Many poor people, however, do not qualify for Medicare or Medicaid. In California, for instance, if you earn more than $210 per month, you can't get Medicaid, according to Ko. If you're one of the working poor, you fall between a rock and a hard place as far as medical care is concerned.

The ranks of the uninsured in America swelled by 2 million in 1992, leaving more than 37.4 million with no health coverage. In the same year, the number of people with health insurance fell 4.2 percent from 1989 levels. A large number of uninsured people manage to pay the rent and put food on the table for their families. As far as health care is concerned, however, they fall in the category of "medically indigent."

For the medically indigent, a variety of medical resources exist. However, they are generally underfunded and stretched to their capacity. For example, many clinics reject patients with diabetes because of the expense involved. Nonetheless, many free clinics and pharmacies, as well as public and university hospitals, make treating people with diabetes a high priority.

Another problem: people with diabetes are often rejected by health insurance programs as a result of their pre-existing condition. This situation won't be remedied for all Americans until comprehensive health-care reform takes place and issues such as portability and universal coverage are addressed.

## Government Assistance

Medicare, Medicaid, and the Veterans Administration offer basic health care. Many wish these programs offered more, but for people in need, the problem is a matter of eligibility, not scope of coverage.

Medicare is a federal medical insurance program designed to assist people over 65 years old. It also serves those who are or have become disabled, as defined by Medicare criteria. In addition, Medicare provides coverage—with limitations—to those with permanent kidney failure. Before the age of 65, you can receive Medicare if you need maintenance dialysis or a kidney transplant. In most cases, your coverage will begin 3 months after you actually begin dialysis treatment. Medicare also has recently added therapeutic footwear as a benefit for recipients with diabetes.

Medicare is divided into two sections, Part A and Part B. Part A covers medically necessary inpatient hospital care, and is subject to deductibles and co-payments. Part B covers doctors services and outpatient hospital and health services, and must be purchased through insurance premiums.

For information on qualifying requirements and coverage, check with your local Social Security office, or call the Medicare Hotline at 1-800-638-6833. The Medicare Hotline will also provide information on Medicare's QMB (Qualified Medical Benefits) and SLMB (Specified Low-income Medicare Beneficiaries) programs which are designed to help people with limited incomes.

Medicare does not currently cover blood glucose testing supplies for people with type II diabetes who are not insulin requiring, but it does cover home blood glucose monitors for people who use insulin *if* a physician has prescribed blood glucose monitoring and has filed the proper forms with Medicare.

Medicaid helps those with medical needs who are under 65 years of age, and it may supplement Medicare costs. While each state is required to cover certain basic services, overall coverage varies from state to state. Check with the public assistance program in your state. You can also receive Medicaid if you receive Aid to Families with Dependent Children (AFDC) or a state supplement such as Old Age Assistance, Aid to the Blind, Aid to the Permanently and Totally Disabled, or Supplemental Security Income. In some cases, you can qualify if you are a nursing-home resident. Apply for assistance at your local or state health and public assistance office.

The Veterans Administration (VA) operates the largest health care system in the United States. The VA primarily serves veterans in two categories: those who have service-related health problems and those who are indigent. Other veterans may or may not qualify, for hospital, outpatient, or nursing home treatment. If they do qualify, they must also pay Medicare-based deductibles and co-payments.

VA spokesperson Linda Stalvey warned that the eligibility rules for VA services are extremely complex. As far as diabetes is concerned, veterans without service-related status are more likely to qualify for care when acute problems require hospitalization. Chances are slim that such a veteran would qualify for outpatient care, even in a VA diabetes clinic, according to Stalvey.

If you are a veteran and have questions about VA health care eligibility, call 1-800-827-1000. The operator will connect you with a regional VA information center.

## Nonprofit Organizations Offering Assistance

In many communities, private, nonprofit groups offer financial support for individual and family medical needs of the poor. If you have a medical need that a governmental agency is unable to fill, check out these possibilities.

The American Academy of Ophthalmology (AAO) has been sponsoring a National Eye Care project for the past 8 years. It's designed to serve people 65 or over (U.S. citizens or legal residents) who do not have access—for financial or other reasons—to an ophthalmologist. The National Eye Care Project number is 1-800-222-EYES. (1-800-222-3937.)

(The cornerstone of this year's National Diabetes Month, which is sponsored by the American Diabetes Association, is a public health campaign to encourage people with diabetes to have eye examinations. The National Eye Institute, the National Institute of Diabetes and Digestive and Kidney Diseases, AAO, the American Optometric Association, and several other groups are joining forces to eliminate preventable blindness through community-based health education. Information on the eye disease initiative will be a special feature of the Association's Diabetes Information and Action Line (DIAL) this month. DIAL's number is 1-800 DIABETES.)

Several fraternal organizations also sponsor eye-care programs for indigent people, including the Benevolent and Protective Order of Elks, and Lions Clubs International.

Your state's hospital association representatives can tell you about local hospital services for those who are uninsured or indigent. Also, local and regional foundations may offer medical, surgical, dental, or rehabilitative assistance to financially distressed local citizens.

Your local library may also be a good source for information on nonprofit organizations.

When you visit a clinic or pharmacy for the first time, go prepared. If possible, take along your identification, evidence of your address (for example, utility bills), medical records (including names and telephone numbers of previous doctors or clinics), prescriptions (or actual vials of insulin or other medications that you are using), and evidence of your income, including government support.

Medicare or Medicaid programs may direct publicly insured clients to a particular clinic or a specific primary care provider. Increasingly, public health care systems are being modeled on a managed care basis; as of early 1993, 35 states and the District of Columbia had launched managed care programs for Medicaid.

Most county or city governments have public health departments that conduct primary care clinics for poor people. According to Carol Brown, a spokesperson at the National Association of County Health Officials, an estimated 98 percent of the nation's 3,000 counties offer some kind of primary care for people in need.

Each municipal government has a different system. For instance, Brown notes that in rural areas several counties may share facilities and personnel. Many facilities specialize in serving specific groups such as the working poor, children, mentally ill people, or the elderly. In some areas, diabetes clinics are under contract to provide care for patients with low incomes.

Unfortunately, not every community government has such public clinics. Many communities, however, have clinics conducted by nonprofit volunteer groups, churches, or charity groups. Your local United Way affiliate may be able to direct you to a treatment facility.

If you visit one of these clinics as a result of being severely ill or because you have run out of medications, tell the receptionist that you have diabetes and politely ask for help or medication now. You will probably be moved to the head of the line, or directed to a walk-in clinic elsewhere.

Healthcare for the Homeless is a federally funded group of over 120 primary care clinics, in 107 cities, for homeless people. To find out if there is a program in your area, call (202) 628-5660. Many private and volunteer groups also offer health-care programs for homeless people.

## Getting Medications and Supplies

Many counties and cities operate prescription drug programs at which people with diabetes can obtain insulin, oral agents, and syringes free of charge or for a low co-payment fee. Other programs offer medications at primary care clinics.

If you visit one of these clinics, take along your insulin vial and your dosage information. Again, tell the receptionist that you have diabetes; often that will move you up the line more quickly.

Many health care programs for indigent people turn away those with diabetes because of the expense of diabetes medications. If you are turned away, ask where you can go for diabetes medications.

Even when public clinics or pharmacies are not available, patients sometimes can get supplies and medications from private physicians. *Tell your doctor if you can't pay for drugs and supplies*, and ask if he or she knows where help is available.

Your doctor or nurse may also be able to contact the parent drug company; many of these companies have drug programs for the medically indigent. For example, major insulin companies and oral medication manufacturers have such programs. However, it may take several weeks for the medication to arrive. It's worth the wait, though, because the company may provide you with several months' worth of medication at a time.

To see whether you might obtain testing strips, your doctor or nurse should call one of the 800 numbers for strip and monitor manufacturers listed in the *Diabetes Forecast* Buyer's Guide, which is published every October.

Because syringes are associated with drug use and the spread of HIV virus, they are often harder to come by than medications. To prevent the spread of the HIV and other diseases, *do not share your syringes with anyone else*. (Ironically, drug addicts can get free syringes in many cities, whereas people with diabetes cannot.)

Sharing needles is always a bad idea, according to Judith Jones, RN, of the Chicago Department of Health needle-exchange program for AIDS prevention. Some financially strapped people with diabetes do it anyway, despite the risk of contracting AIDS and hepatitis. Jones notes that many public health departments run needle-exchange programs to reduce the spread of the HIV, and that these centers provide one-for-one free needles to those who may be at risk. Call your local public health program to determine whether your city has a needle-exchange program.

Most primary care or diabetes clinics carefully guard a store of syringes kept for people in need. Manufacturers donate syringes, like medications, to nurse educators and doctors for such patients.

In addition, many people do reuse their syringes three to four times, or until they get dull. Syringe manufacturers, however, discourage this practice because, after one use, a syringe can no longer be considered sterile.

## Managing Diabetes and Its Complications

The realities of poverty impose limits on the ideals of medicine. For that reason, nurses, dietitians, and doctors are often forced to set different management goals for their homeless and indigent clients than they do for those who carry insurance. If you do not have reliable sources of food, medication, and blood-testing supplies, be sure to have a health-care provider help decide an insulin dosage and schedule that's best for you.

It's just as important to obtain and take your anti-hypertension medicine as your other medications—even if you feel no symptoms. Be sure to make medical appointments well enough in advance to replace medications before you run out. While much else in your life may feel out of your control, this is within your control.

Beatrice Nordberg sees much less foot disease among her working poor clients than in the past. The improvement, she thinks, is largely due to the popularity and design of modern athletic shoes. According to Nordberg, support from a pair of good running shoes will go a long way toward preventing foot problems.

If you have therapeutic footwear prescribed for you, be aware that Medicare now covers limited costs for depth shoes, molded shoes, and various inserts. Unfortunately, few suppliers of therapeutic footwear accept Medicare business because of reimbursement limitations and paperwork. You will need to ask around to find providers who accept reimbursement from Medicare.

A number of charitable groups fund programs for eye surgery and treatments to prevent blindness. Check with your state's Blindness Prevention Program. And over half of the local health departments in the United States offer adult and geriatric well-care. This may or may not include free flu shots. (If flu shots are available, get them in the fall, by November.)

Most programs that provide medical care to indigent people are set up for primary care. Many people, however, aren't able to get treatment until they are dealing with a medical emergency, often in a hospital emergency ward. If you need such immediate help, you are least likely to be rejected in municipal, university, or church-based hospitals.

Indigent people with diabetes face a difficult situation. However, if you are among those struggling to make ends meet, take heart: There are many who are willing and anxious to help.

## Surviving Diabetes and Hunger

Indigent people with diabetes should aim at a balanced diet. They should worry less about diabetic exchanges, and concentrate their energies on getting enough food. If you are indigent and have diabetes, keep the following resources in mind.

**Food Stamps:** If you are poor, you probably are eligible for food stamps, which can be used like cash for groceries. The government is more liberal about dispensing food stamps than many of its other benefits. To apply for food stamps, go to your county or city public assistance office, and bring along the following documentation: identification (such as birth certificates, social security cards or numbers) for *all* family members; verification of all checking or savings accounts; verification of all earned or unearned income for the last 30 days for *all* family members; verification/receipts for household rent or mortgage, utilities, and telephone bills; medical bills/receipts for household members who are over 60 years of age, have a disability, or who are not on Medicaid; and verification of child-care or adult-care expenses.

Normally, people must wait a few weeks for the bureaucratic process to unfold. But if you face a food emergency, tell your food stamp administrator. He or she can issue emergency food stamps. Also, be sure to tell your contact at the food stamp office that you have diabetes.

**Nutrition Advice:** Over half of the country's local health departments employ a full- or part-time nutritionist or dietitian. You may be able to schedule an appointment for advice on your situation.

**Shelters and Soup Kitchens:** If you have diabetes and no money or food, don't let pride get in your way. Find out the times that local churches and shelters open their soup kitchens. Line up for a free, usually well-balanced meal served by volunteers who care about you. Someday in the future, maybe you'll be able to help someone in return.

**Women, Infants and Children (WIC) Programs:** Many local governments have federal grants for programs that provide food subsidies and nutrition counseling for pregnant women and high-risk children to the age of 5. Check with your local health department.

**Government Surplus Foods:** The federal government periodically distributes free surplus foods (such as processed cheese, peanut butter, canned beans, and meat) to the poor. It's not the tastiest fare, but it's nutritious. Call your local public assistance office to find out what organization handles these food distributions and when they take place.

**Food Charities:** Churches and other groups distribute food to poor people from "pantries" or other locations.

**Eating "Out":** Many indigent people eat one meal a day in a fast-food restaurant. One dietitian recommended buying a daily meal in an inexpensive, full-service restaurant instead. These restaurants offer more nutrition for the dollar at breakfast time. Good, hearty breakfasts often cost less than $3.

**Eating at Home:** Avoid junk food. If you have to watch your budget, beans—canned, dried, or fresh—can be a staple of your diet. Beans contain starch, protein, and fiber as well as other nutrients. When you combine beans with rice or corn, you're well on your way to getting enough protein and calories.

Eggs, though somewhat high in fat and cholesterol, are also very nutritional.

Preparing casseroles is also a good way to cut the cost of nutrition. Fill your grocery bag with beans, oatmeal and other grains in bulk, pasta, and greens.

## How Poor Is Poor?

Many medical and financial assistance programs use the federal poverty guidelines in deciding if a person is eligible for assistance.

In February of this year (1994), the federal government defined the poverty level as:

- a single person making $7,360 per year, or
- a family of four making less than $14,800.

Public assistance eligibility workers will make the calculations for your application based on the information you provide and your state's regulations. Be sure to give them as much information as you can. Agencies may adjust these guidelines. If you are receiving other subsidies or if you have extraordinary expenses, the cutoff line may be higher or lower. Local budgets also make a difference.

*—by Leslie Dawson*

Leslie Dawson is a freelance science and medical writer living in Alexandria, Va.

## Chapter 20

# *Self-Monitoring of Blood Glucose*

Self-monitoring of blood glucose (SMBG) is an important component of the treatment plan of patients with diabetes mellitus. Its use was the subject of an American Diabetes Association Consensus Conference in 1986 that dealt with issues regarding the intended and actual use of SMBG, the design, accuracy, and reliability of SMBG devices, how well patients were instructed in SMBG, and how patients and health care providers used the information generated to influence metabolic control. Over the ensuing 7 years, these devices have improved in portability and ease of use. Diabetes educators are teaching an ever-increasing number of people with diabetes to use SMBG. In addition, the recent publication of the results of the Diabetes Control and Complications Trial has given validity to the concept that better metabolic control can significantly reduce the onset and progression of the microvascular and neuropathic complications of insulin-dependent diabetes (IDDM).

Despite these advances, questions remain as to which type(s) of patients might best use SMBG, whether the procedure is accurate, and how the information generated by SMBG should be used. The economics of SMBG also needs to be considered in the context of a changing health-care system. To answer these questions, the American Diabetes Association convened a second Consensus Development Conference on Self-Monitoring of Blood Glucose on 27-29 September 1993.

---

The conference consisted of 24 invited presentations and contributions from a large audience of health-care professionals and representatives from industry. A consensus panel with expertise in the areas of internal medicine, laboratory medicine, nursing, nutrition, pharmacy, endocrinology, and diabetes education, with backgrounds in clinical practice and academic medicine, considered a broad spectrum of issues related to SMBG. The panel reached a consensus on the answers to these questions: 1) What is the epidemiology of SMBG? 2) Who should self-monitor? 3) What is the current technology? 4) How should the data obtained from self-monitoring be used? 5) What is the future of self-monitoring?

## What Is the Epidemiology of SMBG?

Diabetes affects more than 13 million people in the U.S. About 300,000 have IDDM; the remainder have non-insulin-dependent diabetes mellitus (NIDDM). It is estimated that approximately 3 million diabetic patients are being treated with insulin.

A 1989 national sample of nearly 2,500 individuals with diabetes who were over 18 years of age showed that the frequency of self-monitoring varied considerably. Overall, 33% of the diabetic patients self-monitored their blood glucose. Of the IDDM population, 40% monitored once or more a day, 39% monitored less than once a day, and 21% never performed SMBG. Within the NIDDM population using insulin, 26% monitored at least once a day, 27% monitored less than once a day, and 47% never self-monitored. In both of these groups, the proportion of people who self-monitored was found to be directly related to the number of insulin injections per day. For patients with NIDDM not using insulin, only 5% monitored one or more times a day, 19% less than once a day, and 76% never self-monitored.

This survey also showed that the proportion of individuals who self-monitored at least once a day declined with age; the probability of testing decreased 18% with each decade of life in adults. African Americans were 60% less likely than non-Hispanic whites and Hispanics to self-monitor one or more times per day. Factors related to a higher proportion of testing (i.e., 1 or more times a day) included the use of insulin, the frequency of insulin injections, a higher educational level, frequency of physician office visits, and participation in a diabetes education class. This survey did not indicate that health insurance coverage is a determinant of self-monitoring; however, the sampled population was not asked if their insurance covered blood glucose testing equipment, supplies, or education in the use of SMBG.

Community-based intervention programs have increased the proportion of people with diabetes who self-monitor. For example, from 1981 to 1991, in selected communities in Michigan that implemented such programs, the use of SMBG increased from 29 to 85% in the IDDM population, from 6 to 82% in the NIDDM insulin-using population, and from 2 to 31% in the non-insulin-using NIDDM population.

The attitude of physicians regarding the appropriateness of SMBG varies according to the medical specialty. In a recent study, internists and pediatricians expressed a stronger belief in the value of SMBG compared with general practitioners. Younger physicians were found to be more likely to believe that SMBG was useful in achieving glycemic goals.

While self-management is a goal of diabetes care, little information is available concerning how patients use SMBG results. In one study, approximately 70% of IDDM patients thought that SMBG was "very important" in helping them control their diabetes by allowing them to adjust their insulin dosage. Although 60% of insulin-using NIDDM patients thought that monitoring was "very important," only 21% altered their insulin dose based on SMBG results. Further information is needed to determine 1) what frequency of monitoring is optimal for the care of people with IDDM and NIDDM and 2) whether the actions taken in response to SMBG are appropriate.

Future research is also needed to identify and reduce barriers that impede the appropriate use of SMBG and to determine ways to increase the proportion of individuals who initiate a change in self-management in response to SMBG.

## Who Should Self-Monitor?

SMBG is a means of achieving a goal rather than a goal in itself. When properly performed, SMBG permits people with diabetes to determine their blood glucose level. However, the value of SMBG is limited unless it is used as part of an integrated treatment program. The health professional supervising the care of the patient must clearly define the goals of treatment and therefore the reason for performing SMBG. Patients (or designated care providers) must be capable of learning the proper use of SMBG, must be motivated and willing to expend the effort necessary to ensure that the measurements are accurate, and must be committed to constructively modifying their treatment plans in response to the feedback provided by SMBG.

The indications and frequency for monitoring will vary considerably depending on the clinical situation of each patient and the purpose for which SMBG is being used. Potential indications for SMBG include but are not limited to the following areas.

### *Achievement and Maintenance of a Specific Level of Glycemic Control*

Recent clinical trials have demonstrated that when IDDM patients maintain glucose levels in the near-normal range, they both delay the onset and slow the rate of progression of diabetic retinopathy, nephropathy, and neuropathy. These studies also suggest that if normoglycemia cannot be achieved, any improvement in chronic glycemic control likely will be associated with a decrease in microvascular complications. People with NIDDM were not included in these trials. However, since hyperglycemia is associated with the presence or progression of complications in NIDDM, it is likely that lowering blood glucose levels will also decrease microvascular complications in these people. In addition, in women with diabetes, maintenance of blood glucose levels in the near-normoglycemic range before conception and during pregnancy has been shown to decrease rates of fetal malformation, morbidity, and mortality.

Thus SMBG is an essential component of any intensive insulin program directed toward achieving near-normoglycemia. Virtually all intensive therapy programs in insulin-deficient patients depend on the measurement of glucose levels at least four times a day. Knowledge of preprandial, bedtime, and nocturnal blood glucose concentrations is required to determine the appropriate basal and preprandial insulin doses. A decrease in the frequency of monitoring to less than four times a day has been shown to result in a worsening of glycemic control.

A lesser frequency of SMBG may suffice if the patient is still able to secrete substantial amounts of insulin (e.g., recent onset of IDDM, most cases of NIDDM). In these patients glycemic goals often can be met using less complex insulin regimens, oral hypoglycemic agents, and diet. SMBG may be used in these patients to assess temporal patterns (i.e. does glucose concentration rise/fall during the day vs. during the night) so that the morning or evening doses of insulin and/or oral agents can be appropriately increased or decreased. Once therapy is optimized and glycemic control has stabilized, the frequency of monitoring often can be decreased substantially, particularly in people with NIDDM. If the patient's social situation, medical condition, or motivation would discourage or preclude efforts at achieving near-normoglycemia, then the frequency of SMBG or the use of other monitoring systems, e.g. urine glucose measurements, should be utilized in relation to the patient's willingness or ability to obtain the needed information.

## *Prevention and Detection of Hypoglycemia*

Hypoglycemia is a major complication in the treatment of diabetes. The risk of hypoglycemia increases when pharmacological treatments are used to maintain glucose levels in the near-normal range. Hypoglycemia can be a particular problem in people who are unable to recognize the early warning signs of hypoglycemia. People with NIDDM on either insulin or oral agents also are at risk for hypoglycemia. Hypoglycemia, produced by oral agents, may occur more frequently in people with considerable insulin secretory reserve (i.e. hypoglycemia is rare in people in whom oral agents have minimal therapeutic effect) and in the elderly. Appropriately timed SMBG is the only practical means of detecting asymptomatic hypoglycemia in the outpatient setting. By detecting temporal patterns of change in glucose levels, SMBG permits therapy to be modified so as to prevent hypoglycemia. This may be particularly important in individuals in whom hypoglycemia may have serious health consequences (e.g. people with underlying atherosclerotic vascular disease). Glucose levels also should be closely monitored whenever a medication that may decrease recognition of hypoglycemia or impair glucose counter-regulation (e.g., b-blockers) is added to the patient's existing regimen. Hypoglycemia may be particularly dangerous in situations in which impaired mental function may lead to serious bodily harm (e.g. driving). Insulin-taking patients should be instructed to always measure their glucose level before engaging in such activities.

## *Avoidance of Severe Hyperglycemia*

Illness or drugs that alter insulin secretion (e.g., phenytoin, thiazide diuretics) or insulin action (e.g., prednisone) may worsen glycemic control. The risk of severe hyperglycemia and/or ketoacidosis may be increased in individuals with limited insulin secretory reserve (IDDM), limited access to fluids (elderly people with either IDDM or NIDDM), or increased fluid loss due to diarrhea, vomiting, or fever. People with diabetes should be instructed to initiate SMBG or increase the frequency of monitoring in all of these situations, as well as to consult their health-care provider. People using insulin should be provided with guidelines as to how to use SMBG data to appropriately increase their insulin dosage to avoid severe hyperglycemia.

### Adjusting Care in Response to Changes in Life-Style in Individuals Requiring Pharmacological Therapy

Changes in activity and diet can have major effects on blood glucose levels. Regular exercise can increase insulin action, thereby decreasing the dose of either insulin or oral agents required to achieve a given level of glycemia. Exercise can result in an increase, decrease, or no change in glucose levels both during and after exercise, depending on the prevailing insulin concentration. Exercise can alter subcutaneous blood flow and therefore alter the rate of insulin absorption. SMBG can be useful in determining patterns of response to planned or unplanned exercise, permitting pharmacological therapy or diet to be appropriately modified. SMBG may be particularly important in children and adolescents who have wide day-to-day variations in activity.

A reduction in caloric consumption can decrease insulin or oral agent needs. An increase in caloric consumption can have the opposite effect. Regular SMBG may be of assistance in modifying pharmacological therapy during periods of increased or decreased caloric consumption. It also provides the necessary information to determine whether pharmacological therapy should be modified when meal size is altered.

### Determining the Need for Initiating Insulin Therapy in Gestational Diabetes Mellitus (GDM)

Elevation in blood glucose levels in pregnant women influences fetal development. Because of the decrease in insulin action associated with pregnancy, some women not known to have diabetes are found to have abnormal blood glucose concentrations during pregnancy and are therefore diagnosed as having GDM. Untreated, GDM may result in an increased incidence of macrosomia, respiratory distress syndrome, and other abnormalities of fetal metabolism. Women with GDM who have elevated fasting plasma glucose levels are often treated with insulin and perform SMBG frequently each day to achieve near-normoglycemia. (These individuals are included in Goal #1.) However, evolving evidence suggests that SMBG may help identify a subset of women with GDM whose fetal outcome may benefit by earlier initiation of insulin therapy.

SMBG has occasionally been used to document hypoglycemia in nondiabetic individuals. Screening methods must be confirmed by laboratory testing before establishing any medical diagnosis. In some circumstances such as children with hypopituitarism, SMBG may be useful in screening and management of hypoglycemia.

SMBG is only one component of an overall program of diabetes care. Additional studies are needed to determine whether SMBG, as part of a treatment regimen, improves adherence to treatment or quality of life and to determine the associated costs. Until such evidence exists, using SMBG to simply enhance compliance or improve quality of life is of questionable value.

## What Is the Current Technology?

### Measurement Principles and Limitations of SMBG Systems

The operating principles of most self-monitoring systems are the same. Glucose is oxidized enzymatically, followed by a coupled reaction to develop a chromogenic product; the color intensity is proportional to the amount of glucose present, which is quantified by reflectance spectrometry. In other systems, the electrical current generated by glucose oxidation is measured. There is generally good agreement between the glucose concentration measured in whole blood by SMBG systems and that measured in serum or plasma by clinical laboratory procedures. The strength of the correlation varies according to the glucose concentration; a decrease in accuracy is seen at both extremes of glucose concentration. Factors that may influence the results of SMBG include variations in hematocrit, altitude, environmental temperature and humidity, hypotension, hypoxia, and triglyceride concentrations. Drugs taken in pharmacologic dosage do not appear to affect the accuracy of the measurements.

### Performance of SMBG Systems

The overall performance of SMBG systems is a combination of the analytical performance of the instrument, proficiency of the operator(s), and the quality of the test strips. The previous American Diabetes Association Consensus Statement recommended that the performance goal of all SMBG systems should be to achieve a total error (analytical plus user) of less than 10% at glucose concentrations ranging from 30 to 400 mg/dl. Unfortunately, this goal has not been achieved for most SMBG systems. In an assessment of the analytical variability of SMBG systems, the College of American Pathologists recently found that the coefficient of variation ranged within systems from 4 to 33%. Some of this variability may be due to matrix effects, and uniform standards for the determination of the accuracy of SMBG systems are needed. In view of the proven benefits of good metabolic control, it is even more important now than it was in 1986 for SMBG systems to measure glucose accurately. The goal of SMBG device manufacturers should be to make future SMBG systems with an analytic error of +5%.

Operator performance is influenced by the characteristics of the system and the extent and quality of user training. Although some of the commercially available meters have been made less dependent on operator skill, further efforts in this direction are needed. The extent and quality of user training continues to be seriously hampered by current reimbursement policies for diabetes education.

Users are largely dependent on the system manufacturer to ensure the quality of each test strip. There is no way that a user can both verify that a single test strip is satisfactory and at the same time use it to test a blood specimen. In addition, there is significant within-lot and lot-to-lot variation in strips, and their use can be adversely affected by environmental factors. Because of the complexity of the calibration of strips to meters, the use of generic strips should be carefully studied before patients are encouraged to use them. Finally, since control solutions are used in teaching patients SMBG, and to check the functioning of the system, efforts should be made to narrow the acceptable range specified for the solutions.

### *Assessment of Clinically Significant Error*

The reduction of analytic and user errors will result in more accurate glucose measurements. However, it is important to point out that not all errors are clinically significant such that they will result in change in management, e.g., a change in insulin dose. Although the Error Grid developed by Clark and associates is a useful attempt at defining such clinically important errors by defining relatively broad "target ranges," with intensive insulin therapy designed to adjust insulin doses for narrow target ranges, even relatively small errors may cause a change in insulin dosage. Thus, depending upon the therapeutic goals of treatment, outlined above, clinically significant error may in some cases approach analytic plus user error. Efforts should be made to refine the Error Grid target ranges to account for intensive treatment goals. Also, further efforts are needed to link technical error with clinically significant error in future work.

### *Quality Assurance*

All manufacturers define proper quality-assurance practices to be used with their SMBG systems. A quality-assurance program necessitates periodic monitoring of control specimens at both high and low concentrations. If such quality-assurance measurements were performed at frequent intervals it would increase the cost of SMBG, thereby potentially creating a barrier to performance of quality assurance by patients in the home setting. In addition, testing of the instrument with control specimens does not monitor the quality of the collection procedure or the proper application of blood to the test strip. A complete quality-assurance program would address the entire self-monitoring process, from collection of the sample to measurement of the glucose value to application of the result. The development of such a program is recommended by the Panel.

### *Application of SMBG in Hospital Practice*

It is debatable whether patients should perform glucose measurements on their own blood within a hospital, except for training purposes. If this practice is adopted, acceptable conditions under which this is done should be established by each hospital.

### *Further Recommendations*

The Panel recommends the following. 1) Efforts should be made to develop fail-safe SMBG systems. The meter should identify faulty operation and specify the nature of the problem. Also, systems should be less dependent on user skill. 2) Manufacturers should establish a uniform standard for calibration and the determination of the accuracy of SMBG systems. 3) Periodic comparisons should be made between results obtained by the patient with his/her SMBG system and a fasting sample simultaneously obtained and measured by a referenced laboratory.

## How Should the Data Obtained from Self-Monitoring Be Used?

SMBG is a tool used by both health-care providers and patients to monitor therapy. It is important that qualified health-care providers and trained patients have access to this technology. However, it can be of little value without a comprehensive package of diabetes education, counseling, and management. Health-care providers should use SMBG data to 1) set glycemic goals, 2) develop recommendations for pharmacological therapy, 3) evaluate the effectiveness of pharmacological therapy, 4) instruct patients to interpret and respond to blood glucose patterns, 5) evaluate the impact of dietary factors on glycemic control, 6) modify therapy during acute/intercurrent illness or when patients receive medications that affect glycemic control, 7) modify the management plan in response to changes in activity, and 8) identify hypoglycemic unawareness and strategies for treatment.

This information should be conveyed by the health-care provider in a non-pejorative manner that encourages open and honest communication.

People with diabetes should use SMBG data to 1) self-adjust diet, exercise, or pharmacological therapy, 2) identify and properly treat hyper- and hypoglycemia, and 3) improve decision making and problem solving.

The effective use of SMBG encourages the patient to assume a greater responsibility for control, thereby improving confidence and self-management.

Appropriate use of SMBG is dependent on proper processing and interpretation of the data. Manual recording of data in log books has advantages and disadvantages. The advantages include simplicity, familiarity, opportunity to review a written record, and low cost. Disadvantages include difficulty in detecting trends and the integration of large volumes of data. Manual recording is subject to errors in entry and transcription and to falsification of data.

Newer systems, which include a memory meter and a computer with data management software, can potentially avoid many of the problems associated with traditional log books. In addition, these systems provide a variety of methods of data analysis and display. Disadvantages of data management systems include increased expense and complexity. Also, patients may fail to keep personal written logbook records and such decreased direct patient involvement in data analysis may lead to a decrease in self-management and a delay in the implementation of appropriate modifications of therapy. The utility of manual and computer-based systems is likely to vary depending on the expertise and interest of patients and health-care providers.

The Panel recommends that further research be directed toward identifying characteristics of patient/health-care provider relationships that influence interactions and improve glycemic control and health outcomes.

## What Is the Future of Self-Monitoring?

Ideally, SMBG should be a reliable, convenient, safe, closed-loop system easily used by patients. Its cost must be reasonable, and it must show clear benefits when integrated into a comprehensive treatment program. It should be easy to use by children and by people with decreased vision, impaired manual dexterity, or other special needs.

There are a number of areas in which existing SMBG systems should be improved. The systems should be made less dependent on user skill and should decrease the pain associated with monitoring. Also, better methods are needed to detect and prevent analytic, user, and sample collection errors. The cost of monitoring should be reduced. The accuracy and precision of SMBG systems should be increased. Access to and effectiveness of patient and professional education should be a high priority. Appropriate reimbursement for such education and testing supplies must be widely available. Optimal methods of data storage, telecommunication, presentation, and analysis need to be developed further.

Technology now on the horizon has the potential to monitor blood glucose levels on an almost continuous basis. Near-infrared and implantable continuous monitoring systems may decrease or eliminate the pain and inconvenience of testing and thereby facilitate more frequent monitoring. Such increased monitoring is likely to improve glucose control while at the same time decreasing hypoglycemic risk. These new glucose-sensing devices may ultimately allow the development of a closed-loop system. With both of these methods, however, difficulties in miniaturization, mass production, and reliability must be overcome.

The future of SMBG in diabetes care also will be affected by changes in the health-care system. Whatever changes occur, SMBG must be accessible and affordable. Government, third-party payers, manufacturers of diabetes care products, nonprofit organizations, health-care providers, and people with diabetes must work closely together to carry out the activities and research that have been identified at this conference. SMBG is integral to the management of diabetes, and coverage of SMBG should be an important component of any benefits package. The waivered status of SMBG devices under CLIA-88 is an important step in assuring access to this technology, and is endorsed by the Panel.

Advances in computer data analysis for handling the large amounts of data generated by such systems are also forthcoming, including the evolution of "expert" systems, which may aid in the development of individualized, instantly modifiable insulin treatment algorithms.

## Acknowledgements

The conference was sponsored in part by educational grants from Boehringer Mannheim Corporation, LifeScan Inc. (a Johnson & Johnson Company), and Miles Inc. (Diagnostic Division).

## Suggested Reading

1. American Diabetes Association: Consensus statement on self-monitoring of blood glucose. *Diabetes Care* 10:93-99, 1987

2. The Diabetes Control and Complications Trial Research Group: The effect of intensive treatment of diabetes on the development and progression of long-term complications in insulin-dependent diabetes mellitus. *N Engl J Med* 329:977-986, 1993

3. Harris MJ, Cowie CC, Howie LJ: Self-monitoring of blood glucose by adults with diabetes in the United States population. *Diabetes Care* 16:1116-1123, 1993

4. The National Steering Committee for Quality Assurance in Capillary Blood Glucose Monitoring: Proposed strategies for reducing user error in capillary blood glucose monitoring. *Diabetes Care* 16:493-498, 1993

5. Nettles A: User error in blood glucose monitoring. The National Steering Committee for Quality Assurance Report. *Diaetes Care* 16:946-948, 1993

6. Greyson J: Quality control in patient self-monitoring of blood glucose. *Diabetes Care* 16:1306-1308, 1993

7. National Committee for Clinical Laboratory Standards: *Ancillary (Bedside) Blood Glucose Testing Acute and Chronic Care* Facilities. Villanova, PA 1991 (NCCLS Document C30-T)

8. Clarke WL, Cox D, GonderFrederick LA, Carter W, Pohl SL: Evaluating clinical accuracy of systems for self-monitoring of blood glucose. *Diabetes Care* 10:622-628, 1987

9. Walker EA: Quality assurance for blood glucose monitoring. The balance of feasibility and standards. *Nursing Clin N Amer* 28:61-70, 1993

10. Marrero DG, Kronz AA, Golden M, Wright JC, Orr DP, Fineberg NS: Clinical evaluation of computer-assisted self-monitoring of blood glucose system. *Diabetes Care* 12:345-350, 1989

Chapter 21

# Urine Glucose and Ketone Determinations

Historically, urine glucose and ketone determinations were the only practical way for people with diabetes to regularly assess their glycemic control. However, the development of small, convenient, and reasonably accurate blood glucose meters has made urine glucose testing obsolete for most patients. Self-monitoring of blood glucose (SMBG) is now common and is the preferred way to monitor glycemic control. SMBG is recommended for all patients who use insulin [1,2]. Recommendations for testing urine for glucose and ketones as part of diabetes management are described here.

## Urine Glucose Tests

The basis for urine glucose measurements is the fact that glucosuria is roughly correlated with hyperglycemia. Urine testing is painless and less expensive than SMBG. However, the use of urine glucose concentrations to estimate blood glucose concentrations in diabetes management is undesirable for the following reasons:

1. The renal threshold for glucose excretion in healthy adults corresponds to a plasma concentration of ~10 mM (180 mg/dl). In many adults, particularly those with long-standing diabetes, this threshold may increase substantially [3]. Thus, marked hyperglycemia may exist without glucosuria. Conversely, some

Position Statement, *Diabetes Care* Supplement, May 15, 1996, individuals, particularly children and pregnant women, may have very low or variable renal thresholds, resulting in glucosuria with euglycemia [4]. Thus, urine glucose levels imprecisely represent blood glucose concentrations.

2. Fluid intake and urine concentration can affect urine test results.

3. The test reflects an average level of blood glucose during the interval since the last voiding and not the level at the time of the test.

4. A negative urine test does not distinguish between hypoglycemia, euglycemia, and mild or moderate hyperglycemia. Therefore, urine testing is of little help in achieving the management goal of avoiding hypoglycemia and hyperglycemia.

5. Urine testing methodology, which involves comparing the color of a test strip against a printed chart, is less accurate than a digital readout of a blood glucose meter. Furthermore, it poses a problem for patients who are color blind or have other visual impairments.

6. Some drugs may interfere with urine glucose determinations.

Considering these points, the American Diabetes Association recommends that all patients who use insulin should self-monitor their blood not urine glucose. SMBG is also desirable in many patients who do not require insulin. Testing urine for glucose is a less desirable alternative for insulin-using patients only if they are unable or unwilling to perform SMBG. Healthcare professionals should repeatedly encourage the latter group of patients to switch to SMBG.

### *Urine Ketone Tests*

Unlike urine glucose tests, urine ketone determinations remain an important part of monitoring diabetic control, particularly in patients with insulin-dependent diabetes. Urinary ketones may be an indication of impending ketoacidosis, a condition that requires immediate medical attention. Urine must be tested for ketones during acute illness or stress, when blood glucose levels are consistently >13.4 mM

(240 mg/dl), during pregnancy, or when any symptoms of ketoacidosis (e.g., nausea, vomiting, abdominal pain) are present.

## References

1. American Diabetes Association: Standards of medical care for patients with diabetes mellitus (Position statement). *Diabetes Care* 19 (Suppl. 1):S8-S15, 1996

2. American Diabetes Association: Self-monitoring of blood glucose (Consensus statement). *Diabetes Care* 19 (Suppl. 1):S62-S66, 1996

3. Skyler JS: Monitoring diabetes mellitus. In *Diabetes Mellitus*. 9th ed. Galloway JA, Potvin JH, Shuman CR, Eds. Indianapolis, IN, Lilly, 1988, p. 160-173

4. Mogenssen C, Østerby R, Gundersen H: Early functional and morphological vascular renal consequences of the diabetic state. *Diabetologia* 17:71-76, 1979

# Chapter 22

# *Heading Off Heart Disease*

Many people think that heart disease is primarily a man's problem. But despite the fact that estrogen seems to protect women from heart disease until after menopause, heart disease is still the number one killer of women.

Women (and men) with diabetes are more likely to develop the form of heart disease called *coronary artery disease* (the narrowing of the blood vessels that supply the heart with blood) than people who do not have diabetes. And women with diabetes may not ever benefit from the protective action of estrogen.

But it's not all bad news. You can significantly reduce your risk of coronary artery disease by keeping your diabetes in good control, eating a proper diet, exercising, and visiting your doctor regularly.

## *What Is Heart Disease?*

The term heart disease refers to any heart problem, ranging from valve deformities present at birth to problems that occur as we age. Coronary artery disease is the most common type of heart disease.

Tremendous strides have been made in understanding how heart disease develops. Arteries are elastic tubes that bring blood from the heart to each organ of the body. As we age, our arteries become thicker and less elastic and the inner lining weakens. This weakening allows

---

fatty particles in our blood to leak into the walls of the arteries. In response, the body sends out white blood cells called *macrophages* to attack these fatty particles. After destroying the fatty invaders, these cells remain within the wall of the artery and form a plaque, an abnormal patch on the inner fining, which narrows the blood vessel. This is called *atherosclerosis*. Blood platelets can stick to the plaque and form a clot, which in turn may completely block the artery. if this blockage occurs in one of the arteries that supplies the heart with blood, that portion of the heart may die and the person will have a heart attack.

## Diabetes and Heart Disease

Women with diabetes are two to five times more likely to get heart disease than women without diabetes. Over the years, high blood sugar levels cause changes that result in the narrowing of the smaller arteries that supply the heart with blood, ultimately destroying them. This causes tiny scars to form in the heart muscle. Over time, these scars accumulate and can weaken the heart muscle. This is called *diabetic cardiomyopathy*. This process can proceed with few symptoms until a major portion of the heart is damaged.

## Risk Factors

In addition to its direct effect on the heart, diabetes can also increase the severity of several of the risk factors that promote coronary artery disease. People with diabetes are at an increased risk for *hypertension* (high blood pressure), *hyperlipidemia* (high levels of fats in the blood), low levels of high-density lipoprotein (HDL) cholesterol, and obesity.

**Hypertension.** High blood pressure can damage the blood vessels of the heart, brain, eyes, and kidneys. The higher the blood pressure and the longer it stays elevated, the more damage it causes.

People with diabetes are at a much greater risk of developing high blood pressure. By the time people with Type I (insulin-dependent) diabetes reach 40 years of age, more than half have high blood pressure. About half of the people with Type II (non-insulin-dependent) diabetes develop high blood pressure within 10 years of diagnosis. Uncontrolled high blood pressure can set in motion a vicious cycle, with high blood pressure causing kidney damage, which in turn raises blood pressure even more.

**Hyperlipidemia.** High levels of fat and cholesterol in the blood also increase the risk of heart disease. A woman with a total cholesterol level of more than 265 mg/dl is at more than twice the risk for coronary artery disease than a woman whose level is less than 205 mg/dl. Women, especially those with Type II diabetes, are also more likely to have low levels of HDL cholesterol (the "good" cholesterol) and high levels of the fatty acids called *triglycerides*. To protect against heart disease, HDL levels should be greater than 60 mg/dl and triglyceride levels should be less than 190 mg/dl. The best way to raise HDL levels is to lower triglyceride (fat) levels. This can be done by modifying the diet to include less fat and cholesterol.

The high blood sugar levels that occur with poorly controlled diabetes cause the liver to produce extra fat and cholesterol. Because the liver can only store a small portion of this extra fat, the excess then enters the bloodstream. Normally, fat particles in the blood are removed by fat cells. However, in people with poorly controlled diabetes, these particles cannot be removed, and the fats in the blood can rise to very high levels, raising the risk of atherosclerosis.

**Syndrome X.** Scientists have recently discovered a link between Type II diabetes, hypertension, hyperlipidemia, and obesity that they call Syndrome X. Even before being diagnosed with Type II diabetes, people who develop this constellation of symptoms do not respond to the insulin produced by their own pancreas (insulin resistance) and have borderline-high blood sugar levels as a result. It may take two to three times as much insulin in these individuals, who also tend to be overweight, to keep their blood sugar levels normal. These high insulin levels may have potentially harmful side effects, such as promoting salt retention, fat production, and narrowing of the arteries throughout the body. All of these factors promote heart disease.

When risk factors are combined, the chance of having a heart attack is increased dramatically. An extreme example would be a person with diabetes who smokes and has high blood pressure and high cholesterol. This person has almost 100 times the chance of having a heart attack than a person who does not have diabetes or any of these other risk factors.

### *Risk Factors for Heart Disease*

1. High blood pressure
2. Smoking

3. Menopause
4. High levels of fat and cholesterol in the blood
5. Diabetes
6. Excess weight
7. Family history of heart disease
8. Sedentary lifestyle

## Reducing Your Risk

Although women who have diabetes may be at a higher risk for coronary artery disease, the good news is that many of the risk factors described above can be treated. Combining changes in lifestyle and diet with medication, if necessary, can dramatically reduce your risk of heart disease.

**Cigarette smoking.** If you smoke, you must stop now. Diabetes and cigarette smoking is a deadly combination. Heart disease caused by smoking kills many more people than lung cancer does. The nicotine in cigarette smoke is a very powerful drug that narrows the arteries throughout your body and increases the work that your heart has to perform. Nicotine patches may be helpful as part of a smoking-cessation program. However, if you use a nicotine patch and continue to smoke, you increase your intake of nicotine and increase the danger to your heart.

**Hypertension.** Drug therapy to lower blood pressure can dramatically decrease the rate of stroke and heart attack But because most people with high blood pressure don't experience any negative symptoms, they may be tempted to stop taking their medicine because of its cost, side effects, or inconvenience. There are now several new classes of drugs on the market, including ACE inhibitors and calcium channel blockers, that are safe and especially effective for people with diabetes. These drugs cause fewer side effects and usually have to be taken only once a day. With these and other medications, blood pressure can usually be kept under control.

**Dietary modifications.** Eating a healthy diet can dramatically improve diabetes control and lower your levels of cholesterol and triglycerides. A healthy diet should be low in animal fat, dairy fat and refined sugar and should include fish, vegetables, starches, and vegetable oils (such as corn oil and peanut oil). Try substituting low-fat dairy products such as skim milk and reduced-fat cheeses for the high-fat standards such as butter and whole milk. Avoid high-cholesterol foods such as eggs, baked goods, and products containing coconut oil or palm oil. Try to eat a variety of fresh fruits and vegetables, whole grains, and beans. If your fat and cholesterol levels are still high despite following a diet and exercise program, your doctor may prescribe medicine.

**Exercise.** Exercise also plays an important role in reducing the risk of heart disease. Aerobic exercises such as walking, stair-stepping, swimming, cross-country skiing, bicycle riding, and jogging burn calories and fat and can help you lose weight. They also strengthen your heart by increasing its efficiency. Anaerobic exercise, such as weight lifting or resistance work with machines, increases muscle strength and size, but it burns only half the calories of aerobic exercise. Anaerobic exercises may also raise blood pressure, which can be dangerous for some people.

Check with your physician before beginning an exercise program. Your doctor may suggest a stress test to measure your level of fitness and to determine if you already have heart disease. This test is performed on a treadmill or bicycle that increases your level of physical activity while an electrocardiogram (EKG) records the electrical impulses of your heart.

Stress tests are a good idea for everyone with diabetes because diabetes increases your risk of "silent" heart problems—those with no symptoms. *Neuropathy* or nerve damage, a relatively common complication of diabetes that can cause pain, a feeling of pins and needles, or a loss of sensation in the feet can also damage the nerves leading to the heart and the blood vessels that regulate heart rate and blood pressure. This is called *autonomic neuropathy*. People with this type of nerve damage may not feel the chest pain or discomfort that occurs when too little blood reaches the heart (*angina*) or when a heart attack occurs. This is called *silent ischemia* or a silent heart attack. Stress tests can detect heart problems that do not have any warning symptoms.

**Estrogen.** For women who have gone through menopause, estrogen replacement therapy cuts the risk of heart disease in half. In addition, estrogen can increase bone strength and energy levels. However, not all women can take estrogen because of the potential side effects, which can include blood clots in the veins, water retention, and cancer of the uterus. Discuss the pros and cons of estrogen replacement therapy with your doctor to see if it is right for you.

Although women with diabetes may have a higher risk of heart disease than women without diabetes, there are many ways to reduce your risk significantly. By keeping your diabetes in good control, keeping your blood pressure at normal levels, lowering your cholesterol, starting an exercise program, maintaining a healthy diet, and taking medicine if necessary, the progression of heart disease can be slowed and even stopped.

*—by Harvey L. Katzeff, M.D.*

Dr. Harvey L. Katzeff is Director of the Diabetes Treatment and Education Program and Associate Professor of Medicine at North Shore University Hospital—University Medical School in Manhasset, New York.

Chapter 23

# Skin Care for People with Diabetes

Diabetes can affect every part of the body, including the skin. As many as a third of people with diabetes will have a skin disorder caused or affected by diabetes at some time in their lives. In fact, such problems are sometimes the first sign that a person has diabetes. Luckily, most skin conditions can be prevented or easily treated if caught early.

Some of these problems are skin conditions that anyone can have, but that people with diabetes get more easily.

These include bacterial infections, fungal infections, and itching. Other skin problems happen mostly or only to people with diabetes. These include diabetic dermopathy, necrobiosis lipoidica diabeticorum, diabetic blisters, and eruptive xanthomatosis.

## Bacterial Infections

Several kinds of bacterial infections occur in people with diabetes. One common one is styes. These are infections of the glands of the eyelid.

Another kind of infection is boils, infections of the hair follicles. Carbuncles are deep infections of the skin and the tissue underneath. Infections can also occur around the nails.

Inflamed tissues are usually hot, swollen, red, and painful. Several different organisms can cause infections. The most common ones are the *Staphylococcus* bacteria, also called staph.

Once, bacterial infections were life threatening, especially for people with diabetes. Today, death is rare, thanks to antibiotics and better methods of glucose control.

But even today, people with diabetes have more bacterial infections than other people do. Doctors believe people with diabetes can reduce their chances of these infections in several ways.

If you think you have a bacterial infection, see your doctor.

## Fungal Infections

The culprit in fungal infections of people with diabetes is often *Candida albicans*. This yeast-like fungus can create itchy rashes of moist, red areas surrounded by tiny blisters and scales.

These infections often occur in warm, moist folds of the skin. Problem areas are under the breasts, around the nails, between fingers and toes, in the corners of the mouth, under the foreskin (in uncircumcised men), and in the armpits and groin.

Common fungal infections include jock itch, athlete's foot, ringworm (a ring-shaped itchy patch), and vaginal infection that causes itching.

If you think you have a yeast or fungal infection, call your doctor. You will need a prescription medicine to cure it.

## Itching

Localized itching is often caused by diabetes. It can be caused by a yeast infection, dry skin, or poor circulation. When poor circulation is the cause of itching, the itchiest areas may be the lower parts of the legs.

You may be able to treat itching yourself. Limit how often you bathe, particularly when the humidity is low. Use mild soap with moisturizer and apply skin cream after bathing.

## Diabetic Dermopathy

Diabetes can cause changes in the small blood vessels. These changes can cause skin problems called diabetic dermopathy. Dermopathy often looks like light brown, scaly patches.

These patches may be oval or circular. Some people mistake them for age spots. This disorder most often occurs on the front of both legs. But the legs may not be affected to the same degree. The patches do not hurt, open up, or itch.

Dermopathy is harmless. You do not need to be treated.

## Necrobiosis Lipoidica Diabeticorum

Another disease that may be caused by changes in the blood vessels is necrobiosis lipoidica diabeticorum (NLD). NLD is similar to diabetic dermopathy. The difference is that the spots are fewer, but larger and deeper.

NLD often starts as a dull red raised area. After a while, it looks like a shiny scar with a violet border. The blood vessels under the skin may become easier to see. Sometimes, NLD is itchy and painful. Sometimes, the spots crack open.

NLD is a rare condition. Adult women are the most likely to get it. As long as the sores do not break open, you do not need to have it treated. But if you get open sores, see your doctor for treatment.

## Atherosclerosis

Thickening of the arteries (atherosclerosis) can affect the skin on the legs. People with diabetes tend to get atherosclerosis at younger ages than other people do.

As atherosclerosis narrows the blood vessels, the skin changes. It becomes hairless, thin, cool, and shiny. The toes become cold. Toenails thicken and discolor. And exercise causes pain in the calf muscles because the muscles are not getting enough oxygen.

Because blood carries the infection-fighting white cells, affected legs heal slowly when the skin in injured. Even minor scrapes can result in open sores that heal slowly.

People with neuropathy are more likely to suffer foot injuries. These occur because the person does not feel pain, heat, cold, or pressure as well. The person can have an injured foot and not know about it. The wound goes uncared for, and so infections develop easily. Atherosclerosis can make things worse. The reduced blood flow can cause the infection to become severe.

## Allergic Reactions

Allergic skin reactions can occur in response to medicines, such as insulin or diabetes pills. You should see your doctor if you think you are having a reaction to a medicine. Be on the lookout for rashes, depressions, or bumps at the sites where you inject insulin.

## Diabetic Blisters (Bullosis Diabeticorum)

Rarely, people with diabetes erupt in blisters. Diabetic blisters can occur on the backs of fingers, hands, toes, and feet and, sometimes, on legs or forearms.

These sores look like burn blisters. They sometimes are large. But they are painless and have no redness around them. They heal by themselves, usually without scars, in about three weeks. They often occur in people who have diabetic neuropathy. The only treatment is to bring glucose levels under control.

## Eruptive Xanthomatosis

Eruptive xanthomatosis is another condition caused by diabetes out of control. It consists of firm yellow pea-like enlargements in the skin. Each bump has a red halo and may itch. This condition occurs most often on the backs of hands, feet, arms, legs, and buttocks.

The disorder usually occurs in young men with type 1 diabetes. The person often has high levels of cholesterol and fat in the blood. Like diabetic blisters, these bumps disappear when diabetes control is restored.

## Digital Sclerosis

Sometimes, people with diabetes develop tight, thick, waxy skin on the backs of their hands. Sometimes skin on the toes and forehead also becomes thick. The finger joints become stiff and no longer can move the way they should. Rarely, knees, ankles, or elbows also get stiff.

This condition happens to about a third of people who have type 1 diabetes. The only treatment is to bring glucose levels under control.

## Disseminated Granuloma Annulare

In disseminated granuloma annulare, the person has sharply defined ring-shaped or arc-shaped raised areas on the skin. These rashes occur most often on parts of the body far from the trunk (for example, the fingers or ears). But sometimes the raised areas occur on the trunk. They can be red, red-brown, or skin colored.

See your doctor if you get rashes like this. There are drugs that can help clear up this condition.

## Acanthosis Nigricans

Acanthosis nigricans is a condition in which tan or brown raised areas appear on the sides of the neck, armpits, and groin. Sometimes they also occur on the hands, elbows, and knees.

Acanthosis nigricans usually strikes people who are very overweight. The best treatment is to lose weight. Some creams can help the spots look better.

## Good Skin Care

There are several things you can do to head off skin problems:

1. Keep your diabetes well controlled. People with high glucose levels tend to have dry skin and less ability to fend off harmful bacteria. Both conditions increase the risk of infection.

2. Keep skin clean and dry. Use talcum powder in areas where skin touches skin, such as armpits and groin.

3. Avoid very hot baths and showers. If your skin is dry, don't use bubble baths. Moisturizing soaps, such as Dove or Basis, may help. Afterward, use an oil-in-water skin cream, such as Lubriderm or Alpha-Keri. But don't put lotions between toes. The extra moisture there can encourage fungus to grow.

4. Prevent dry skin. Scratching dry or itchy skin can open it up and allow infection to set in. Moisturize your skin to prevent chapping, especially in cold or windy weather.

5. Treat cuts right away. Wash minor cuts with soap and water. Do not use Mercurochrome antiseptic, alcohol, or iodine to clean skin because they are too harsh. Only use an antibiotic cream or ointment if your doctor says it's okay. Cover minor cuts with sterile gauze. See a doctor right away if you get a major cut, burn, or infection.

6. During cold, dry months, keep your home more humid. Bathe less during this weather, if possible.

7. Use mild shampoos and unscented soaps. Do not use feminine hygiene sprays.

8. See a dermatologist (skin doctor) about skin problems if you are not able to solve them yourself.

9. Take good care of your feet. Check them every day for sores and cuts. Wear broad, flat shoes that fit well. Check your shoes for foreign objects before putting them on.

## Chapter 24

# Foot Care and Diabetes

### Why Your Feet Require Special Care

People with diabetes are at increased risk of serious foot problems. Foot disease is the most common diabetes complication leading to hospitalization. Major causes of foot disease are ulcers or sores on the feet or ankles caused by infection and minor injuries. Studies show that the prevalence of these problems increases with age, especially among persons whose diabetes was diagnosed before age 30. Starting preventive measures early is the best way to avoid trouble later.

#### *How Diabetes Affects the Feet*

If you have diabetes, your feet are more vulnerable to infection for any or all of the following reasons:

- *Decreased Circulation.* Diabetes can damage the walls of blood vessels, which reduces circulation to the lower legs and feet. If the foot is cut or injured in any way, healing may be slowed and infection risk increases.
- *Nerve Damage.* Diabetic neuropathy, or nerve damage, can make the feet feel numb—insensitive to hot or cold or pain. A

---

 The information in this chapter is not intended to take the place of medical advice. For guidance on topics discussed, consult your health care professional.

person with diabetes may not feel an injury to the foot and not be aware when an infection sets in.

- *Reduced Resistance to Infection.* When blood sugar is above normal, the white blood cells that fight infection do not work as they should. Therefore, bacteria and other organisms invade more rapidly and cause more damage.

### Prevention Is the Key

A person with diabetes should view all foot problems as potentially dangerous, take care to prevent foot problems whenever possible, and seek medical assistance as soon as problems occur. If you are the parent of a child with diabetes, be alert to the early signs of damage.

- In 1994, 67,000 people in the U.S. with diabetes had one or more amputations in their feet and legs.
- Prevention of foot problems and their proper treatment could have made amputation unnecessary in up to 50 percent of these cases.

The point is clear: Foot care makes a difference. Two people have major responsibility for preventing foot problems and treating them before they become serious: you and your doctor or health care provider.

## How to Take Care of Your Feet, Step-by-Step

- *Take care of your diabetes.* Work with your doctor to keep your blood sugar levels in a good range. A national study, the Diabetes Control and Complications Trial, has shown that improved blood sugar control reduces and slows the progression of nerve and vascular damage that can lead to serious foot problems.
- *Check your feet every day.* To prevent infection and identify trouble spots early, examine your bare feet every day for cuts, blisters, red spots, swelling, changes in the shape of your feet, color changes, hard or "hot" spots, and ingrown toenails. Use a mirror to check the bottom of your feet or (if you have trouble seeing) ask a family member for help. See your health care provider at the first sign of a problem.

- *Wash your feet every day*. Wash your feet in warm, not hot, water every day and dry them well, especially between the toes. Test the water temperature with your elbow before taking a bath to be sure it isn't too hot.

- *Keep the skin of your feet soft and smooth*. After drying, rub a thin coat of skin lotion or petroleum jelly over the tops and bottoms of your feet, but not between the toes. Use talcum powder to keep the skin between the toes dry.

- *Smooth corns and calluses gently*. Use a pumice stone to smooth corns and calluses after bathing; never use razors or cutting tools or do-it-yourself corn and callus plasters to remove them. If you have trouble with corns and calluses, check with your doctor or podiatrist (foot care specialist).

- *Trim your toenails each week or when needed*. Trim your toenails straight across and file the edges with an emery board or nail file. Don't cut into the corners. Toenails are easier to trim after bathing. If you can't see well or if your toenails are thick or yellowed, they should be trimmed by a podiatrist.

- *Wear shoes and socks at all times*. Never walk barefoot, even indoors. Choose comfortable shoes or slippers and always wear socks or stockings to help avoid blisters and sores. Choose socks made of cotton or wool to keep your feet dry and change your socks every day. Avoid tight legwear that might restrict circulation. Your shoes should fit well and protect your feet. Athletic or walking shoes made of canvas or leather are good for daily wear—they support your feet and allow them to "breathe." New shoes should be comfortable from the start and have enough room for your toes. Avoid shoes with pointed toes or high heels and shoes made of vinyl or plastic. Feel inside your shoes before putting them on to make sure the lining is smooth and there are no objects inside.

- *Protect your feet from hot and cold*. Wear shoes at the beach or on hot pavements. Put sunscreen on the tops of your feet to avoid sunburn, and check your feet often in cold weather for frostbite. Wear socks at night if your feet get cold; don't use heating pads or hot water bottles.

- *Keep the blood flowing to your feet.* Put your feet up when sitting and don't cross your legs for any period of time. Wiggle your toes and move your ankles up and down for five minutes, two or three times a day. Don't smoke—smoking constricts blood vessels—and, if you have high blood pressure or high cholesterol, work with your doctor to lower it.

- *Be more active.* Get involved with exercise, but be sure to check with your doctor first. If you have foot problems avoid activities that are hard on the feet such as running and jumping, and be sure to wear shoes that fit properly and provide good support.

- *Check with your doctor.* Ask your doctor to check the sense of feeling and pulses in your feet at least once a year and to tell you if you are likely to have serious foot problems. If so, your feet should be checked at every visit. Ask your doctor to refer you to a podiatrist if you need help caring for your feet. If you need special shoes or inserts and have Medicare Part B insurance, some of the costs may be covered. Your doctor or podiatrist can give you a prescription if you qualify.

- *Get started now.* Begin taking good care of your feet today. Here's a list of what you'll need: nail clippers, pumice stone, emery board, skin lotion, talcum powder, mirror, socks, athletic shoes, and slippers. Remember, daily foot care is your responsibility!

## The Role of Your Doctor

On your first visit, your doctor should examine your feet thoroughly. This is the first step in defining current problems and averting future ones. As part of the exam, your doctor should:

- Determine whether you have any diabetes complications.

- Ask you about foot or leg pain when sitting, standing, or walking.

- Physically examine your feet for any corns, calluses, bruises, ulcers, deformities, or any other problems.

- Check the pulse in your groin, behind your knees, and on top of your feet.

- Listen to the blood vessels in your legs with a stethoscope.
- Perform a sensory exam to check the response of your feet and toes to touch, vibrations, and pain.
- Check the kind of shoes you are wearing.

You are considered at high risk for developing severe foot problems and your feet should be examined at every visit if any examination shows you have one or more of the conditions listed below:

- No protective feeling in your feet
- No pulse in your feet
- A severe foot deformity
- A history of foot ulcer
- Prior amputation.

## Your Role

You have responsibilities, too.

- Make sure your doctor examines your feet annually. If you are at high risk for foot problems, your feet should be examined at every visit. If necessary, remove your shoes and socks to remind your doctor to examine your feet.
- Consult your doctor at the first sign of foot problems. Prompt attention could mean the difference between antibiotics and amputation.

*Prevention, detection, and proper treatment are key to avoiding serious foot problems. You and your doctor should work as a team. Together, you can make the difference.*

## Additional Information

The following Juvenile Diabetes Foundation International brochures provide additional information about the topics discussed in this chapter:

- What You Should Know About Diabetes
- Monitoring Your Blood Sugar

- Information About Insulin
- Oral Medications and Type 2 Diabetes

Juvenile Diabetes Foundation International
120 Wall Street
New York, NY 10005-4001
(800) JDF CURE
www.jdfcure.com

Chapter 25

# Overcoming Impotence

Impotence. Just mentioning the word can make the mightiest of men uncomfortable. But did you know that nearly 50% of all men with diabetes will develop it? That's the bad news. The good news is that nearly all men who suffer from impotence can be helped. Today, no one needs to simply endure it in silence.

This chapter will review how a normal erection occurs, the mechanisms that cause impotence in men with diabetes, and the simple diagnostic steps your doctor can use to determine the best treatment. And finally, we will look at the treatments currently available for this common, but devastating problem.

## What Causes a Normal Erection?

Think of a man's penis as a tire being inflated by an air compressor. To fill the tire with air, many conditions must be met. The compressor must be in good working order. It must be plugged into an energy source and the power switch must be on. The tubing from the compressor to the tire must be attached and unblocked, and the tire cannot have any leaks. If there is a problem with any one of these conditions, the tire will not fill with air. A similar series of complex,

---

 Appended section on Viagra from "FDA Approves Impotence Pill, Viagra," *Talk Paper*, U. S. Food and Drug Administration, March 27, 1998.

interconnected events is required to create an erection. When a man is aroused, his brain sends a message to the blood vessels supplying his penis to open up so that blood can rush in. His heart pumps in blood that fills the widened arteries and saturates the spaces between the muscle fibers. Meanwhile, the veins that normally allow blood to flow out of the penis close off. The blood becomes trapped and the penis becomes enlarged and hard. All this occurs under the influence of a hormone, testosterone, that is produced in the testicles.

## What Is Impotence?

Impotence is the inability to obtain and maintain an erection that is adequate for sexual intercourse. Of course, every man, if he is honest, can admit to an occasional failure in the bedroom. For example, if a man is fatigued, distracted by a problem at work, and has had a few drinks, he may have difficulty achieving an erection. But this occasional misfortune does not constitute a problem that requires medical attention. However, if a man notices the problem is getting progressively worse, and that he has more failures than successes, he needs to see a doctor for an evaluation and appropriate treatment.

Impotence can affect men in a variety of ways. Some men will complain that they cannot maintain an erection, some will complain they cannot get an erection at all, and others will notice that their penis does not get hard enough to sustain penetration. Many men will experience all three problems at one time or another. And all men with an impotence problem are frustrated that their erection is not predictable, as it was in their younger years.

## Why Does Diabetes Affect Impotence?

Just a few years ago, most cases of impotence were thought to be caused by psychological problems. "It's in your head," doctors told their patients. Today we know that in most men over 50, regardless of whether they have diabetes, impotence has physical roots. Nerve damage, narrowed blood vessels, hormone deficiencies, and the side effects of some drugs can all wreak havoc on the intricate machinery involved in creating an erection. And since diabetes appears to accelerate the aging process, impotence can often occur at a much younger age. Although men with diabetes have the same risk of developing impotence caused by emotional issues as the rest of the population, their impotence is usually brought on by physical factors.

According to many reports in the medical literature, 50% of all men with diabetes will develop an impotence problem within 10 years after their diabetes is diagnosed. In fact, it is not uncommon for diabetes to be first diagnosed when the man seeks help for impotence. Impotence affects men with Type I (insulin-dependent) and Type II (non-insulin-dependent) diabetes with equal frequency. And neither the severity of the diabetes nor the use of insulin, pills, or diet alone has any effect on whether impotence will occur. The only factors that are predictive for the development of impotence are age, the degree of blood glucose control, and the appearance of retinal disease or other neurological symptoms. High blood pressure also adds to the risk of impotence, possibly because the blood vessels throughout the body, including those that supply blood to the penis, become narrow.

In men under age 50 who do not have diabetes, impotence is often psychological in nature. For example, a man may suffer from fear of failure or performance anxiety. These fears can develop after he has had a few failures at intercourse. Eventually he becomes frightened that he will fail every time he tries to engage in sexual intercourse, so much so that the fear becomes a self-fulfilling prophecy and he does fail every time. Next, he accelerates the process by losing interest in sex and complaining of a lack of desire. Actually, he isn't experiencing a lack of desire at all, but a lack of interest. After all, who wants to stand at the plate and try to hit the ball if you're going to strike out every time you come to bat?

Unfortunately, diabetes is a major cause of impotence in men in their 20's and 30's. Diabetes causes impotence in two ways. First, hardening of the arteries is accelerated in diabetic men. As a result, blood flow to the penis is restricted. Second, nerve damage prevents the normal transmission of nerve impulses to the blood vessels in the penis. This complication is referred to as neuropathy, the same problem that can cause loss of sensation or pain in the legs, or difficulty with stomach emptying.

Drugs can also cause impotence. Certain drugs used to treat high blood pressure and various heart problems are the most common offenders. Examples of the cardiovascular drugs associated with the side effect of impotence include the thiazide diuretics, reserpine, spironolactone, propanolol, and methyldopa. No one knows for certain why these drugs produce impotence. One idea is that the drug interrupts the normal transmission of information from the nerves to the blood vessels that are responsible for dilating and increasing the blood flow to the penis. The cardiovascular drugs that are least likely to produce impotence are the angiotensin-converting enzyme (ACE) inhibitors, and the calcium channel blockers. Other drugs that can affect a man's ability to have an erection include sedatives, tranquilizers, and pain killers. In many cases, if a drug is causing the problem, your doctor can either decrease the dose or substitute a different class of drug that is equally effective but does not cause impotence.

Aggravating factors that can also affect a man's erection include smoking, drinking alcohol, and using illegal drugs such as marijuana and cocaine. In most instances alcohol and illicit drugs will impair a man's erection only temporarily. However, long-standing alcohol abuse, which also results in severe liver damage, can cause permanent impotence.

Smoking tobacco—even just 2 cigarettes before sex—will also affect a man's erection. Tobacco is thought to constrict the blood vessels to the penis and to promote narrowing of the blood vessels. Smokers are found to be impotent twice as often as nonsmokers of the same age. Often, just making a man aware of this statistic is enough to convince him to give up cigarettes.

## Testing for Impotence

A large number of tests are available to pinpoint the exact cause of impotence. For the vast majority of men with diabetes, extensive testing is not necessary. The evaluation consists of a medical history, a physical examination, a blood test, and one or two other tests that can be done in the office or in the privacy of the man's home. The blood test measures the level of testosterone. Although this is not a common cause of impotence in men with diabetes, it is a simple test with an easy treatment, so it makes sense to check.

The next test determines whether or not a vascular problem is causing the impotence. The doctor injects a drug, usually papaverine, phentolamine, or prostaglandin, directly into the penis to stimulate the blood vessels to dilate. This injection tests the blood supply to the penis and the ability of the veins to trap the blood in the penis to allow the penis to fill with blood and become firm enough for intercourse.

If these two tests can't make the diagnosis or if there is a chance the impotence has psychological roots, a nocturnal penile tumescence test (NPT) can be performed. This test is based on the fact that a man normally has three to five involuntary erections during the night, each lasting 20 to 30 minutes. By using the NPT test, the presence or absence of these nighttime erections can be determined.

The test consists of two ribbons or strings that are placed around the base and tip of the penis when the man prepares to go to sleep.

These are attached to a small computer box at the bedside. The test is usually done for two consecutive nights. If a man has nighttime erections, the penis increases in length and girth, and these changes are recorded in the computer. If a man experiences normal erections in his sleep, it is safe to assume that the nerves, hormones, and blood vessels are functioning properly; in other words, the cause is most likely psychological in origin, and a referral to a counselor or sex therapist is in order. The absence of nighttime erections confirms that the problem is due to physical causes. However, the NPT test is often unnecessary. In most situations the history, physical exam, the blood test, and the injection of the drugs into the penis can determine if the problem is due to physical or psychological causes.

## What Are the Treatments?

Back when the prevailing wisdom was that impotence was just a natural part of aging, or a symptom of psychological troubles, little beyond a session with the psychiatrist was offered for treatment. Today however, there are a number of successful treatments that can help nearly every man with diabetes achieve an erection that is adequate for sexual intercourse.

### *Vacuum Constriction Therapy*

The easiest and least expensive treatment is the vacuum constriction device. This simple device can fill the penis with blood to create a natural erection without surgery. It works by creating a vacuum, that is, negative pressure around the penis, so that blood will rush in to fill the vascular chambers. To achieve this effect, the man places his penis inside a plastic cylinder and removes the air from the chamber with either a manual or electric pump. The man can then trap the blood inside his penis using a special elastic band before removing the vacuum chamber.

This technique has been used successfully by thousands of men for the long-term treatment of impotence. It is easily available, can be used frequently, and does not require medicine or surgery. In addition, the vacuum constriction device is relatively inexpensive ($170 to $450) and in most states, it is reimbursed by Medicare.

Like all treatments, vacuum constriction devices do have some disadvantages. The elastic band can only be left in place for up to 30 minutes. Since the ring acts like a tourniquet to stop the blood flow, leaving it on too long can cause tissue damage. The penis can become cold, too, which may feel unpleasant for some men or their partners. Also, ejaculation may be painful if the elastic band is applied too tightly. Finally, the vacuum constriction device can be cumbersome and can detract from the spontaneity of sex.

Vacuum constriction devices can be purchased through several mail-order catalogs or from a physician. The advantage of buying the device from a doctor is that he can fit the man properly and provide instructions for using it. However, most devices come with excellent written instructions, and several come with videos that show the proper use of the device.

### *Injection Therapy*

This approach is one of the most popular methods of treating impotence in diabetic men. The man simply injects a small amount of medicine directly into the shaft of his penis, using a tiny needle (27 gauge). The drug dilates the arteries and increases the overall blood flow through the penis to create a natural and rigid erection, with only minimal discomfort from the injection. The erection usually occurs within 10 minutes and lasts 30 to 45 minutes. Injection therapy works in approximately 70% of men who select this method of treatment.

Before beginning injection therapy, it is very important to determine the exact amount of medicine to inject. To find the proper dosage, a urologist administers a series of test injections. During the testing procedure, the man is instructed on how to give himself sterile injections.

Several drugs are available for self-injection therapy. Tri-mix, which contains a combination of papaverine, phentolamine, and prostaglandin, is used most often. By using this triple-drug therapy, the dose of each drug can be reduced, resulting in a good erection with few, if any complications.

The most common complication is priapism, a sustained, painful erection that will not become soft or flaccid. This is considered a medical emergency and the man must return to his doctor or go to an emergency room and have another drug injected into the penis to reverse the effect of Tri-mix. This complication only occurs in a few men who use the injection therapy, and it is less likely if the proper dose of medication is used. However, if the priapism is left untreated, the end result can be a scarred penis that is incapable of any further erections. Other complications are a slight bruising and discoloration of the skin at the injection site and the development of scar tissue inside the penis. Scar formation can be reduced by alternating the injection sites similar to alternating the sites on the abdomen or thighs for insulin injections. In the past, scar formation occurred more frequently when only papaverine was used as a treatment. Since the amount of papaverine is reduced in Tri-mix, scar formation is less of a problem. Finally, men who take monoamine oxidase inhibitors (used to treat high blood pressure and as a tranquilizer) should not use injection therapy because the treatment could raise blood pressure to extremely dangerous levels.

Although none of these drugs are approved by the Federal Drug Administration (FDA) for the specific purpose of creating an erection, they have been used successfully by thousands of men who are impotent. Most men are very satisfied with the results and are willing to take the small risks associated with their use. The advantages are that they produce results almost immediately, they are inexpensive ($3.00 to $5.00 for each injection), and do not require any surgery. At the present time, injection therapy is not reimbursed by Medicare or most other insurance companies. (Editor's note: The Upjohn Company has applied for FDA approval on a drug to be used in injection therapy. If approval is granted, this may change reimbursement policies.)

### *Penile Implants*

Finally, if all else fails, you may want to consider penile implants. This procedure requires surgery and is quite expensive ($12,000 to $15,000). However, the erection is more natural and less cumbersome than those from injection therapy or vacuum devices. The success rate is approximately 85% and most insurance companies will pay for the operation if the impotence has organic causes. Two companies that make penile implants, American Medical Systems and Mentor Corporation, offer a life-time guarantee on the prosthesis. If the device fails, for whatever reason, they will replace it without charge. If the implant is removed, usually for infection, the man can still use a vacuum device after he has recovered from surgery.

### *Other Options*

There are many other treatments for impotence, although they are not as applicable to men who have diabetes. These treatments include yohimbine, testosterone injections, and vascular surgery.

Yohimbine is an extract from the bark of an African tree that is effective in 15% to 20% of men who have impotence that is psychological in origin or of unknown cause. Hormone replacement therapy with testosterone is only effective in men with severe testosterone deficiency. It is rarely effective in men with normal hormone levels and it should be avoided by all men with a history of prostate cancer or heart, kidney, or liver disease. Testosterone can be administered through an intramuscular injection every 2 to 3 weeks or through skin patches worn on the scrotum. These patches must be changed every day to be effective. Although they are inconvenient to use, they have the advantage of providing a constant level of medicine.

Trazodone is an antidepressant medication that has been observed to cause prolonged erections in some patients who take it for emotional problems. The drug has been used in small doses to treat impotence and has been used in combination with yohimbine. It may improve the quality of the erection in a small number of cases. However, there are no reported studies of the efficacy of Trazodone in impotent men with diabetes.

Vascular bypass surgery and venous ligation (tying off or removing abnormal veins) are surgical procedures that are similar in technical complexity to heart bypass operations. However, they are not as risky as heart bypass operations. Still, only a small number of men are candidates for these types of surgery. Most diabetic men cannot have vascular bypasses because the diabetes affects the tiny blood vessels in the penis. The techniques of performing this surgery on the small blood vessels in the penis are improving, but available data demonstrate that only 20% of the operations are successful, and even the successes fail in two years after the surgery.

## What's on the Horizon?

A tremendous amount of research is being done in the area of impotence. In the near future drugs will be available that can be inserted into the end or the tip of the urethra (the tube that transports urine from the bladder to the outside of the body) just before intercourse, patches that can be applied on the penis that will deliver the drugs into the penis without an injection, and even a pill that a man can take that will increase the blood supply to the penis.

One treatment option that is currently being evaluated is nitroglycerin paste. This paste would be applied to the skin of the penis just before intercourse. The problem with this drug is that it can cause headaches as it is absorbed into the man's vascular system—not the best prelude to an evening of romance. In addition, the drug can affect the man's partner, so he may have to wear a condom.

Minoxidil cream, which would be used similarly to the way nitroglycerin paste is applied, is another option that is currently under investigation. So far, researchers report that minoxidil cream produces a better erection with fewer side effects than nitroglycerin paste.

To date, no pill has been found to be totally effective in improving erections. Papaverine tablets are currently being investigated, but they are not yet ready for clinical testing. A painkiller called apomorphine is also being researched. Unfortunately, although 8 out of 12 men who took the drug in a trial developed erections, many of the men also suffered the rather unromantic side effect of nausea. [Note: The first oral pill to treat impotence, Viagra (sildenafil citrate), was approved by the FDA on March 27, 1998. Additional information about Viagra can be found at the end of this chapter.]

Several years ago, a report in *The New England Journal of Medicine* mentioned that nitrous oxide was identified as "the neurotransmitter responsible for erection." Many men were under the impression that the same nitrous oxide used by the dentist to reduce the pain associated with dental work was the magic pill or gas that could restore a man's erection. But the report only indicated that minute amounts of nitrous oxide are necessary to transmit the message from the nerves to the tissue in the penis that open up and allow more blood to enter the penis. Although this is an important research finding, it does not currently have any applicability to treating the problem of impotence.

## Getting Help

Admitting that you have a problem with impotence, even to your doctor, can be embarrassing and difficult. But with all the treatment options available, there is no need to suffer in silence. Contact your family doctor or the endocrinologist who treats your diabetes and ask for a referral to a urologist who specializes in treating impotence.

If you prefer more anonymity, you can also contact the Impotence Institute of America (1-800-669-1603) or the Impotence Foundation (1-800-221-5517) and they will provide you with a name of a doctor in your area who specializes in impotence. These organizations, which have over 100 chapters throughout the United States, also have support groups for impotent men and their partners. These groups usually meet each month and provide a forum for people to discuss their different ways of coping with impotence. They also address the emotional effects of impotence on the man and his partner. These meetings provide reassurance in a positive but serious setting. Usually they are conducted by a urologist and a mental-health professional. Often, several members who have already sought treatment for impotence are available to share their experiences. There is no question that sharing experiences helps many to overcome their fear and loss of self-esteem. Often, men feel confident enough to seek treatment after attending a meeting.

Above all, support groups let men and their partners know that it is okay to feel the way that they do and that they are not the only ones who have this problem. Part of the battle with impotence is the resulting depression and feeling of hopelessness. Sharing their thoughts and experiences in support groups, as well as national media attention to the condition, has helped millions of men realize that the problem is not "all in your head."

At the present time, many treatment options are available for men who suffer from impotence. Contact your doctor or one of the support groups and start to reverse this very treatable problem. Today, no one needs to suffer in silence any longer.

## Where to Go for Help

Several foundations can offer advice, doctor recommendations, and support services for impotent men and their partners.

**Impotence Institute of America**
P.O. Box 6020
Santa Barbara, CA 93160
1-800-669-1603 (Impotence Anonymous hotline)

**The Impotence Foundation**
2020 Pennsylvania Avenue, N.W., Suite 292
Washington, D.C. 20006
1-800-221-5517

To read more about impotence, check out these publications:

*Ecnetopmi Impotence—It's Reversible*, by Dr. Steve Wilson and Dr. Neil Baum. (The Impotence Foundation of New Orleans, New Orleans, Louisiana, 1992); for a copy, call 1-504-883-6090

*Men's Health Advisor*, by Michael Lafavore. (Rodale Press, Emmaus, Pennsylvania, 1995)

*The Male*, by Dr. Sherman Silber. (Scribners, New York, 1981)

### Vacuum Constriction Devices

To learn more about vacuum constriction devices, contact the following manufacturers for information and brochures.

- Encore, Inc. (1-800-221-6603)
- Mentor Corporation (1-800-235-5731)
- Mission Pharmacal Company (1-800-531-3333 and in Texas 1-800-292-7364)
- Osbon Medical Systems, Ltd. (1-800-438-8592)
- Pos-T-Vac (1-800-279-7434)
- Vet-co (1-800-827-8382)

*—by Neil Baum, MD*

Dr. Neil Baum is a Clinical Assistant Professor of Urology at Tulane Medical School and Louisiana State University Medical School and a urologist in private practice in New Orleans, Louisiana.

## FDA Approves Impotence Pill, Viagra

On March 27, 1998, the Food and Drug Administration announced the approval of Viagra (sildenafil citrate), the first oral pill to treat impotence, a dysfunction that affects millions of men in the United States.

Unlike previously approved treatments for impotence, Viagra does not directly cause penile erections, but affects the response to sexual stimulation. The drug acts by enhancing the smooth muscle relaxant effects of nitric oxide, a chemical that is normally released in response to sexual stimulation. This smooth muscle relaxation allows increased blood flow into certain areas of the penis leading to an erection.

Viagra was evaluated in numerous randomized, placebo controlled trials involving more than 3000 men with varying degrees of impotence associated with diabetes, spinal cord injury, history of prostate surgery, and no identifiable organic cause of impotence. Patients also had a wide range of other concomitant illnesses including hypertension and coronary artery disease.

The drug's effectiveness was assessed primarily using a sexual function questionnaire. Patients were asked to report at the beginning, and periodically throughout the studies, how often they were able to achieve an erection adequate for intercourse, and how often that erection was maintained after penetration. In addition, patients kept diaries of their sexual histories. In all trials, men on Viagra reported success more often than did men on placebo, and rates of success increased with dose. The findings were consistent in men representing a wide range of severity and etiology of their erectile dysfunction (impotence). Men with diabetes or radical prostate surgery had somewhat less improvement than did other groups.

The recommended dose is 50mg taken one hour before sexual activity; individuals may need more (100mg) or less (25 mg) and dosing should be determined by a physician depending on effectiveness and side effects. The drug should not be used more than once a day.

The most common side effects reported in clinical trials included headache, flushing, and indigestion, which occurred at a slightly higher rate in patients taking the drug than among those taking placebo. Some patients on Viagra (about 3 percent) also reported changes in vision, principally altered color perception.

The drug should not be used with organic nitrates such as nitroglycerin patches or sublingual tablets because the combination may lower blood pressure. The safety and efficacy of using Viagra with other treatments for impotence has not been studied, and the use of such combinations is not recommended.

Viagra confers no resistance to AIDS or other sexually transmitted diseases.

Before taking Viagra, patients are advised to:

- Have a thorough medical history and physical examination to diagnose impotence, determine underlying causes and identify appropriate treatment, and
- Discuss the cardiac risk associated with sexual activity prior to initiating any treatment for impotence.

Viagra is manufactured by Pfizer Pharmaceuticals, New York, NY. The product was approved by FDA in less than six months after submission. The FDA's clinical review of the studies, approval letter and labeling can be found on the internet at http://www.fda.gov/cder/news/viagra.htm.

# Chapter 26

# *Raising a Child with Diabetes*

Raising a child, with or without diabetes, is never easy. Diabetes doesn't change the basics of parenting. However, it adds new challenges at every stage, from birth to the teenage years.

Remember, diabetes is only one part of your child's life. Most often, families do better if they try to fit diabetes into their lifestyles rather than fitting their lifestyles around diabetes.

Do not let diabetes run your life. It's all too easy to use diabetes as an excuse. Bobby wants to sleep over at a friend's house. A nervous Dad doesn't want him to go. When Bobby asks why, Dad can't think of a good answer. "Your blood sugar was too high tonight," he says.

Dad is using diabetes to solve another problem. Children learn by example. Later on Bobby may start to use diabetes as an easy excuse or a way to get special treatment.

The problems diabetes poses will change as your child grows and matures. This chapter gives some basics. Many other resources provide detailed information on each of these topics and more.

You might try talking to your child's health care team, reading books and articles, calling your local American Diabetes Association chapter, taking a parenting course, or joining or starting a parents' support group.

As your child grows, he or she will have questions about diabetes. You will learn along with your child, and you will share what you learn. Your goal is to instill knowledge and a positive attitude in your child.

---

These tools will prepare your child for diabetes self-care. You want to ensure that your child is healthy, both mentally and physically. This doesn't always mean perfect blood glucose levels. It means doing the best you can at each age and stage.

## Infants and Toddlers

Children under age two are too young to know why they need fingersticks and insulin shots. They may think that sticks or shots are a sign of anger or punishment. They also pick up their parents' worries. Seeing an upset parent can frighten a baby or toddler.

To help your child adjust to diabetes care, be calm. Let diabetes care be as normal as giving a bottle. Things will go more smoothly if you get all the supplies ready ahead of time.

Do the stick and shot quickly and gently. Hold the child gently but securely. Say something soothing, like, "It's time for your insulin. This keeps you healthy."

Comfort and reassure your child afterward. Hold your toddler closely with a special blanket or stuffed animal.

## Preschool Children

At age 3 and 4, children have very imaginative ideas about how their bodies work and heal. For example, they may think that taking drops of blood from the finger will cause them to lose all their blood. Having trouble getting a big enough drop of blood for a test strip may seem to prove this notion.

Children of all ages have a hard time understanding how and why illness happens. They may think that they caused diabetes. Children also have a hard time sensing low blood glucose and understanding why it happens.

Explain diabetes-related tasks in simple terms, and do this often. "Nothing you did made you get diabetes," you might say. "You don't get sick because you did something bad."

Help your child learn how to recognize low blood glucose. Try pretending you are having a reaction, so your child can see the signs and symptoms. Show your child cartoon pictures of what it feels like to have a reaction. Name the symptoms when you spot them in your child. Say, for example, "You're shaky. You are having a low blood glucose reaction."

Work closely with your child's health care team. Parents must learn to balance the demands of diabetes care against the normal needs of any growing child.

"Acceptable" diabetes control is not always "perfect" control. Your health care team can help you devise flexible rules and guidelines. Also talk to the parents of other children with diabetes. Chances are they are working through the same problems.

## Children Five to Twelve

Through elementary school, children often adapt well to diabetes, especially right off the bat. They are at the peak of their desire to learn new things. They do not easily envision the future.

Later on, children may feel that diabetes care takes too much time. Because they compare themselves with their peers, they come to see that diabetes makes special, tough demands. They begin to realize that diabetes will never go away.

You can help by slowly letting your child take on diabetes care tasks. By encouraging the child's gradual involvement in self-care, you let the child know that in the future you will expect him or her to take most of the responsibility. Of course, you also need to show that you will be there to help.

Let your child's maturity, skills, and interests guide you. No school-aged child should be expected to take on all, or even most, of diabetes self-care. Some limited rewards for your child's involvement may be a good idea.

A child will often want to "do it myself" when there is a benefit such as being allowed to spend the night at a friend's house.

As your child takes on more responsibility for diabetes self-care, don't expect perfection. Make it easier by leaving reminders. Set the insulin on the kitchen table, for example. Use simple encouragements, but avoid lectures.

While there are no vacations from diabetes care, you can give your child a breathing spell if you are creative. Talk to the health care team about ways to work in splurges from time to time. Ask about how to handle special events such as overnight trips and birthday parties.

Share some of the chores of diabetes self-care. Maybe you can give your child the morning shot and your child can do the evening one. Chore charts can help. When your child does a task, draw a star. Set up game rules that lead to a small reward.

## The Teen Years

Teenagers are changing physically and emotionally. They worry about being different, they test limits, and they make choices and mistakes. Priorities change, and diabetes is often low on the list. Teens often rebel against their parents' rules, so they may take serious risks with their health.

You can help your teen through this time by being honest, sensitive, and supportive. Teens need to learn about making decisions and living with the outcome. To make good decisions, they need the facts about diabetes. They need to know how the choices they make about diabetes will affect them. Topics of special concern for teens are:

1. How to reduce the risk of short-term and long-term complications.
2. Alcohol and drug use and abuse.
3. Social and sexual relationships.

Your teen's health care team can provide some of this information. Teen support groups and diabetes camps may also help.

Watch your own actions and feelings. Know the difference between being supportive and being nagging. Don't try to take over if there are a few days of high blood glucose levels.

Instead, try to solve the problem together and ask your teen how you can help. Be patient, honest, and consistent, though flexible.

Keep clear lines of communication open. Share your feelings; when things are going well, praise your teen for good judgement. When things are rough, recognize your teen's frustrations.

## Third Parties

It's a great challenge to work with your child on diabetes care. What about the other people who take care of your child? You will need to work with them, too: babysitters, teachers, and coaches. The more they know about diabetes, the better they can watch out for your child.

**Babysitters.** Even if you find an experienced, mature sitter, you may worry about how he or she will handle diabetes care. Having someone else watch your child need not be stressful if you know that your child and your sitter know enough about diabetes.

Help educate your sitter about diabetes. You may even want to arrange for him or her to take a diabetes education class.

Leave a clear list of instructions for the sitter. The brochure, A Word to Teachers and Child-Care Providers, available from the American Diabetes Association, has a sample checklist. The list should include:

1. A simple definition of diabetes.
2. The symptoms of an insulin reaction, particularly those your child tends to show.
3. How to treat low blood glucose in your child.
4. What to do if the reaction keeps up 10 to 15 minutes after it's treated.
5. A list of approved snacks and off-limits foods.
6. Telephone numbers for you, the doctor, and perhaps a neighbor or friend who will be home.

If your sitter will be giving a shot, be sure to plan ahead. Arrange a time well in advance of the date you'll go out so that you can teach your sitter in a relaxed setting. To make things easier, you could consider prefilling your child's syringe.

If your sitter will need to do a blood test, also arrange to teach the testing method ahead of time. Write down the times and situations when you want your child to test.

With some careful thought and planning, you can make leaving your child with the babysitter easier and safer for everyone.

**The school.** Your role in talking to the staff of your child's school depends, of course, on your child's age.

The parent of a first grader plays a different role than the parent of a high school student. If you are the parent of a teen, your child will probably want to assume more of the responsibility of talking to teachers or coaches.

Although parents are responsible for informing the adults in a school setting about diabetes, children have the right to choose which peers they tell and how they tell them.

Before the start of the school year, plan a friendly, relaxed meeting with the school staff. You may want to get advice from your health care team about what topics to cover and how to present them. Talk in an upbeat, positive way.

The meeting with the school staff should include the school nurse, teachers, the principal, and any other adults who supervise your child, such as bus drivers and extended day staff.

Teachers, not the school nurse, will most often be the first ones to observe symptoms of low blood glucose in your child. Because exercise can change blood glucose levels, be sure that the gym teacher and/or coach attend. Give the same information to everyone during the meeting:

1. A brief, simple explanation of diabetes.
2. A list of the signs of low blood glucose.
3. Steps for treating low blood glucose.
4. Other information, depending on the age of your child (snack and meal times, foods to avoid, special precautions).

Make sure that the school personnel know that your child has diabetes but is not to be labeled as “diabetic”. Federal law requires that school districts provide certain “aids and services” for any child to be able to fully participate in an education program.

Regulations based on Section 504 of the Federal Rehabilitation Act of 1973 say that children are entitled to “participate fully and without discrimination” in school programs. Children with diabetes must not be separated from their peers more than needed.

This also means that schools must provide health services that the child needs during the day if they can be given by a qualified school nurse or other trained person.

For example, giving medication and testing blood for glucose are services prescribed by a doctor, but they can be provided by a school nurse or other responsible adult.

You may worry about how peers will accept your child’s diabetes. Keep in mind that other children will tend to take their cues about diabetes from your child’s attitude. If your child accepts diabetes, most friends will too.

Some children are embarrassed about having diabetes. Teachers can help by giving support—not by increasing restrictions. If a teacher senses that a child is having trouble coping with diabetes, he or she and the school counselor can suggest more help.

Your local ADA chapter or parents’ support group may also provide names of counselors with experience working with children with diabetes. If a problem comes up, get help early on rather than waiting for it to become serious.

When you, your child, and the school staff have done their homework, your child will be able to enjoy school to the fullest, without undue worry or restriction.

## How to Explain Low Blood Glucose

Any adult who spends time with your child should know something about low blood glucose, or hypoglycemia. When the amount of insulin injected is too much for the food or exercise your child has gotten that day, low blood glucose often follows.

Most times, low blood glucose levels in children cause only mild symptoms that are easy to spot: shakiness, sweating, nervousness, or drowsiness. Children with a mild reaction get better quickly after having a snack that has sugar, such as juice, milk, or raisins.

For a more serious reaction, you will be better able to cope if you plan ahead. Write down the situations that worry you. Go through the list with your doctor or nurse educator; ask all the "what ifs" you can think of. Talk to your child's dietitian about good snack choices.

You may want to ask your health care team:

1. What if my child has a seizure from low blood glucose?
2. Why doesn't my child know when her blood glucose is going low?
3. How can I prevent her from getting low blood glucose during or after hard exercise?
4. What can I do to avoid low blood glucose when my child is asleep?
5. What should I do after the reaction?

Keeping good records of blood test results is the best way to learn what's going on with diabetes care. Discussing these records with your child's health care team puts this important information to work for your child's health.

Be sure to let the pediatrician know if your child has had a severe insulin reaction. You may need to change the treatment plan.

## Loving Care

At times, the challenges of diabetes care can seem endless as you try to maintain adequate control while continuing a normal family life.

Take things step by step, and get support from your health care team, your child's school, and other parents who share your concerns. Diabetes is about the health of your child. Don't let it control the happiness of your family.

# Part Four

# The Role of Diet and Exercise in Diabetes Management

# Chapter 27

# *Nutrition Recommendations and Principles for People with Diabetes Mellitus*

Medical nutrition therapy is integral to total diabetes care and management. Although adherence to nutrition and meal planning principles is one of the most challenging aspects of diabetes care, nutrition therapy is an essential component of successful diabetes management.

Achieving nutrition-related goals requires a coordinated team effort that includes the person with diabetes. Because of the complexity of nutrition issues, it is recommended that a registered dietitian, knowledgeable and skilled in implementing current principles and recommendations for diabetes, be a member of the treatment team.

Effective self-management training requires an individualized approach, appropriate for the personal lifestyle and diabetes management goals of the individual with diabetes. Monitoring of glucose and glycated hemoglobin, lipids, blood pressure, and renal status is essential to evaluate nutrition-related outcomes. If goals are not met, changes must be made in the overall diabetes care and management plan.

Nutrition assessment is used to determine what the individual with diabetes is able and willing to do. A major consideration is the likelihood of adherence to nutrition recommendations. To facilitate adherence, sensitivity to cultural, ethnic, and financial considerations is of prime importance.

---

This text reflects scientific nutrition and diabetes knowledge as of 1994. However, there are limited published data for some recommendations and, under these circumstances, recommendations are based on clinical experiences and consensus. This position paper is based on the concurrent technical review paper, which discusses published research and issues that remain unresolved[1].

## Goals of Medical Nutrition Therapy

Although the overall goal of nutrition therapy is to assist people with diabetes in making changes in nutrition and exercise habits leading to improved metabolic control, there are additional specific goals.

1. Maintenance of as near-normal blood glucose levels as possible by balancing food intake with insulin (either endogenous or exogenous) or oral glucose-lowering medications and activity levels.

2. Achievement of optimal serum lipid levels.

3. Provision of adequate calories for maintaining or attaining reasonable weights for adults, normal growth and development rates in children and adolescents, increased metabolic needs during pregnancy and lactation, or recovery from catabolic illnesses. Reasonable weight is defined as the weight an individual and health care provider acknowledge as achievable and maintainable, both short- and long-term. This may not be the same as the traditionally defined desirable or ideal body weight.

4. Prevention and treatment of the acute complications of insulin-treated diabetes such as hypoglycemia, short-term illnesses, and exercise-related problems, and of the long-term complications of diabetes such as renal disease, autonomic neuropathy, hypertension, and cardiovascular disease.

5. Improvement of overall health through optimal nutrition. *Dietary Guidelines for Americans*[2] and the *Food Guide Pyramid*[3] summarize and illustrate nutritional guidelines and nutrient needs for all healthy Americans, and can be used by people with diabetes and their family members.

## Nutrition Therapy and Type I Diabetes

A meal plan based on the individual's usual food intake should be determined and used as a basis for integrating insulin therapy into the usual eating and exercise patterns. It is recommended that individuals using insulin therapy eat at consistent times synchronized with the time-action of the insulin preparation used. Further, individuals need to monitor blood glucose levels and adjust insulin doses for the amount of food usually eaten. Intensified insulin therapy, such as multiple daily injections or use of an insulin pump, allows considerable flexibility in when and what individuals eat. With intensified therapy, insulin regimens should be integrated with lifestyle and adjusted for deviations from usual eating and exercise habits.

## Nutrition Therapy and Type II Diabetes

The emphasis for medical nutrition therapy in type II diabetes should be placed on achieving glucose, lipid, and blood pressure goals. Weight loss and hypocaloric diets usually improve short-term glycemic levels and have the potential to increase long-term metabolic control. However, traditional dietary strategies, and even very-low calorie diets, have usually not been effective in achieving long-term weight loss; therefore, emphasis should be placed instead on glucose and lipid goals. Although weight loss is desirable, and some individuals are able to lose and maintain weight loss, several additional strategies can be implemented to improve metabolic control. There is no one proven strategy or method that can be uniformly recommended.

An initial strategy is improvement in food choices, as illustrated by *Dietary Guidelines for Americans* and the *Food Guide Pyramid*. A nutritionally adequate meal plan with a reduction of total fat, especially saturated fats, can be employed. Spacing meals (spreading nutrient intake throughout the day) is another strategy that can be adopted. Mild to moderate weight loss (5-10 kg [10-20 pounds]) has been shown to improve diabetes control, even if desirable body weight is not achieved. Weight loss is best attempted by a moderate decrease in calories and an increase in caloric expenditure. Moderate caloric restriction (250-500 calories less than average daily intake) is recommended.

Regular exercise and learning new behaviors and attitudes can help facilitate long-term lifestyle changes. Monitoring blood glucose levels, glycated hemoglobin, lipids, and blood pressure is essential. However, if metabolic control has not improved after employment of better nutrition and regular exercise, an oral glucose-lowering medication or insulin may be needed.

Many individuals with refractory obesity may have limited success with the above strategies. Newer pharmacological agents, i.e., the serotonergic appetite suppressants, as well as gastric reduction surgery (for people with a body mass index >35 kg/M[2]), May prove to be potentially beneficial to this group. Studies on the long-term efficacy and safety of these methods are, however, unavailable.

## Protein

There is limited scientific data upon which to establish firm nutritional recommendations for protein intake for individuals with diabetes. At the present time, there is insufficient evidence to support protein intakes either higher or lower than average protein intake for the general population. For people with diabetes, this translates into ~10-20% of the daily caloric intake from protein. Dietary protein should be derived from both animal and vegetable sources.

With the onset of nephropathy, lower intakes of protein should be considered. A protein intake similar to the adult Recommended Dietary Allowance (0.8 g.kg body $wt^{-1}$ $day^{-1}$), ~10% of daily calories, is sufficiently restrictive and is recommended for individuals with evidence of nephropathy.

## Total Fat

If dietary protein contributes 10-20% of the total caloric content of the diet, then 80-90% of calories remain to be distributed between dietary fat and carbohydrate. Less than 10% of these calories should be from saturated fats and up to 10% calories from polyunsaturated fats, leaving 60-70% of the total calories from monounsaturated fats and carbohydrates. The distribution of calories from fat and carbohydrate can vary and be individualized based on the nutrition assessment and treatment goals.

The recommended percentage of calories from fat is dependent on desired glucose, lipid, and weight outcomes. For individuals who have normal lipid levels and maintain a reasonable weight (and for normal growth and development in children and adolescents) the *Dietary Guidelines for Americans* recommendations of 30% or less of the calories from total fat and <10% of calories from saturated fat can be implemented.

If obesity and weight loss are the primary issues, a reduction in dietary fat intake is an efficient way to reduce caloric intake and weight, particularly when combined with exercise.

If elevated low-density lipoprotein (LDL) cholesterol is the primary problem, the National Cholesterol Education Program Step II diet guidelines, in which <7% of total calories are from saturated fat, 30% or fewer of the calories are from total fat, and dietary cholesterol is <200 mg/day, should be implemented.

If elevated triglycerides and very low density lipoprotein cholesterol are the primary problems, one approach that may be beneficial, other than weight loss and increased physical activity, is a moderate increase in monounsaturated fat intake, With <10% of calories each from saturated and polyunsaturated fats, monounsaturated fats up to 20% of calories, and a more moderate intake of carbohydrate. However, in obese individuals, the increase in fat intake may perpetuate or aggravate the obesity. In addition, patients with triglyceride levels >1,000 mg/dl may require reduction of all types of dietary fat to reduce levels of plasma dietary fat in the form of chylomicrons.

Monitoring glycemic and lipid status and body weight, on any diet, is essential to asses the effectiveness of the nutrition recommendations.

## Saturated Fat and Cholesterol

A reduction in saturated fat and cholesterol consumption is an important goal to reduce the risk of cardiovascular disease (CVD). Diabetes is a strong independent risk factor for CVD, over and above the adverse effects of an elevated serum cholesterol. Therefore, <10% of the daily calories should be from saturated fats, and dietary cholesterol should be limited to 300 mg or less daily. However, even these recommendations must be incorporated with consideration of an individual's cultural and ethnic background.

Polyunsaturated fat of the omega-3 series are provided naturally in fish and other seafood, and the intake of these foods need not be curtailed in people with diabetes mellitus.

## Carbohydrate and Sweeteners

The percentage of calories from carbohydrate will also vary, and is individualized based on the patient's eating habits and glucose and lipid goals. For most of this century, the most widely held belief about the dietary treatment of diabetes has been that "simple" sugars should be avoided and replaced with complex carbohydrates. This belief appears to be based on the assumption that sugars are more rapidly digested and absorbed than are starches and thereby aggravate hyperglycemia to a greater degree. There is, however, very little scientific evidence that supports this assumption. Fruits and milk have been shown to have a lower glycemic response than most starches, and sucrose produces a glycemic response similar to that of bread, rice, and potatoes. Although various starches do have different glycemic responses, from a clinical perspective first priority should be given to the total amount of carbohydrate consumed rather than the source of the carbohydrate.

### Sucrose

Scientific evidence has shown that the use of sucrose as part of the meal plan does not impair blood glucose control in individuals with type I or type II diabetes. Sucrose and sucrose-containing foods must be substituted for other carbohydrates and foods and not simply added to the meal plan. In making such substitutions, the nutrient content of concentrated sweets and sucrose-containing foods, as well as the presence of other nutrients frequently ingested with sucrose such as fat, must be considered.

### Fructose

Dietary fructose produces a smaller rise in plasma glucose than isocaloric amounts of sucrose and most starchy carbohydrates. In that regard, fructose may offer an advantage as a sweetening agent in the diabetic diet. However, because of potential adverse effects of large amounts of fructose (i.e., double the usual intake [20% of calories]) on serum cholesterol and LDL cholesterol, fructose may have no overall advantage as a sweetening agent in the diabetic diet. Although people with dyslipidemia should avoid consuming large amounts of fructose, there is no reason to recommend that people avoid consumption of fruits and vegetables, in which fructose occurs naturally, or moderate consumption of fructose-sweetened foods.

### Other Nutritive Sweeteners

Nutritive sweeteners other than sucrose and fructose include corn sweeteners such as corn syrup, fruit juice or fruit juice concentrate, honey, molasses, dextrose, and maltose. There is no evidence that these sweeteners have any significant advantage or disadvantage over sucrose in terms of improvement in caloric content or glycemic response.

Sorbitol, mannitol, and xylitol are common sugar alcohols (polyols) that produce a lower glycemic response than sucrose and other carbohydrates. Starch hydrolysates are formed by the partial hydrolysis and hydrogenation of edible starches, thus becoming polyols. The exact caloric value of the polyols is difficult to determine. There appear to be no significant advantages of the polyols over other nutritive sweeteners. Excessive amounts of polyols may, however, have a laxative effect.

### *Nonnutritive Sweeteners*

Saccharin, aspartame, and acesulfame K are approved for use by the Food and Drug Administration (FDA) in the United States. The FDA also determines an acceptable daily intake for approved food additives, including nonnutritive sweeteners. Nonnutritive sweeteners approved by the FDA are safe to consume by all people with diabetes.

## *Fiber*

Dietary fiber may be beneficial in treating or preventing several gastrointestinal disorders, including colon cancer, and large amounts of soluble fiber have a beneficial effect on serum lipids. There is no reason to believe that people with diabetes would be more or less amenable to these effects than those without diabetes. Although selected soluble fibers are capable of delaying glucose absorption from the small intestine, the effect of dietary fiber on glycemic control is probably insignificant. Therefore, fiber intake recommendations for people with diabetes are the same as for the general population. Daily consumption of a diet containing 20-35 g dietary fiber from a wide variety of food sources is recommended.

## *Sodium*

People differ greatly in their sensitivity to sodium and its effect on blood pressure. Because it is impractical to assess individual sodium sensitivity, intake recommendations for people with diabetes are the same as for the general population. Some health authorities recommend no more than 3,000 mg/day of sodium for the general population, while other authorities recommend no more than 2,400 mg/day. For people with mild to moderate hypertension, 2,400 mg or less per day of sodium is recommended.

## Alcohol

The same precautions regarding the use of alcohol that apply to the general public also apply to people with diabetes. Under normal circumstances, however, blood glucose levels will not be affected by moderate use of alcohol when diabetes is well controlled. For people using insulin, 1-2 alcoholic beverages (1 alcoholic beverage = 12 oz beer, 5 oz wine, or 1½ oz distilled spirits) can be ingested with and in addition to the usual meal plan.

Special considerations for further modification of alcohol intake include the following. Abstention from alcohol should be advised for people with a history of alcohol abuse or during pregnancy. Alcohol may increase the risk for hypoglycemia in people treated with insulin or sulfonylureas. If alcohol is consumed by such people, it should only be ingested with a meal. Reduction of or abstention from alcohol intake may be advisable for people with diabetes with other medical problems such as pancreatitis, dyslipidemia, or neuropathy. When calories from alcohol need to be calculated as part of the total caloric intake, alcohol is best substituted for fat exchanges or fat calories (1 alcoholic beverage = 2 fat exchanges).

## Micronutrients: Vitamins and Minerals

When dietary intake is adequate, there is generally no need for additional vitamin and mineral supplementation for the majority of people with diabetes. Although there are theoretical reasons to supplement with antioxidants, there is little confirmatory evidence at present that such therapy has any benefits.

The only known circumstance in which chromium replacement has any beneficial effect on glycemic control is for people who are chromium deficient as a result of long-term chromium-deficient parenteral nutrition. However, it appears that most people with diabetes are not chromium deficient and, therefore, chromium supplementation has no known benefit.

Similarly, although magnesium deficiency may play a role in insulin resistance, carbohydrate intolerance, and hypertension, the available data suggest that routine evaluation of serum magnesium levels is recommended only in patients at high risk for magnesium deficiency. Levels of magnesium should be repleted only if hypomagnesium can be demonstrated.

Potassium loss may be sufficient to warrant dietary supplementation in patients taking diuretics. Hyperkalemia sufficient to warrant dietary potassium restriction may occur in patients with renal insufficiency or hyporeninemic hypodosteronism or in patients taking angiotensin-converting enzyme inhibitors.

## *Pregnancy*

Nutrition recommendations for women with preexisting and gestational diabetes mellitus should be based on a nutrition assessment. Monitoring blood glucose levels, urine ketones, appetite, and weight gain can be a guide to developing and evaluating an appropriate individualized meal plan and to making adjustments to the meal plan throughout pregnancy to ensure desired outcomes.

## *Summary*

A historical perspective of nutrition recommendations is provided in Table 27.1. Today there is no **one** "diabetic" or "ADA" diet. The recommended diet can only be defined as a dietary prescription based on nutrition assessment and treatment goals.

**Table 27.1.** Historical perspective of nutrition recommendations.

| | Distribution of Calories | | |
|---|---|---|---|
| Year | %Carbohydrate | %Protein | %Fat |
| Before 1921 | Starvation diets | | |
| 1921 | 20 | 10 | 70 |
| 1950 | 40 | 20 | 40 |
| 1971 | 45 | 20 | 35 |
| 1986 | up to 60 | 12-20 | <30 |
| 1994 | * | 10-20 | *, † |

*Based on nutritional assessment and treatment goals. †Less than 10% of calories from saturated fats.

Medical nutrition therapy for people with diabetes should be individualized, with consideration given to usual eating habits and other lifestyle factors. Nutrition recommendations are then developed to meet treatment goals and desired outcomes. Monitoring metabolic parameters including blood glucose, glycated hemoglobin, lipids, blood pressure, and body weight, as well as quality of life, is crucial to ensure successful outcomes.

## References


1. Franz MJ, Horton ES, Bantle JP, Beebe CA, Brunzell JD, Coulston AM, Henry RR, Hoogwerf BJ, Stacpoole PW: Nutrition principles for the management of diabetes and related complications (Technical review). *Diabetes Care* 17:490-518, 1994.

2. U.S. Department of Agriculture, U.S. Department of Health and Human Services: *Nutrition and Your Health—Dietary Guidelines for Americans*. 3rd Ed. Hyattsville MD, USDA's Human Nutrition Information Service, 1990.

3. U.S. Department of Agriculture: *The Food Guide Pyramid*. Hyattsville, MD. USDA's Human Nutrition Information Service, 1992.

Chapter 28

# The New Food Label: Important Information for People with Diabetes

Pat Coyle, of Rockville, Md., is a 67year-old woman with diabetes, vitamin $B_{12}$-deficiency anemia, and osteoporosis. So she has to pay attention to her diet. But ask her what she likes most about the new food label, and you won't hear much about serving sizes, names of nutrients, and %Daily Values. Instead, you'll get rave reviews about the print size and background color.

The nutrition information on the new label is in bigger type, and FDA requires that it appear on a white or other neutral contrasting background, when practical.

Those are benefits for Coyle because she has diabetic retinopathy, an eye condition that can lead to blindness. She already has had two surgeries to correct poor eyesight. Before the surgeries, she had trouble reading food labels.

"I needed a magnifying glass to read [the nutrition information]," she recalls, referring to the small type and shaded backgrounds on the old labels. "I'm looking forward to not having to read the teeny tiny print."

For people with diabetes, easily readable labeling information is vital because diet is important in managing diabetes.

## Other Label Benefits

New food labeling regulations that went into effect May 1994 now require labels on most packaged foods to provide nutrition information.

---

Reprinted from *FDA Consumer* November 1994, Pub. No. (FDA) 95-2289.

That previously was voluntary and appeared on only about 60 percent of such foods.

Also, nutrition information for fresh fruits and vegetables and raw meat and fish may appear at the point of purchase.

The nutrition information is now more complete. Labels continue to provide information about calories, fat, carbohydrate, sodium, protein, iron, calcium, and vitamins A and C. But now they also contain additional information about saturated fat and cholesterol. These two nutrients are important to people with diabetes because diabetes increases the risk of heart disease, and heart disease is also linked to high intakes of saturated fat and cholesterol.

## Diet for Diabetes

How beneficial the new label will be for people with diabetes depends on the type of meal plan they follow. Today, diabetes experts no longer recommend a single diet for all people with diabetes. Instead, they advocate dietary regimes that are flexible and take into account a person's lifestyle and particular health needs.

The American Diabetes Association (ADA) described some common options in a 1994 position paper. A first step, for example, is to encourage people with diabetes to follow the government's Dietary Guidelines for Americans and Food Guide Pyramid.

According to Phyllis Barrier, a registered dietitian and director of council affairs for ADA, this step alone may be enough to maintain normal blood glucose, or sugar, levels. Maintaining these levels helps reduce the risks of retinopathy and other diabetes-related complications, such as kidney and heart disease.

Other people use the Exchange Lists for Meal Planning, she said. This system, established by the American Dietetic and American Diabetes associations, separates foods into six categories based on their nutritional makeup. People following this plan choose a set amount of servings from each category daily, depending on their nutritional needs.

A more sophisticated method of meal planning is "carbohydrate counting," in which grams of carbohydrate consumed are monitored and adjusted daily according to blood glucose levels. Some people count protein and fat grams, too. These two nutrients also can affect blood sugar levels, although to a lesser extent.

Whatever method used, ADA recommends these general dietary guidelines for people with diabetes:

- Limit fat to 30 percent or less of daily calories.
- Limit saturated fat to 10 percent or less of daily calories.
- Limit protein to 10 to 20 percent of daily calories. For those with initial signs of diabetes-induced kidney disease, restrict protein to 10 percent of daily calories.
- Limit cholesterol to 300 milligrams or less daily.
- Consume about 20 to 35 grams of fiber daily.

Most of these guidelines are a good idea for the general population, as well.

Those who are overweight also may moderately restrict calories. ADA recommends a calorie reduction of 250 to 500 calories less than normally eaten per day. That should result in a weight loss of about 0.2 to 0.5 kilograms (one-half to 1 pound) a week, ADA's Barrier said. The calorie restriction, along with increased exercise, should help an overweight person achieve a weight loss of 5 to 10 kilograms (11 to 22 pounds) in about six months to one year. The weight loss, although moderate, can help improve diabetes control.

Carbohydrate intake can vary, but, contrary to popular belief, the type of carbohydrate is not a factor. As ADA points out in its position paper, people with diabetes have for years been told to avoid "simple" sugars, such as table sugar and those found in sugary snacks, because they were thought to elevate blood glucose more quickly and more severely than other carbohydrates.

"There is, however, very little scientific evidence that supports this assumption," ADA wrote in its position paper. The organization recommended that the focus be on total carbohydrate—not source of carbohydrate. If sugar and sugar-containing foods are eaten, the amounts must be figured into the daily allotment of carbohydrate.

## *Get the Nutrition Facts*

Considering these factors, how should people with diabetes go about using the new food label?

They can begin with the Nutrition Facts panel, usually on the side or back of the package. A column headed %Daily Values shows whether a food is high or low in many of the nutrients listed.

People with diabetes should check the %Daily Values for fat, saturated fat, and cholesterol. As a rule of thumb, if the number is 5 or less, the food may be considered low in that nutrient.

The goal for most people with diabetes is to pick foods that have low %Daily Values for fat, saturated fat, and cholesterol and high %Daily Values for fiber. Other label nutrition information can help people with diabetes see if and how a food fits into their meal plan.

## Serving Sizes

The serving size information gives the amount of food to which all other numbers on the Nutrition Facts panel apply.

Serving sizes now are more uniform among similar products and reflect the amounts people actually eat. For example, the reference amount for a serving of snack crackers is 30 g. Thus, the serving size for soda crackers is 10 crackers and for Goldfish Tiny Crackers, 55, because these are the amounts that come closest to 30g.

The similarity makes it easier to compare the nutritional qualities of related foods.

People who use the Exchange Lists should be aware that the serving size on the label may not be the same as that in the Exchange Lists. For example, the label serving size for orange juice is 8 fluid ounces (240 milliliters). In the Exchange Lists, the serving size is 4 ounces (one-half cup) or 120 mL. So, a person who drinks one cup of orange juice has used two fruit exchanges.

## Calorie and Other Information

The Nutrition Facts panel also gives total calories and calories from fat per serving of food. This is helpful for people who count calories and monitor their daily percentage of calories from fat.

Here's how to use calories from fat information: At the end of the day, add up total calories and then calories from fat eaten. Divide calories from fat by total calories. The answer gives the percentage of calories from fat eaten that day. For example, 450 calories from fat divided by 1,800 total calories = 0.25 (25 percent), an amount within the recommended level of not more than 30 percent calories from fat.

The label also gives grams of total carbohydrate, protein and fat, which can be used for carbohydrate counting.

The values listed for total carbohydrate include all carbohydrate, including dietary fiber and sugars listed below it. Not singled out is complex carbohydrates, such as starches.

The sugars include naturally present sugars, such as lactose in milk and fructose in fruits, and those added to the food, such as table sugar, corn syrup, and dextrose.

The listing of grams of protein also is helpful for those restricting their protein intake, either to reduce their risk of kidney disease or to manage the kidney disease they have developed.

## Front Label Info

Elsewhere on the label, consumers may find claims about the food's nutritional benefits. Often, they appear on the front of the package, where shoppers can readily see them. These claims signal that the food contains desirable levels of certain nutrients.

Some claims, such as "low-fat " "no saturated fat," and "high-fiber," describe nutrient levels. Some of these are particularly interesting to people with diabetes because they highlight foods containing nutrients at beneficial levels. (See "Nutrient Claims Guide." at end of this chapter.)

Other claims, called health claims, show a relationship between a nutrient or food and a disease or health condition. FDA has authorized eight such claims; they are the only ones about which there is significant scientific agreement.

Two that relate to heart disease are of particular interest to people with diabetes:

- A diet low in saturated fat and cholesterol may help reduce the risk of coronary heart disease.
- A diet rich in fruits, vegetables and grain products that contain fiber, particularly soluble fiber, and are low in saturated fat and cholesterol may help reduce the risk of coronary heart disease.

Both claims also must state that heart disease depends on many factors.

Nutrient and health claims can be used only under certain circumstances, such as when the food contains appropriate levels of the stated nutrients. So now, when consumers see the claims, they can believe them.

The intent, though, is not just to ensure the label information is truthful, but also to enable the consumer to use it to choose healthier foods. For people with diabetes, that's especially important because of the increased risk of other chronic diseases. Pat Coyle is one person with diabetes who realizes this.

"I'm looking forward to greater health because I won't have any excuses," she says. "The information . . . is right there." And, she adds, "I especially like the large print."

## Nutrient Claims Guide for Individual Foods

### Fat

- *Fat-free*: less than 0.5 grams (g) fat per serving
- *Low-fat*: 3 g or less per serving and, if the serving size is 30 g or less or 2 table spoons or less, per 50 g of the food
- *Reduced or less fat*: at least 25 percent less per serving than reference food

### Saturated Fat

- *Saturated fat free*: less than 0.5 g and less than 0.5 g of *trans* fatty acids per serving
- *Low saturated fat*: 1 g or less per serving and not more than 15 percent of calories from saturated fatty acids
- *Reduced or less saturated fat*: at least 25 percent less per serving than reference food

### Cholesterol

- *Cholesterol-free*: less than 2 milligrams (mg) and 2 g or less of saturated fat per serving
- *Low-cholesterol*: 20 mg or less and 2 g or less of saturated fat per serving and, if the serving is 30 g or less or 2 tablespoons or less, per 50 g of the food
- *Reduced or less cholesterol*: at least 25 percent less than reference food and 2 g or less of saturated fat per serving

The following claims can be used to describe meat, poultry, seafood, and game meats:

- *Lean*: less than 10 g fat, 4.5 g or less saturated fat, and less than 95 mg cholesterol per serving and per 100 g
- *Extra lean*: less than 5 g fat, less than 2 g saturated fat, and less than 95 mg cholesterol per serving and per 100 g

### Healthy

- "low fat," "low saturated fat," with 60 mg or less cholesterol per serving (or, if raw meat, poultry and fish, "extra lean")

- at least 10 percent of Daily Value for one or more of vitamins A and C, iron, calcium, protein, and fiber per serving
- 480 mg or less sodium per serving, and, if the serving is 30 g or less or 2 tablespoons or less, per 50 g of the food. (After Jan. 1, 1998, maximum sodium levels drop to 360 mg.)

### Calories

- *Calorie-free*: fewer than 5 calories per serving
- *Low-calorie*: 40 or fewer calories per serving and, if the serving size is 30 g or less or 2 tablespoons or less, per 50 g of the food
- *Reduced or fewer calories*: at least 25 percent fewer calories per serving than the reference food

### Light (two meanings)

- one-third fewer calories or half the fat of the reference food—if the food derives 50 percent or more of its calories from fat, the reduction must be 50 percent of the fat
- a "low-calorie," "low-fat" food whose sodium content has been reduced by 50 percent from the reference food ("Light in sodium" means the food has 50 percent or less sodium than the reference food and may be used on foods that are not "low-calorie" and "low-fat.")

### Fiber

- *High-fiber*: 5 g or more per serving
- *Good source of fiber*: 2.5 g to 4.9 g per serving
- *More or added fiber*: at least 2.5 g more per serving than the reference food. (Label will say 10 percent more of the Daily Value for fiber.)

Foods making claims about increased fiber content also must meet the definition for "low-fat" or the amount of total fat per serving must appear next to the claim.

### Sugar

- *Sugar-free*: less than 0.5 g per serving

- *No added sugar, without added sugar, no sugar added*:
  - no sugar or ingredients that functionally substitute for sugar (for example, fruit juices) added during processing or packing
  - no ingredients made with added sugars, such as jams, jellies, or concentrated fruit juice

  ("Sugar-free" and "No added sugar" signal a reduction in calories from sugars only, not from fat, protein and other carbohydrates. If the total calories are not reduced or the food is not "low-calorie," a statement will appear next to the "sugar-free" claim explaining that the food is "not low-calorie," "not reduced calorie," or "not for weight control." If the total calories are reduced, the claim must be accompanied by a "low-calorie" or "reduced-calorie" claim.)

- *Reduced sugar*: at least 25 percent less sugar than the reference food.

*—by Paula Kurtzweil*

Paula Kurtzweil is a member of FDA's public affairs staff.

## Chapter 29

# When Should I Eat?

## Why Should I Keep My Blood Sugar at a Healthy Level?

You should keep your blood sugar (also called blood glucose) at a healthy level to prevent or slow down diabetes problems. Ask your doctor or diabetes teacher what a healthy blood sugar level is for you.

Your blood sugar can go too high if you eat too much. If your blood sugar goes too high, you can get sick.

Your blood sugar can also go too high if you do not take the right amount of diabetes medicine.

If your blood sugar stays high too much, you can get diabetes problems. These can be heart, eye, foot, kidney, and other problems.

You can also get sick if your blood sugar gets too low.

## How Can I Keep My Blood Sugar at a Healthy Level?

- Eat about the same amounts of food each day.
- Eat your meals and snacks at about the same times each day.
- Do not skip meals or snacks.
- Take your medicines at the same times each day.
- Exercise at about the same times each day.

---

National Institute of Diabetes and Digestive and Kidney Diseases (NIDDK), NIH Pub. No. 98-4242, November 1997.

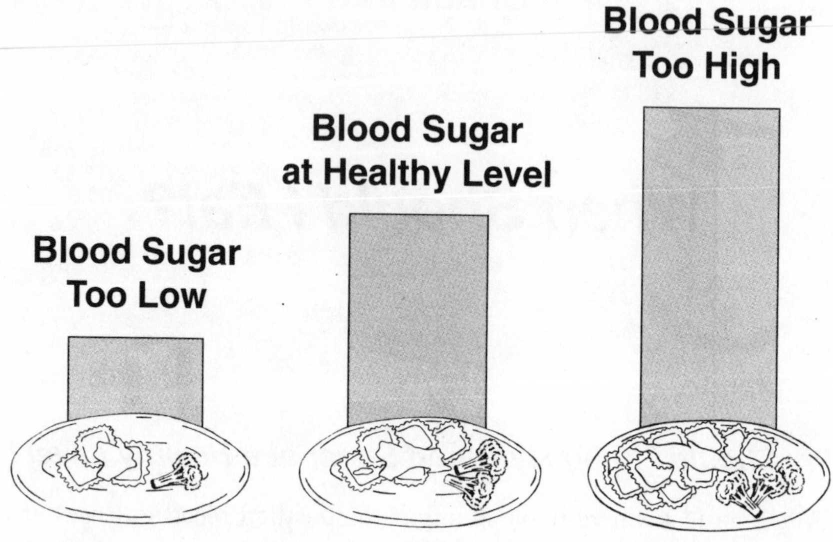


***Figure 29.1.*** *Eat about the same amounts of food each day to keep your blood sugar at a healthy level.*

## *Why Should I Eat about the Same Amount Each Day?*

The food you eat turns into sugar and travels to your blood. This is called blood sugar. Your blood sugar goes up after you eat.

Keep your blood sugar at a healthy level by eating about the same amounts of food at about the same times each day.

Your blood sugar will not stay at a healthy level if you eat a big lunch one day and a small lunch the next day.

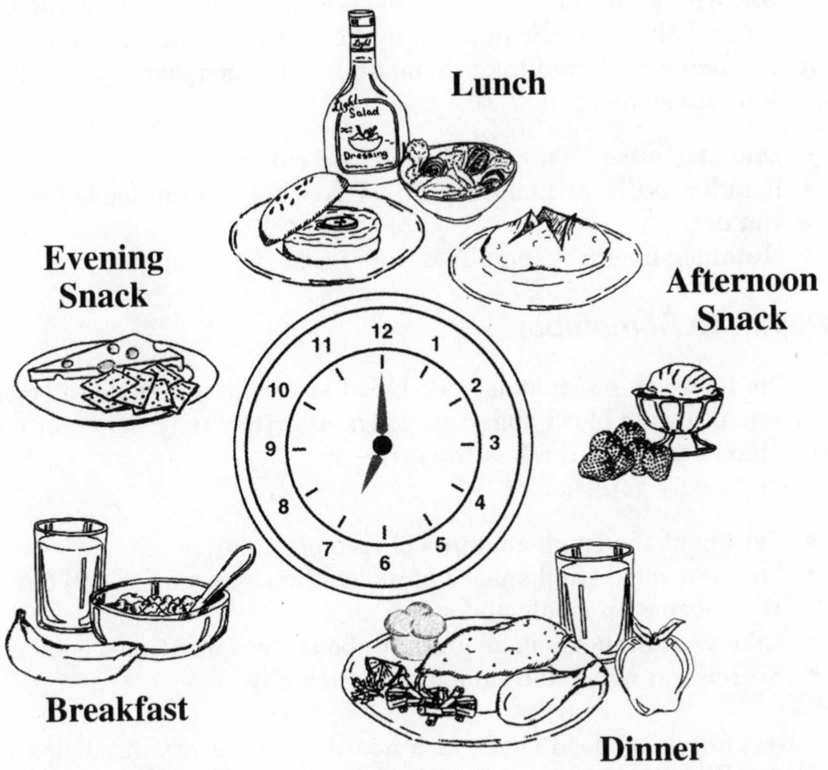


***Figure 29.2.*** *Eat your meals and snacks at about the same times each day.*

## *Why Should I Eat at about the Same Times Each Day?*

Eating at about the same times each day helps you keep your blood sugar from getting too high or too low.

Eating at about the same times each day also helps your diabetes medicine keep your blood sugar at a healthy level.

## What Times Should I Take My Diabetes Medicines?

Talk with your doctor or diabetes teacher about the best times to take your diabetes medicines. Fill in the names of your diabetes medicines, when you should take them, and how much you should take.

Here are some hints:

- Diabetes pills: Take these before you eat.
- Regular, NPH, or Lente insulin: Take this 30 minutes before you eat.
- Humalog insulin lispro: Take this just before you eat.

## Points to Remember

The food you eat makes your blood sugar go up. Diabetes medicines make your blood sugar go down. Together they help you keep your blood sugar at the healthy level.

That's why you should:

- Eat about the same amounts of food each day.
- Eat your meals and snacks at about the same times each day.
- Try not to skip meals and snacks.
- Take your diabetes medicines at about the same times each day.
- Exercise at about the same times each day.

Keeping your blood sugar at a healthy level every day helps you prevent diabetes problems for a long time.

Two other booklets can help you learn more about food and diabetes:

- *I Have Diabetes: What Should I Eat?*
- *I Have Diabetes: How Much Should I Eat?*

For your convenience they are included in this volume. For free copies of these booklets:

- Call the National Diabetes Information Clearinghouse (NDIC) at (301) 654-3327.
- Write to NDIC, 1 Information Way, Bethesda, MD 20892-3560.
- E-mail NDIC at <ndic@info.niddk.nih.gov>.
- Look at these booklets online at <http://www.niddk.nih.gov> under "Health Information."

## Chapter 30

# What Should I Eat?

### How Can I Control My Diabetes?

You can help control your blood sugar (also called blood glucose) and diabetes when you eat healthy, get enough exercise, and stay at a healthy weight.

A healthy weight also helps you control your blood fats and lower your blood pressure.

Many people with diabetes also need to take medicine to help control their blood sugar.

### How Can I Eat Healthy?

Using the food pyramid helps you eat a variety of healthy foods. When you eat different foods, you get the vitamins and minerals you need.

Eat different foods from each group each day. See how to do this in Table 30.1.

### What Are Starches?

Starches are bread, grains, cereal, pasta, or starchy vegetables. Eat some starches at each meal. People might tell you not to eat many starches, but that is no longer correct advice. Eating starches is healthy for everyone, including people with diabetes.

---

National Institute of Diabetes and Digestive and Kidney Diseases (NIDDK), NIH Pub. No. 98-4192, November 1997.

**Table 30.1.** Examples of different foods from same group.

| | Day 1 | Day 2 |
|---|---|---|
| Fruit: | apple<br>orange | banana<br>mango |
| Vegetable: | broccoli | salad<br>green beans |

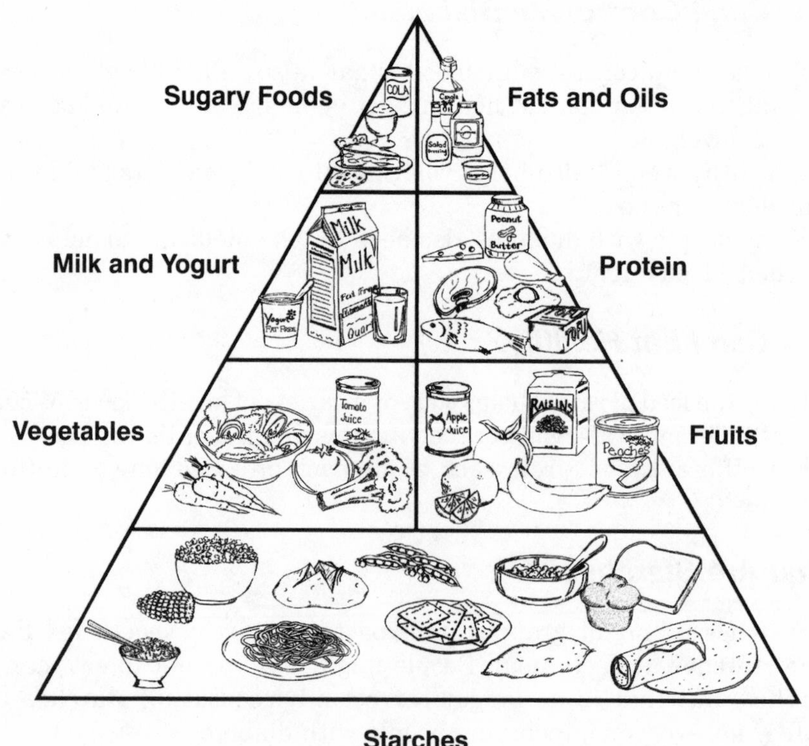


*Figure 30.2. The Food Pyramid*

The number of servings you should eat each day depends on:

- The calories you need.
- Your diabetes treatment plan.

Starches give your body energy, vitamins and minerals, and fiber. Whole grain starches are healthier because they have more vitamins, minerals, and fiber. Fiber helps you have regular bowel movements.

## How Much Is a Serving of Starch?

### *1 Serving*

- 1 slice of bread or
- 1 small potato or
- ½ cup cooked cereal or
- ¾ cup dry flakes of cereal or
- 1 small tortilla

### *2 Servings*

- 2 slices of bread or
- 1 small potato plus 1 small ear of corn

### *3 Servings*

- 1 small roll plus ½ cup of peas plus 1 small potato or
- 1 cup of rice

You might need to eat one, two, or three starch servings at a meal. If you need to eat more than one serving at a meal, choose several different starches or have two or three servings of one starch.

## What Are Healthier Ways to Buy, Cook, and Eat Starches?

- Buy whole grain breads and cereals.
- Eat fewer fried and high-fat starches such as regular tortilla chips and potato chips, french fries, pastries, biscuits, or muffins.
- Use low-fat or fat-free yogurt or fat-free sour cream instead of regular sour cream on a baked potato.

- Use mustard instead of mayonnaise on a sandwich.
- Use the low-fat or fat-free substitutes such as low-fat mayonnaise or light margarine on bread, rolls, or toast.
- Use vegetable oil spray instead of oil, shortening, butter, or margarine.
- Cook or eat cereal with fat-free (skim) or low-fat (1%) milk.
- Use no-sugar jelly, low-fat or fat-free cottage cheese, nonfat yogurt, or salsa.

## What Are Vegetables?

Vegetables are healthy for everyone, including people with diabetes. Eat raw and cooked vegetables every day. Vegetables give you vitamins, minerals, and fiber, with very few calories.

The number of servings you should eat each day depends on:

- The calories you need.
- How you take care of your diabetes.

## How Much Is a Serving of Vegetables?

### 1 Serving

- ½ cup carrots or
- ½ cup cooked green beans

### 2 Servings

- ½ cup carrots plus 1 cup salad or
- ½ cup vegetable juice plus ½ cup cooked green beans

### 3 Servings

- ½ cup cooked greens plus ½ cup cooked green beans and 1 small tomato or
- ½ cup broccoli plus 1 cup tomato sauce

You might need to eat one, two, or three vegetable servings at a meal. If you need to eat more than one serving at a meal, choose a few different types of vegetables or have two or three servings of one vegetable.

## What Are Healthier Ways to Buy, Cook, and Eat Vegetables?

Eat raw and cooked vegetables with little or no fat. You can cook and eat vegetables without any fat.

- Try low-fat or fat-free salad dressing on raw vegetables or salads.
- Steam vegetables using a small amount of water or low-fat broth.
- Mix in some chopped onion or garlic.
- Use a little vinegar or some lemon or lime juice.
- Add a small piece of lean ham or smoked turkey.
- Sprinkle with herbs and spices. These flavorings add almost no fat or calories.

If you do use a small amount of fat, use canola oil, olive oil, or tub margarine instead of fat from meat, butter, or shortening.

## What Are Fruits?

Fruit is healthy for everyone, including people with diabetes. Fruit gives you energy, vitamins and minerals, and fiber.

The number of servings you should eat each day depends on:

- The calories you need.
- How you take care of your diabetes.

## How Much Is a Serving of Fruit?

### *1 Serving*

- 1 small apple or
- ½ cup juice or
- ½ grapefruit

### *2 Servings*

- 1 banana or
- ½ cup orange juice plus 1¼ cup whole strawberries

You might need to eat one or two fruit servings at a meal. If you need to eat more than one serving at a meal, choose different types of fruits or have two servings of one fruit.

## How Should I Eat Fruit?

Eat fruits raw, as juice with no sugar added, canned in their own juice, or dried.

- Buy smaller pieces of fruit.
- Eat pieces of fruit rather than drinking fruit juice. Pieces of fruit are more filling.
- Buy fruit juice that is 100-percent juice with no added sugar.
- Drink fruit juice in small amounts.
- Save high-sugar and high-fat fruit desserts such as peach cobbler or cherry pie for special occasions.

## What Are Milk and Yogurt Foods?

Fat-free and low-fat milk and yogurt are healthy for everyone, including people with diabetes. Milk and yogurt give you energy, protein, calcium, vitamin A, and other vitamins and minerals.

Drink fat-free (skim or nonfat) or low-fat (1%) milk each day. Eat low-fat or fat-free yogurt. They have less total fat, saturated fat, and cholesterol.

The number of servings you should eat each day depends on:

- The calories you need.
- How you take care of your diabetes.

**Note:** If you are pregnant or breastfeeding, eat four to five servings of milk and yogurt each day.

## How Much Is a Serving of Milk and Yogurt?

### *1 Serving*

- 1 cup fat-free plain yogurt or
- 1 cup skim milk

## What Are Protein Foods?

Protein foods are meat, poultry, eggs, cheese, fish, and tofu. Eat small amounts of some of these foods each day.

Protein foods help your body build tissue and muscles. They also give your body vitamins and minerals.

The number of servings you should eat each day depends on:

- The calories you need.
- How you take care of your diabetes.

## How Much Is a Serving of Protein Food?

### *1 Serving*

- 2 to 3 ounces of cooked fish or
- 2 to 3 ounces of cooked chicken or
- 2 ounces of cheese or
- 4 ounces (½ cup) of tofu

The serving size you eat now may be too big. One serving should weigh between 2 and 3 ounces after cooking, about the size of a deck of cards.

## What Are Healthier Ways To Buy, Cook, and Eat Protein Foods?

- Buy cuts of beef, pork, ham, and lamb that have only a little fat on them. Trim off extra fat.
- Eat chicken or turkey without the skin.
- Cook protein foods in low-fat ways:
    - Broil
    - Grill
    - Stir-fry
    - Roast
    - Steam
    - Stew
- To add more flavor, use vinegars, lemon juice, soy or teriyaki sauce, salsa, ketchup, barbecue sauce, and herbs and spices.
- Cook eggs with a small amount of fat.
- Eat small amounts of nuts, peanut butter, fried chicken, fish, or shellfish. They are high in fat.

## What Are Fats and Oils?

You find the fats and oils section at the tip of the food pyramid. This tells you to eat small amounts of fats and oils because they have lots of calories. Some fats and oils also contain saturated fats and cholesterol that are not good for you.

You also get fat from other foods such as meats and some dairy foods.

High-fat food is tempting. But eating small amounts of high-fat food will help you lose weight, keep your blood sugar and blood fats under control, and lower your blood pressure.

## How Much Is a Serving of Fat or Oil?

### 1 Serving

- 1 strip of bacon or
- 1 teaspoon oil

### 2 Servings

- 1 tablespoon regular salad dressing or
- 2 tablespoons light salad dressing plus 1 tablespoon light mayonnaise

Your meals may include one or two servings of fat.

## What Are Sugary Foods?

You find the sugary foods and sweets section at the tip of the food pyramid. This tells you to eat small amounts of sugary foods.

Sugary foods have calories and do not have much nutrition. Sugary foods have lots of calories. Some sugary foods are also high in fat—like cakes, pies, and cookies. They also may contain saturated fats and cholesterol.

Sugary foods and sweets are tempting. But eating small amounts of sugary foods will help you lose weight, keep your blood sugar under control, control your blood fats, and lower your blood pressure.

## How Much Is a Serving of Sugary Foods and Sweets?

### 1 Serving

- 3" diameter cookie or
- 1 plain cake doughnut or
- 4 chocolate kisses or
- 1 tablespoon maple syrup

Once in a while you can eat a serving of a sugary food. Talk to your diabetes teacher about how to fit sugary foods into your meal plan.

## *How Can I Satisfy My Sweet Tooth?*

Eat a serving of sugar-free popsicles, diet soda, fat-free ice cream or yogurt, or sugar-free hot cocoa mix once in a while.

Remember, fat-free and low sugar foods still have some calories. Eat them as part of your meal plan.

## *Points to Remember*

To follow a healthy eating plan:

- Choose foods from all six food groups each day
- Eat a wide variety of foods from each group to get all your vitamins and minerals.
- Eat enough starches, vegetables, fruits, and low-fat milk and yogurt.
- Eat smaller amounts of lower fat protein foods.
- Eat fewer fats, oils, and sugary foods.

## *How To Find More Help*

**Diabetes Teachers** (nurses, dietitians, pharmacists, and other health professionals)

- To find a diabetes teacher near you, call the American Association of Diabetes Educators toll-free at 1-800 TEAMUP4 (1-800-832-6874).

**Recognized Diabetes Education Programs** (teaching programs approved by the American Diabetes Association)

- To find a program near you, call 1-800-DIABETES (1-800-342-2383) or look at its Internet home page <http://www.diabetes.org> and click on “Diabetes Info.”

**Dietitians**

- To find a dietitian near you, call The American Dietetic Association’s National Center for Nutrition and Dietetics at 1-800-366-1655 or look at its Internet home page <http://www. eatright. org> and click on “Find a Dietitian.”

Two other booklets can help you learn more about food and diabetes:

- *I Have Diabetes: How Much Should I Eat?*
- *I Have Diabetes: When Should I Eat?*

For your convenience these two booklets are included in this volume. For free copies of these booklets:

- Call the National Diabetes Information Clearinghouse (NDIC) at (301) 654-3327.
- Write to NDIC, 1 Information Way, Bethesda, MD 20892-3560.
- E-mail NDIC at <ndic@info.niddk.nih.gov>
- Look at these booklets online at <http://www.niddk.nih.gov> under "Health Information."

## Chapter 31

# How Much Should I Eat?

### How Much Should I Eat?

How much you should eat depends on:

- Whether you are a man or woman.
- How much you weigh.
- How tall you are.
- Your age.
- How much you exercise.
- The type of work or other activity you do every day.
- If you are pregnant or breastfeeding.

### How Can I Eat Healthy?

- Eat healthy foods like fruits, vegetables, breads and cereals, low-fat dairy foods, and lean meats.
- Eat healthy foods in the proper amounts for you.

Remember, even healthy foods can cause problems if you eat too much of them. A diabetes teacher can help you decide how much food you should eat.

---

National Institute of Diabetes and Digestive and Kidney Diseases (NIDDK), NIH Pub. No. 98-4243, November 1997.

## What Measuring Tools Can Help Me Eat the Right Amount of Food?

- Measuring cups.
- Measuring spoons.
- A food scale.
- The Nutrition Facts labels on food packages help you learn how much food is in one serving.

## How Can I Find Out How Much to Eat Each Day?

Ask yourself these questions:

- Am I a small woman who exercises? Yes or No.
- Am I a small woman who wants to lose weight? Yes or No.
- Am I a medium woman who wants to lose weight? Yes or No.
- Am I a medium woman who does not exercise much? Yes or No.

If your answer to every question is No, go to the next "How Can I Find Out How Much to Eat Each Day?" section. If you answered Yes to any of these questions, eat between 1,200 and 1,600 calories a day.

Eat these numbers of servings to eat 1,200 to 1,600 calories a day:

- 6 starches
- 3 vegetables
- 2 fruits
- 2 milk and yogurt
- 2 protein foods
- 4 to 6 fats
- 0 to 1 sugary foods

You may continue at "The Food Pyramid" section.

## How Can I Find Out How Much to Eat Each Day?

Ask yourself these questions:

- Am I a large woman who needs to lose weight? Yes or No.
- Am I a small man at a healthy weight? Yes or No.
- Am I a medium man who needs to lose weight? Yes or No.

- Am I a medium man who does not exercise much? Yes or No.

If your answer to every question is No, go to the next "How Can I Find Out How Much to Eat Each Day?" section. If you answer Yes to any of these questions, eat between 1,600 and 2,000 calories a day.

Eat these numbers of servings from these food groups to eat 1,600 to 2,000 calories a day:

- 8 starches
- 4 vegetables
- 3 fruits
- 2 milk and yogurt
- 2 protein foods
- 6 to 8 fats
- 0 to 1 sugary foods

You may continue at "The Food Pyramid" section.

## How Can I Find Out How Much to Eat Each Day?

Ask yourself these questions:

- Am I a large man who does not need to lose weight? Yes or No.
- Am I a large man who needs to lose weight? Yes or No.
- Am I a medium to large man who does a lot of exercise or has an active job? Yes or No.
- Am I a large woman who does a lot of exercise or has an active job? Yes or No.

If you answer Yes to any of these questions, eat between 2,000 and 2,400 calories a day.

Eat these numbers of servings from these food groups to eat 2 000 to 2,400 calories a day:

- 10 starches
- 4 vegetables
- 3 fruits
- 2 milk and yogurt
- 2 protein foods
- 8 to 10 fats
- 0 to 1 sugary foods

## The Food Pyramid

Seven food groups make up the food pyramid. The food pyramid helps you decide how many servings of each food group to eat. It shows that you should eat the most servings from the starches, vegetables, and fruits—the largest sections of the food pyramid. You should eat small amounts from the sugary foods and fats and oils sections of the pyramid.

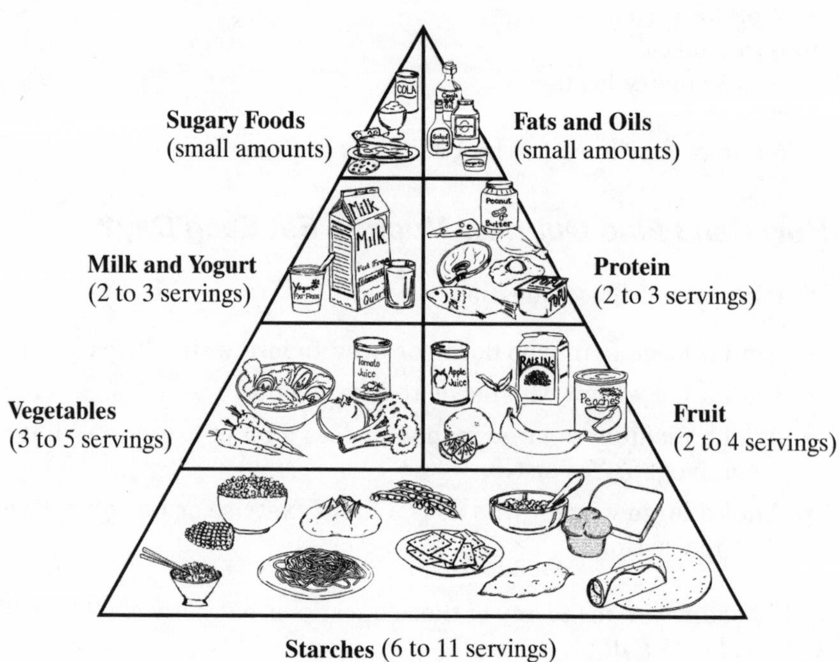


***Figure 31.1.*** *The Food Pyramid*

## How Many Servings of Starches Should I Eat?

The grains, cereal, rice, pasta, and starchy vegetables group is the largest part of the food pyramid. Examples of one serving of food from this group are:

- 1 slice of bread or
- 1/3 cup rice or
- ½ cup cooked cereal or
- ¾ cup dry flakes of cereal or
- 1 small baked potato

Do you eat starches that are not listed? Ask your diabetes teacher how much and how often to eat them. Also ask the healthiest ways to eat them.

Remember, you might need more than one serving at a meal. If you need two servings, eat double the amount or eat one serving each of two starches.

Every time you eat foods like dry cereal, hot cereal, pasta, or rice, use the same type of bowl or plate. Measure the correct serving with a measuring tool.

When you eat the food again, fill the bowl to the same level. Use a measuring tool to measure foods once in a while to make sure your servings are still correct.

## How Many Servings of Vegetables Should I Eat?

Vegetables are in the next level of the food pyramid. Examples of one serving of food from the vegetable group are:

- ½ cup tomato juice or
- ½ cup cooked green beans or
- 1 cup tossed salad or
- 1 cup raw spinach or
- ½ cup cooked carrots

Do you eat vegetables that are not listed? Ask your diabetes teacher how much and how often to eat them. Also ask the healthiest ways to eat them.

Remember, you might need more than one serving at a meal. If you need two servings, eat double the amount or eat one serving each of two vegetables.

If you buy fresh vegetables, buy the vegetables you like in the serving size you should eat. For example, buy small tomatoes or small squashes. If you buy vegetables in servings that are larger than you need, you might eat too much.

## How Many Servings of Fruit Should I Eat?

Fruits are on the same level of the food pyramid as the vegetable group. Examples of one serving of food from the fruit group are:

- 1 small apple or
- ½ cup apple juice or
- 2 tablespoons raisins or
- ½ cup canned fruit

Do you eat fruits that are not listed? Ask your diabetes teacher how much and how often to eat them. Also ask the healthiest ways to eat them.

Remember, you might need more than one serving at a meal. If you need two servings, eat double the amount or eat one serving each of two fruits.

If you buy fresh fruits, buy small to medium pieces. If the pieces of fruit you buy are too big, you might eat too much.

## How Many Servings of Milk and Yogurt Should I Eat?

Milk and yogurt are on the next level of the food pyramid. One serving of food from the milk and yogurt group is:

- 1 cup fat-free milk or
- 1 cup buttermilk or
- 1 cup nonfat yogurt

Do you eat milk and yogurt-type foods that are not listed? Ask your diabetes teacher how much and how often to eat them. Also ask the healthiest ways to eat them.

Always drink milk out of the same size of glass. Fill a 1-cup measuring cup with milk. Pour the milk into your glass. See how high it fills the glass.

Measure the amount of milk in a measuring cup once in a while to make sure your servings are still correct.

## How Many Servings of Protein Foods Should I Eat?

Protein foods are on the same level of the food pyramid as milk and yogurt. Examples of one serving (about 2 to 3 ounces) of food from the protein food group are:

- 2 to 3 ounces cooked fish or
- 2 to 3 ounces cooked chicken or
- 2 ounces cheese or
- 2 to 3 ounces cooked hamburger

Do you eat protein foods that are not listed? Ask your diabetes teacher how much and how often to eat them. Also, ask the healthiest ways to eat them.

If you cannot weigh the food, make sure the serving is about the size and thickness of the palm of your hand or a deck of cards.

Remember, meats weigh more before they are cooked. For example: 4 ounces of raw meat weighs 3 ounces after cooking. If the meat has bone, like a pork chop or a chicken leg, then cook 5 ounces raw to get 3 ounces cooked.

## How Many Servings of Fats and Oils Should I Eat?

Fats and oils are part of the smallest section of the food pyramid. This means you should eat fats and oils only in small amounts. Examples of one serving of fats and oils are:

- 1 tablespoon regular salad dressing or
- 1 teaspoon regular margarine or
- 2 tablespoons light salad dressing or
- 1 teaspoon oil or
- 1 tablespoon light mayonnaise or
- 6 whole peanuts

Do you eat fats or oils that are not listed? Ask your diabetes teacher how much and how often to eat them. Also ask the healthiest way to eat them.

Use measuring spoons to learn how much fat or oil to use. Then, when you do not have measuring spoons, like in a restaurant, you will know how much to use. It is easy to eat too much fat and oil.

## How Many Servings of Sugary Foods Should I Eat?

Sugary foods are part of the smallest section of the food pyramid. This means you should eat sugary foods only once in a while. Examples of one serving of sugary foods and sweets are:

- 1 plain cake doughnut or
- 1/12 piece of angel food cake or

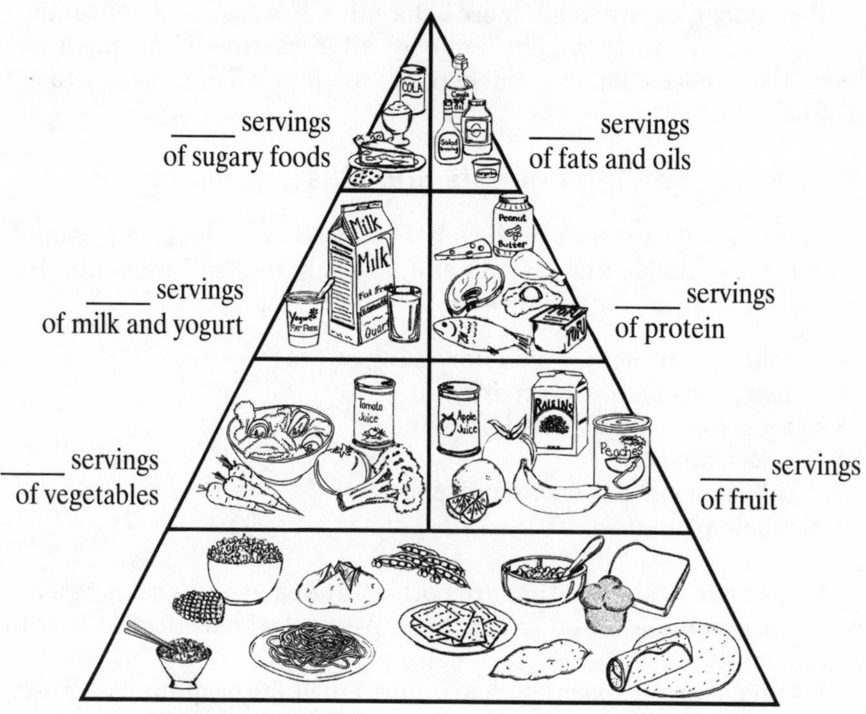


***Figure 31.2.*** *Make your own food pyramid.Use your own food pyramid to plan meals and snacks. (Work with your diabetes teacher if you need help.)*

- 1 3" diameter cookie or
- 1 tablespoon maple syrup

Do you eat sugary foods that are not listed? Ask your diabetes teacher how much and how often to eat them. Also ask the healthiest ways to eat them.

Here are ways to eat small portions of sugary foods:

- Split and share desserts in restaurants.
- Order small or child-size servings of ice cream or frozen yogurt.
- Divide homemade desserts into small servings and wrap each piece separately.
- Freeze the extra servings.
- Do not have candy dishes around the house or near you at work.

## Points to Remember

To follow a healthy eating plan:

- Eat the right number of servings of food from each of the food groups.
- Eat these foods in the right amounts.
- Use your measuring tools.
- Choose foods in the proper serving size when you shop.

## How To Find More Help

**Diabetes Teachers** (nurses, dietitians, pharmacists, and other health professionals). To find a diabetes teacher near you, call the American Association of Diabetes Educators toll-free at 1-800-TEAMUP4 (1-800-832-6874).

**Recognized Diabetes Education Programs** (teaching programs approved by the American Diabetes Association). To find a program near you, call 1-800-DIABETES (1-800-342-2383) or look at its Internet home page <http://www.diabetes.org> and click on "Diabetes Info."

**Dietitians.** To find a dietitian near you, call The American Dietetic Association's National Center for Nutrition and Dietetics at 1-800-366-1655 or look at its Internet home page <http://www.eatright.org> and click on "Find a Dietitian."

Two other booklets can help you learn more about food and diabetes:

- *I Have Diabetes: What Should I Eat?*
- *I Have Diabetes: When Should I Eat?*

For your convenience they are included in this volume. For free copies of these booklets:

- Call the National Diabetes Information Clearinghouse (NDIC) at (301) 654-3327.
- Write to NDIC, 1 Information Way, Bethesda, MD 20892-3560.
- E-mail NDIC at <ndic@info.niddk.nih.gov>.
- Look at these booklets online at <http://www.niddk.nih.gov> under "Health Information."

## Chapter 32

# *Can I Drink Alcoholic Beverages?*

Alcohol is everywhere when the family gathers, at cookouts, after the softball game, at parties. "What will you have?"; someone asks. If you have diabetes, what do you say?

It all depends. Start by asking yourself three basic questions:

1. Is my diabetes under control?
2. Does my doctor agree that I am free from health problems that alcohol can make worse, for example, diabetic nerve damage or high blood pressure?
3. Do I know how alcohol can affect me and my diabetes?

If you said yes to all three, it's okay to have an occasional drink. What does occasional mean? The American Diabetes Association suggests that you have no more than two drinks a day.

### *Your Body and Alcohol*

Alcohol moves very quickly into the blood without being broken down (metabolized) in your stomach. Within five minutes of having a drink, there's enough alcohol in your blood to measure. Thirty to 90 minutes after having a drink, the alcohol in your bloodstream is at its highest level.

---

Your liver does most of the job of breaking down the alcohol once it's in your body. But it needs time. If you weigh 150 pounds, it will take about 2 hours to metabolize a beer or mixed drink.

If you drink alcohol faster than your liver can break it down, the excess alcohol moves through your bloodstream to other parts of your body. Brain cells are easy targets. When someone talks about getting a buzz from alcohol, this is what they are feeling.

## Risk of Low Blood Glucose

If you have diabetes and take insulin shots or oral diabetes pills, you risk low blood glucose when you drink alcohol. To protect yourself, never drink on an empty stomach. Plan to have your drink with a meal or after eating a snack that contains protein, fat, or both.

How does alcohol add to your chances of having low blood glucose? It has to do with your liver.

Normally, when your blood glucose level starts to drop, your liver steps in. It goes to work changing stored carbohydrate into glucose. Then it sends the glucose out into the blood, which helps you avoid or slow down a low blood glucose reaction.

However, when alcohol enters your system, this changes. Alcohol is a toxin. Your body reacts to alcohol like a poison. The liver wants to clear it from the blood quickly. In fact, the liver won't put out glucose again until it has taken care of the alcohol. If your blood glucose level is falling, you can quickly wind up with very low blood glucose.

This is why drinking as little as 2 ounces of alcohol (about 2 drinks) on an empty stomach can lead to very low blood glucose.

When you mix alcohol and exercise, you increase the risk of going low. This can happen because exercise helps lower your blood glucose levels.

Let's say you've just played a couple of hard sets of tennis. You have a beer after the match. But in the hours after the game, your body is still working.

It replaces the energy your muscles used up. To do this, it clears glucose from the blood and adds it to the muscles' store. This is why hard exercise can cause your blood glucose level to go down.

If you take insulin or diabetes pills, they too are working to clear glucose from your blood. Unless you eat or your liver adds glucose to your blood, you could be heading for a very low blood glucose level. If you drink a beer, the alcohol will stop your liver from sending out any glucose. Your chances of going low are even greater.

If you take diabetes pills that work over a long period of time, such as chlorpropamide, you are at risk for very low blood glucose when drinking. This is because alcohol changes how the diabetes pill works. It makes the pill stronger and longer lasting. Hopefully, your doctor warned you about mixing long-lasting diabetes pills with alcohol.

Low blood glucose when drinking is less of a risk for those with type 2 diabetes who control their diabetes by diet and exercise alone. Still, alcohol is a wild card when it is mixed with diet plans.

## *Don't Go Low*

**Follow these guidelines to avoid low blood glucose levels when you drink:**

1. Never drink alcohol on an empty stomach.
2. Limit yourself to 1 or 2 drinks.
3. If you just finished hard exercise, test your blood glucose before you drink and at least once while you're drinking. Watch for falling blood glucose levels in the hours after exercise.

Alcohol also affects your body's ability to get over a low blood glucose level. If you have low blood glucose, you may need to treat it more than once as time goes by. If you've been drinking, check your blood glucose before you go to sleep. You may need to have a snack before you retire to avoid a low blood glucose reaction while you sleep.

**A warning:** glucagon shots don't help severe low blood glucose caused by drinking. Glucagon shots treat very severe low blood glucose reactions caused by too much insulin.

Glucagon works by getting your liver to release more glucose into your blood. But alcohol stops this process. You need to be able to treat your reaction with a carbohydrate, such as oral glucose tablets or gels. So you need to avoid letting a low blood glucose level become severe. If you pass out, you will need glucose injected into your bloodstream by a health care professional.

Heavy drinking over time can hurt your liver. It won't be able to make glucose as well. When this happens, your diabetes is harder to control.

Some of the signs of drinking too much, such as confusion or slurred speech, are similar to the effects of a low blood glucose reaction or ketoacidosis (most common in people with type 1 diabetes who have taken too little insulin).

You may be asked to take a blood or a breath test for alcohol if you have some of these signs. Don't worry. Diabetes will not affect the results of a test for alcohol, even if you are having a reaction or have a fruity smell to your breath because of high ketone levels.

If you are asked to take a test for alcohol and you have a choice, choose a blood test. That way, doctors can check your levels of glucose and ketones, too.

## Beer Belly Blues

Although an occasional drink may not hurt your blood glucose control, it can harm your eating plan if your goal is weight loss.

Two light beers equal about 200 extra calories. Alcohol is called empty calories because it does not give you any nutrients.

When you drink, you have to add the calories from alcohol to your daily calorie count. You don't want to bump out other calories that supply vital nutrients.

Talk to your dietitian or doctor about ways to work alcohol into your meal plan. If you are on a low-calorie diet, think twice about adding alcohol. In general, alcohol counts as fat and starch/bread exchanges.

## Wise Drink Choices

Some drinks are better choices for people with diabetes. Select drinks that are lower in alcohol and sugar. Avoid sweet dessert wines, port and liqueurs, which can cause a sharp rise in blood glucose.

If you use mixers in your drinks, choose ones that are low in sugar or sugar free, such as diet soft drinks, diet tonic, club soda, seltzer, or water. This will help keep your blood glucose levels in your target range. Light beer and dry wines are good choices. They have less alcohol and carbohydrates and fewer calories.

To make drinks last longer, try a spritzer. Mix wine with sparkling water, club soda, or diet soda. Try a virgin Bloody Mary made without alcohol. Or sample a nonalcoholic beer or wine. (These drinks are not calorie free. You need to add them to your meal plan.)

## When Alcohol Is a Poor Choice

Some people with diabetes should not drink alcohol. Alcohol can make some diabetic problems worse.

If you have nerve damage from diabetes in your arms or legs, drinking can make it worse. Alcohol is toxic to nerves. Drinking can increase the pain, burning, tingling, numbness, and other symptoms found with nerve damage. Some studies show that even regular light drinking (less than two drinks per week) can bring on nerve damage.

Heavy drinking (3 or more drinks per day) may make diabetic eye disease worse. If you have high blood pressure, you can lower it if you stop drinking alcohol.

Many people with diabetes have high levels of the fat called triglyceride in their blood. If you do, you should not drink alcohol. Alcohol affects how the liver clears fat from the blood. Alcohol also spurs the liver on to make more triglycerides. Even light drinking (two 4-ounce glasses of wine a week) can raise triglyceride levels.

## Chapter 33

# *Exercise and Diabetes Management*

During exercise, whole-body oxygen consumption may increase by as much as 20-fold, and even greater increases may occur in the working muscles. To meet its energy needs under these circumstances, skeletal muscle uses, at a greatly increased rate, its own stores of glycogen and triglycerides, as well as free fatty acids (FFAs) derived from the breakdown of adipose tissue triglycerides and glucose released from the liver. To preserve central nervous system function, blood glucose levels are remarkably well maintained during exercise. Hypoglycemia during exercise rarely occurs in nondiabetic individuals. The metabolic adjustments that preserve normoglycemia during exercise are in large part hormonally mediated. A decrease in plasma insulin and the presence of glucagon appear to be necessary for the early increase in hepatic glucose production during exercise, and during prolonged exercise, increases in plasma glucagon and catecholamines appear to play a key role. These hormonal adaptations are essentially lost in insulin-deficient patients with type 1 diabetes. As a consequence, when such individuals have too little insulin in their circulation due to inadequate therapy, an excessive release of counterinsulin hormones during exercise may increase already high levels of glucose and ketone bodies and can even precipitate diabetic ketoacidosis. Conversely, the presence of high levels of insulin, due to exogenous insulin administration, can attenuate or even prevent the increased mobilization of glucose and other substrates induced by exercise, and

---

hypoglycemia may ensue. Similar concerns exist in patients with type 2 diabetes on insulin or sulfonylurea therapy; however, in general, hypoglycemia during exercise tends to be less of a problem in this population. Indeed, in patients with type 2 diabetes, exercise may improve insulin sensitivity and assist in diminishing elevated blood glucose levels into the normal range.

The purpose of this position statement is to update and crystallize current thinking on the role of exercise in patients with types 1 and 2 diabetes. With the publication of new clinical reviews, it is becoming increasingly clear that exercise may be a therapeutic tool in a variety of patients with, or at risk for diabetes, but that like any therapy its effects must be thoroughly understood. [(1-3)] From a practical point of view, this means that the diabetes health care team will be required to understand how to analyze the risks and benefits of exercise in a given patient. Furthermore, the team, consisting of but not limited to the physician, nurse, dietitian, mental health professional, and patient, will benefit from working with an individual with knowledge and training in exercise physiology. Finally, it has also become clear that it will be the role of this team to educate primary care physicians and others involved in the care of a given patient.

## Evaluation of the Patient Before Exercise

Before beginning an exercise program, the individual with diabetes mellitus should undergo a detailed medical evaluation with appropriate diagnostic studies. This examination should carefully screen for the presence of macro- and microvascular complications that may be worsened by the exercise program. Identification of areas of concern will allow the design of an individualized exercise prescription that can minimize risk to the patient. Most of the following recommendations are excerpts from *The Health Professional's Guide to Diabetes and Exercise.* [(3)]

A careful medical history and physical examination should focus on the symptoms and signs of disease affecting the heart and blood vessels, eyes, kidneys, and nervous system.

### Cardiovascular System

A graded exercise test may be helpful if a patient, about to embark on a moderate- to high-intensity exercise program,[(4-6)] is at high risk for underlying cardiovascular disease, based on one of the following criteria:

- age >35 years
- type 2 diabetes of >10 years' duration
- type 1 diabetes of >15 years' duration
- presence of any additional risk factor for coronary artery disease
- presence of microvascular disease (retinopathy or nephropathy, including microalbuminuria)
- peripheral vascular disease
- autonomic neuropathy

In some patients who exhibit nonspecific electrocardiogram (ECG) changes in response to exercise, or who have nonspecific ST and T wave changes on the resting ECG, alternative tests such as radionuclide stress testing may be performed. In patients planning to participate in low-intensity forms of exercise (<60% of maximal heart rate) such as walking, the physician should use clinical judgment in deciding whether to recommend an exercise stress test. Patients with known coronary artery disease should undergo a supervised evaluation of the ischemic response to exercise, ischemic threshold, and the propensity to arrhythmia during exercise. In many cases, left ventricular systolic function at rest and during its response to exercise should be assessed.

### *Peripheral Arterial Disease*

Evaluation of peripheral arterial disease (PAD) is based on signs and symptoms, including intermittent claudication, cold feet, decreased or absent pulses, atrophy of subcutaneous tissues, and hair loss. The basic treatment for intermittent claudication is nonsmoking and a supervised exercise program. The presence of a dorsalis pedis and posterior tibial pulse does not rule out ischemic changes in the forefoot. If there is any question about blood flow to the forefoot and toes on physical examination, toe pressures as well as Doppler pressures at the ankle should be carried out.

### *Retinopathy*

The eye examination schedule should follow the American Diabetes Association's Clinical Practice Guidelines. For patients who have proliferative diabetic retinopathy (PDR) that is active, strenuous activity may precipitate vitreous hemorrhage or traction retinal detachment. These individuals should avoid anaerobic exercise and exercise that involves straining, jarring, or Valsalva-like maneuvers.

On the basis of the Joslin Clinic experience, the degree of diabetic retinopathy has been used to stratify the risk of exercise, and to individually tailor the exercise prescription.

### Nephropathy

Specific exercise recommendations have not been developed for patients with incipient (microalbuminuria >20 mg/min albumin excretion) or overt nephropathy (>200 mg/min). Patients with overt nephropathy often have a reduced capacity for exercise, which leads to self-limitation in activity level. Although there is no clear reason to limit low- to moderate-intensity forms of activity, high-intensity or strenuous exercises should probably be discouraged in these individuals.

### Neuropathy: Peripheral

Peripheral neuropathy (PN) may result in loss of protective sensation in the feet. Significant PN is an indication to limit weight-bearing exercise. Repetitive exercise on insensitive feet can ultimately lead to ulceration and fractures. Evaluation of PN can be made by checking the deep tendon reflexes, vibratory sense, and position sense. Touch sensation can best be evaluated by using monofilaments. The inability to detect sensation using the 5.07 (10 g) monofilament is indicative of the loss of protective sensation. Table 33.1 lists contraindicated and recommended exercises for patients with loss of protective sensation in the feet.

**Table 33.1.** Exercises for diabetic patients with loss of protective sensation

| Contraindicated exercise | Recommended exercise |
|---|---|
| Treadmill | Swimming |
| Prolonged walking | Bicycling |
| Jogging | Rowing |
| Step exercises | Chair exercises |
| | Arm exercises |
| | Other non-weight-bearing exercise |

### Neuropathy: Autonomic

The presence of autonomic neuropathy may limit an individual's exercise capacity and increase the risk of an adverse cardiovascular event during exercise. Cardiac autonomic neuropathy (CAN) may be indicated by resting tachycardia (>100 beats per minute), orthostasis (a fall in systolic blood pressure >20 mmHg upon standing), or other disturbances in autonomic nervous system function involving the skin, pupils, gastrointestinal, or genitourinary systems. Sudden death and silent myocardial ischemia have been attributed to CAN in diabetes. Resting or stress thallium myocardial scintigraphy is an appropriate noninvasive test for the presence and extent of macrovascular coronary artery disease in these individuals. Hypotension and hypertension after vigorous exercise are more likely to develop in patients with autonomic neuropathy, particularly when starting an exercise program. Because these individuals may have difficulty with thermoregulation, they should be advised to avoid exercise in hot or cold environments and to be vigilant about adequate hydration.

## Preparing for Exercise

Preparing the individual with diabetes for a safe and enjoyable exercise program is as important as exercise itself. The young individual in good metabolic control can safely participate in most activities. The middle-aged and older individual with diabetes should be encouraged to be physically active. The aging process leads to a degeneration of muscles, ligaments, bones, and joints, and disuse and diabetes may exacerbate the problem. Before beginning any exercise program, the individual with diabetes should be screened thoroughly for any underlying complications as described above.

A standard recommendation for diabetic patients, as for nondiabetic individuals, is that exercise includes a proper warm-up and cool-down period. A warm-up should consist of 5-10 min of aerobic activity (walking, cycling, etc.) at a low-intensity level. The warm-up session is to prepare the skeletal muscles, heart, and lungs for a progressive increase in exercise intensity. After a short warm-up, muscles should be gently stretched for another 5-10 min. Primarily, the muscles used during the active exercise session should be stretched, but warming up all muscle groups is optimal. The active warm-up can either take place before or after stretching. Following the activity session, a cool-down should be structured similarly to the warm-up. The cool-down should last about 5-10 min and gradually bring the heart rate down to its pre-exercise level.

There are several considerations that are particularly important and specific for the individual with diabetes. Aerobic exercise should be recommended, but taking precautionary measures for exercise involving the feet is essential for many patients with diabetes. The use of silica gel or air midsoles as well as polyester or blend (cotton-polyester) socks to prevent blisters and keep the feet dry is important for minimizing trauma to the feet. Proper footwear is essential and must be emphasized for individuals with peripheral neuropathy. Individuals must be taught to monitor closely for blisters and other potential damage to their feet, both before and after exercise. A diabetes identification bracelet or shoe tag should be clearly visible when exercising. Proper hydration is also essential, as dehydration can effect blood glucose levels and heart function adversely. Exercise in heat requires special attention to maintaining hydration. Adequate hydration prior to exercise is recommended (e.g., 17 ounces of fluid consumed 2 h before exercise). During exercise, fluid should be taken early and frequently in an amount sufficient to compensate for losses in sweat reflected in body weight loss, or the maximal amount of fluid tolerated. Precautions should be taken when exercising in extremely hot or cold environments. High-resistance exercise using weights may be acceptable for young individuals with diabetes, but not for older individuals or those with long-standing diabetes. Moderate weight training programs that utilize light weights and high repetitions can be used for maintaining or enhancing upper body strength in nearly all patients with diabetes.

## Exercise and Type 2 Diabetes

The possible benefits of exercise for the patient with type 2 diabetes are substantial, and recent studies strengthen the importance of long-term exercise programs for the treatment and prevention of this common metabolic abnormality and its complications. Specific metabolic effects can be highlighted as follows.

### Glycemic Control

Several long-term studies have demonstrated a consistent beneficial effect of regular exercise training on carbohydrate metabolism and insulin sensitivity, which can be maintained for at least 5 years. These studies used exercise regimens at an intensity of 50-80% $VO_{2max}$ three to four times a week for 30-60 min a session. Improvements in $HbA_{1c}$ were generally 10-20% of baseline and were most marked in patients with mild type 2 diabetes and in those who are likely to be the most insulin resistant. It remains true, unfortunately, that most of these studies suffer from inadequate randomization and controls, and are confounded by associated lifestyle changes. Data on the effects of resistance exercise are not available for type 2 diabetes although early results in normal individuals and patients with type 1 disease suggest a beneficial effect.

It now appears that long-term programs of regular exercise are indeed feasible for patients with impaired glucose tolerance or uncomplicated type 2 diabetes with acceptable adherence rates. Those studies with the best adherence have used an initial period of supervision followed by relatively informal home exercise programs with regular, frequent follow-up assessments. A number of such programs have demonstrated sustained relative improvements in $VO_{2max}$ over many years with little in the way of significant complications.

### *Prevention of Cardiovascular Disease*

In patients with type 2 diabetes, the insulin resistance syndrome continues to gain support as an important risk factor for premature coronary disease, particularly with concomitant hypertension, hyperinsulinemia, central obesity, and the overlap of metabolic abnormalities of hypertriglyceridemia, low HDL, altered LDL, and elevated FFA. Most studies show that these patients have a low level of fitness compared with control patients, even when matched for levels of ambient activity, and that poor aerobic fitness is associated with many of the cardiovascular risk factors. Improvement in many of these risk factors has been linked to a decrease in plasma insulin levels, and it is likely that many of the beneficial effects of exercise on cardiovascular risk are related to improvements in insulin sensitivity.

### *Hyperlipidemia*

Regular exercise has consistently been shown to be effective in reducing levels of triglyceride-rich VLDL. However, effects of regular exercise on levels of LDL cholesterol have not been consistently documented. With one major exception, most studies have failed to demonstrate a significant improvement in levels of HDL in patients with type 2 diabetes, perhaps because of the relatively modest exercise intensities used.

### *Hypertension*

There is evidence linking insulin resistance to hypertension in patients. Effects of exercise on reducing blood pressure levels have been demonstrated most consistently in hyperinsulinemic subjects.

### Fibrinolysis

Many patients with type 2 diabetes have impaired fibrinolytic activity associated with elevated levels of plasminogen activator inhibitor-1 (PAI-1), the major naturally occurring inhibitor of tissue plasminogen activator (TPA). Studies have demonstrated an association of aerobic fitness and fibrinolysis. There is still no clear consensus on whether physical training results in improved fibrinolytic activity in these patients.

### Obesity

Data have accumulated suggesting that exercise may enhance weight loss and in particular weight maintenance when used along with an appropriate calorie-controlled meal plan. There are few studies specifically dealing with this issue in type 2 diabetes, and much of the available data is complicated by the simultaneous use of unusual diets and other behavioral interventions. Of particular interest are studies suggesting a disproportionate effect of exercise on loss of intra-abdominal fat, the presence of which has been associated most closely with metabolic abnormalities. Data on the use of resistance exercise in weight reduction are promising, but studies in patients with type 2 diabetes in particular are lacking.

### Prevention of Type 2 Diabetes

A great deal of evidence has been accumulated supporting the hypothesis that exercise, among other therapies, may be useful in preventing or delaying the onset of type 2 diabetes. Currently, a large randomized prospective National Institutes of Health (NIH) study is under way to clarify the feasibility of this approach.

## Exercise and Type 1 Diabetes

All levels of exercise, including leisure activities, recreational sports, and competitive professional performance, can be performed by people with type 1 diabetes who do not have complications and are in good blood glucose control (note previous section). The ability to adjust the therapeutic regimen (insulin and diet) to allow safe participation and high performance has recently been recognized as an important management strategy in these individuals. In particular, the important role played by the patient in collecting self-monitored blood glucose data of the response to exercise and then using these data to improve performance and enhance safety is now fully accepted.

Hypoglycemia, which can occur during, immediately after, or many hours after exercise, can be avoided. This requires that the patient have both an adequate knowledge of the metabolic and hormonal responses to exercise and well-tuned self-management skills. The increasing use of intensive insulin therapy has provided patients with the flexibility to make appropriate insulin dose adjustments for various activities. The rigid recommendation to use carbohydrate supplementation, calculated from the planned intensity and duration of exercise, without regard to glycemic level at the start of exercise, the previously measured metabolic response to exercise, and the patient's insulin therapy, is no longer appropriate. Such an approach not infrequently neutralizes the beneficial glycemic lowering effects of exercise in patients with type 1 diabetes.

General guidelines that may prove helpful in regulating the glycemic response to exercise can be summarized as follows:

*1. Metabolic control before exercise*

- Avoid exercise if fasting glucose levels are >250 mg/dl and ketosis is present or if glucose levels are >300 mg/dl, irrespective of whether ketosis is present.
- Ingest added carbohydrate if glucose levels are <100 mg/dl.

*2. Blood glucose monitoring before and after exercise*

- Identify when changes in insulin or food intake are necessary.
- Learn the glycemic response to different exercise conditions.

*3. Food intake*

- Consume added carbohydrate as needed to avoid hypoglycemia.
- Carbohydrate-based foods should be readily available during and after exercise.

Since diabetes is associated with an increased risk of macrovascular disease, the benefit of exercise in improving known risk factors for atherosclerosis is to be highly valued. This is particularly true in that exercise can improve the lipoprotein profile, reduce blood pressure, and improve cardiovascular fitness. However, it must also be appreciated that several studies have failed to show an independent effect of exercise training on improving glycemic control as measured by $HbA_{1c}$ in patients with type 1 diabetes. Indeed, these studies have been valuable in changing the focus for exercise in diabetes from glucose control to that of an important life behavior with multiple benefits. The challenge is to develop strategies that allow individuals with type 1 diabetes to participate in activities that are consistent with their lifestyle and culture in a safe and enjoyable manner.

In general, the principles recommended for dealing with exercise in adults with type 1 diabetes, free of complications, apply to children, with the caveat that children may be prone to greater variability in blood glucose levels. In children, particular attention needs to be paid to balancing glycemic control with the normalcy of play, and for this the assistance of parents, teachers, and athletic coaches may be necessary. In the case of adolescents, hormonal changes can contribute to the difficulty in controlling blood glucose levels. Despite these added problems, it is clear that with careful instructions in self-management and the treatment of hypoglycemia, exercise can be a safe and rewarding experience for the great majority of children and adolescents with insulin-dependent diabetes mellitus.

## Exercise in the Elderly

Evidence has accumulated suggesting that the progressive decrease in fitness and muscle mass and strength with aging is in part preventable by maintaining regular exercise. The decrease in insulin sensitivity with aging is also partly due to a lack of physical activity. Lower levels of physical activity are especially likely in the population at risk for type 2 diabetes. A number of recent studies of exercise training have included significant numbers of older patients. These patients have done well with good training and metabolic responses, levels of adherence at least as good as the general population, and an acceptable incidence of complications. It is likely that maintaining better levels of fitness in this population will lead to less chronic vascular disease and an improved quality of life.

## Conclusions

The recent Surgeon General's Report on Physical Activity and Health [4] underscores the pivotal role physical activity plays in health promotion and disease prevention. It recommends that individuals accumulate 30 min of moderate physical activity on most days of the week. In the context of diabetes, it is becoming increasingly clear that the epidemic of type 2 diabetes sweeping the globe is associated with decreasing levels of activity and an increasing prevalence of obesity. Thus, the importance of promoting exercise as a vital component of the prevention, as well as management of type 2 diabetes must be viewed as a high priority. It must also be recognized that the benefit of exercise in improving the metabolic abnormalities of type 2 diabetes is probably greatest when it is used early in its progression from insulin resistance to impaired glucose tolerance to overt hyperglycemia requiring treatment with oral glucose-lowering agents and finally to insulin.

For people with type 1 diabetes, the emphasis must be on adjusting the therapeutic regimen to allow safe participation in all forms of physical activity consistent with an individual's desires and goals. Ultimately, all patients with diabetes should have the opportunity to benefit from the many valuable effects of exercise.

### *About This Position Statement*

Originally approved February 1990. Revised in 1997. The initial draft of this revision was prepared by Bernard Zinman, MD (co-chair); Neil Ruderman, MD, DPhil (co-chair); Barbara N. Campaigne, PhD; John T. Devlin, MD; and Stephen H. Schneider, MD. The paper was peer-reviewed, modified, and approved by the Professional Practice Committee and the Executive Committee, June 1997, as well as by the American College of Sports Medicine's Pronouncements Committee and Board of Trustees, July 1997.

The recommendations in this paper are based on the evidence reviewed in the following publications: Exercise and NIDDM. *Diabetes Care* 13:785-789, 1990, and Exercise in individuals with NIDDM. *Diabetes Care* 17:924-937, 1994.

Abbreviations: CAN, cardiac autonomic neuropathy; ECG, electrocardiogram; FFA, free fatty acid; PDR, proliferative diabetic retinopathy; PN, peripheral neuropathy.

## References

1. Schneider SH, Ruderman NB: Exercise and NIDDM (Technical Review). *Diabetes Care* 13:785-789, 1990

2. Wasserman DH, Zinman B: Exercise in individuals with IDDM (Technical Review). *Diabetes Care* 17:924-937, 1994

3. American Diabetes Association: Diabetes and exercise: the risk-benefit profile. In *The Health Professional's Guide to Diabetes and Exercise*. Devlin JT, Ruderman N, Eds. Alexandria, VA, American Diabetes Association, 1995, p. 34

4. U.S. Department of Health and Human Services: *Physical Activity and Health: A Report of the Surgeon General*. Centers for Disease Control and Prevention, National Center for Chronic Disease Prevention and Health Promotion, Washington, DC, U.S. Govt. Printing Office, 1996

5. Centers for Disease Control and Prevention and the American College of Sports Medicine: Physical activity and public health: a recommendation. *JAMA* 273:402-407, 1995

6. American College of Sports Medicine: The recommended quantity and quality of exercise for developing and maintaining cardiorespiratory and muscular fitness in healthy adults (Position Statement). *Med Sci Sports Exercise* 22:265-274, 1990

# *Part Five*

# *Insulin and Other Diabetes Medicines*

# Chapter 34

# *Medicines for People with Diabetes*

## *Do I Need to Take Diabetes Medicine?*

### *What if I have type 1 diabetes?*

Type 1 is the type of diabetes that people most often get before 30 years of age. All people with type 1 diabetes need to take insulin (*IN-suh-lin*) because their bodies do not make enough insulin. Insulin helps turn sugar from food into energy for the body to work.

### *What if I have type 2 diabetes?*

Type 2 is the type of diabetes most people get as adults after the age of 40. But you can get diabetes at a younger age.

Healthy eating, exercise, and losing weight may help you lower your blood sugar (also called blood glucose) when you find out you have type 2 diabetes. If these treatments do not work, you may need one or more types of diabetes pills to lower your blood sugar. After a few more years, you may need to take insulin shots because your body is not making enough insulin.

You, your doctor, and your diabetes teacher should always find the best diabetes plan for you.

---

"Medicines for People with Diabetes," National Institute of Diabetes and Digestive and Kidney Diseases (NIDDK), NIH Pub. No. 98-4222, November 1997.

## *Why Do I Need Medicines for Type 1 Diabetes?*

Most people make insulin in their pancreas. **If you have type 1 diabetes,** your body does not make insulin. Insulin helps sugar from the foods you eat get to all parts of your body to use for energy.

Because your body no longer makes insulin, you need to take insulin in shots. Take your insulin as your doctor tells you.

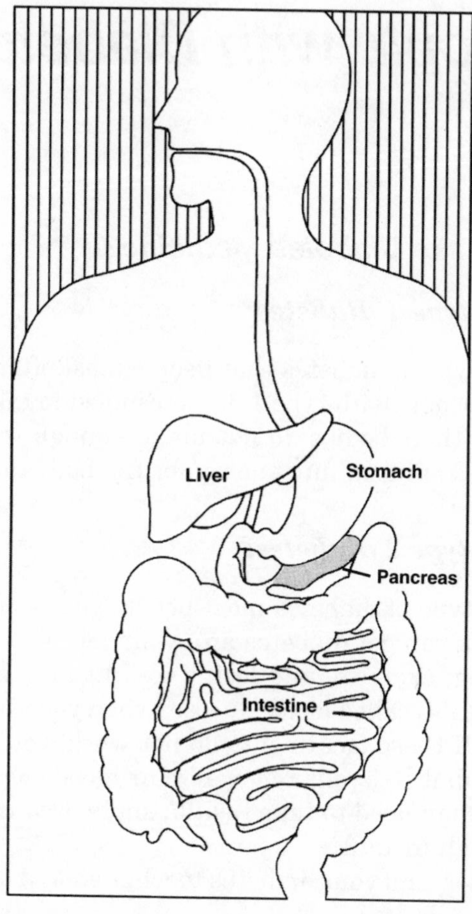


***Figure 34.1.*** *The pancreas is where your body makes insulin.*

## Why Do I Need Medicines for Type 2 Diabetes?

**If you have type 2 diabetes,** your pancreas usually makes plenty of insulin. But your body cannot correctly use the insulin you make. You might get this type of diabetes if members of your family have or had diabetes. You might also get type 2 diabetes if you weigh too much or do not exercise enough.

After you have had type 2 diabetes for a few years, your body may stop making enough insulin. Then you will need to take diabetes pills or insulin.

### You Need To Know

- Diabetes medicines that lower blood sugar never take the place of healthy eating and exercise.
- If your blood sugar gets too low more than a few times in a few days, then call your doctor.
- Take your diabetes pills or insulin even if you are sick. If you cannot eat much, call your doctor.

## What Are the Four Types of Diabetes Pills?

Four types of diabetes pills can help people with type 2 diabetes lower their blood sugar. Each type of pill helps lower blood sugar in a different way. The diabetes pill you take is from one of these groups. You might know your pills by a different name.

- **Sulfonylureas** (*SUL-fah-nil-YOO-ree-ahz*).
- **Biguanides** (*by-GWAN-ides*).
- **Alpha-glucosidase inhibitors** (*AL-fa gloo-KOS-a-dayss in-HIB-it-erz*).
- **Thiazolidinediones** (*THEE-ah-ZAH-la-deen-DYE-owns*).

Your doctor might prescribe one pill. If the pill does not lower your blood sugar, your doctor may

- Ask you to take more of the same pills, or
- Add a new pill or insulin, or
- Ask you to change to another pill or insulin.

### *Questions to Ask about Your Diabetes Medicines*

Ask these questions when your doctor prescribes a medicine.

- When do I take the medicine—before a meal, with a meal, or after a meal?
- How often should I take the medicine?
- Should I take the medicine at the same time every day?
- What should I do if I forget to take my medicine?
- What side effects may happen?
- What should I do if I get side effects?

## *What Are Side Effects?*

- Side effects are changes that may happen in your body when you take a medicine. When your doctor gives you a new medicine, ask what the side effects might be.
- Some side effects happen just when you start to take the medicine. Then they go away.
- Some side effects happen only once in a while. You may get used to them or learn how to manage them.
- Some side effects will cause you to stop taking the medicine. Your doctor may try another one that doesn't cause you side effects.

## Sulfonylureas

These pills do two things:

- They help your pancreas make more insulin, which then lowers your blood sugar.
- They help your body use the insulin it makes to better lower your blood sugar.

For these pills to work, your pancreas has to make some insulin. Sulfonylureas can make your blood sugar too low, which is called hypoglycemia (*HY-po-gly-SEE-mee-ah*).

### *How often should I take sulfonylureas?*

Some sulfonylureas work all day, so you take them only once a day. Others you take twice a day. Your doctor will tell you how many times a day you should take your diabetes pill(s). Ask if you are not sure.

### *When should I take sulfonylureas?*

The time you take your pill depends on which pill you take and what your doctor tells you. If you take the pill once a day, you will likely take it just before the first meal of the day (breakfast). If you take the medicine twice a day, you will likely take the first pill just before your first meal, and the second pill just before the last meal of the day (supper). Take the medicine at the same times each day. Ask your doctor when you should take your pills.

### *What are possible side effects?*

Taking sulfonylureas might cause:

- A low blood sugar reaction (hypoglycemia).
- An upset stomach.
- A skin rash or itching.
- Weight gain.

**Table 34.2.** Other Names for Sulfonylureas

| Generic Name | Brand Name |
|---|---|
| acetohexamide | Dymelor |
| chlorpropamide | Diabinese |
| glimepiride | Amaryl |
| glipizide | Glucotrol, Glucotrol XL |
| glyburide | DiaBeta,Glynase PresTab, Micronase |
| tolazamide | Tolinase |
| tolbutamide | Orinase |

## *Biguanides*

Biguanides are another type of diabetes medicine. Metformin (*met-FOR-min*) is a biguanide that helps lower blood sugar by making sure your liver does not make too much sugar. Metformin also lowers the amount of insulin in your body.

You may lose a few pounds when you start to take metformin. This weight loss can help you control your blood glucose. Metformin can also improve blood fat and cholesterol levels, which are often not normal if you have type 2 diabetes.

Do not take metformin if you have kidney disease.

If you drink alcohol, talk to your doctor about whether you should take metformin.

A good thing about metformin is that it does not cause blood sugar to get too low (hypoglycemia) when it is the only diabetes medicine you take.

***How often should I take metformin?***

Two or three times a day.

***When should I take metformin?***

With a meal. Your doctor should tell you which meals to take it with.

***What are possible side effects?***

Taking metformin might cause:

- Nausea, diarrhea, and some other stomach symptoms (these usually go away after you take the medicine for a while).
- A metallic taste in your mouth.

**Table 34.3.** Names for Biguanides

| Generic Name | Brand Name |
|---|---|
| metformin | Glucophage |

### *You Need to Know:*

- Do not change or stop taking your diabetes medicine without first talking to your doctor.
- Your doctor might ask you to switch from pills to insulin shots if your pancreas stops making enough insulin.

## *Alpha-glucosidase Inhibitors*

There are now two alpha-glucosidase inhibitors, acarbose (*AK-er-bose*) and miglitol (*MIG-leh-tall*). Both medicines block the enzymes that digest the starches you eat. This action causes a slower and lower rise of blood sugar through the day, but mainly right after meals.

Neither acarbose nor miglitol causes blood sugar to get too low (hypoglycemia) when it is the only diabetes medicine you take.

***How often should I take acarbose or miglitol?***

Three times a day, at each meal. Your doctor might ask you to take the medicine less often at first.

***When should I take acarbose or miglitol?***

With the first bite of a meal.

***What are possible side effects?***

Taking this pill may cause stomach problems (gas, bloating, and diarrhea) that most often go away after you take the medicine for a while.

**Table 34.4.** Names for Alpha-glucosidase inhibitors

| Generic Name | Brand Name |
|---|---|
| acarbose | Precose |
| miglitol | Glyset |

## Thiazolidinediones

This type of medicine helps your muscles make better use of your insulin. The only medicine now in this group is called troglitazone (*tro-GLIT-uh-zone*). Troglitazone doesn't cause blood sugar to go too low when it is the only diabetes medicine you take.

***How often should I take troglitazone?***

Usually once a day.

***When should I take troglitazone?***

With the same meal at the same time each day. Ask your doctor when you should take it. Your body uses this medicine best if you take it with your largest meal of the day.

***What are possible side effects?***

Most people can take troglitazone without any side effects. However, if you take birth control pills, you should know that troglitazone might make your birth control pills less effective. Make sure your doctor knows that you take birth control pills.

**Table 34.5.** Names for Thiazolidinediones

| Generic Name | Brand Name |
|---|---|
| troglitazone | Rezulin |

## What Do I Need to Know about Insulin?

If your pancreas no longer makes enough insulin, then you need to take insulin as a shot. You inject the insulin just under the skin with a small, short needle. You cannot take insulin as a pill.

### Why can't I take insulin as a pill?

Insulin is a protein. If you took insulin as a pill, your body would break it down and digest it before it got into your blood to lower your blood sugar.

### How does insulin work?

Insulin lowers blood sugar by moving sugar from the blood into the cells of your body. Once inside the cells, sugar provides energy. Insulin lowers your blood sugar whether you eat or not. You should eat on time if you take insulin.

### How often should I take insulin?

Most people with diabetes need at least two insulin shots a day for good blood sugar control. Some people take three or four shots a day to have a more flexible diabetes plan.

### When should I take insulin?

You should take insulin 30 minutes before a meal if you take regular insulin alone or with a longer-acting insulin. If you take insulin lispro (Humalog), an insulin that works very quickly, you should take your shot just before you eat.

### Are there several types of insulin?

Yes. There are five main types of insulin. They each work at different speeds. Many people take two types of insulin.

## What are the five types of insulin?

*Quick acting, insulin lispro (Humalog)*

- **Starts** working in 5 to 15 minutes.
- **Lowers** blood sugar most in 45 to 90 minutes.
- **Finishes** working in 3 to 4 hours.

*Short acting, Regular (R) insulin*

- **Starts** working in 30 minutes.
- **Lowers** blood sugar most in 2 to 5 hours.
- **Finishes** working in 5 to 8 hours.

*Intermediate acting, NPH (N) or Lente (L) insulin*

- **Starts** working in 1 to 3 hours.
- **Lowers** blood sugar most in 6 to 12 hours.
- **Finishes** working in 16 to 24 hours.

*Long acting, Ultralente (U) insulin*

- **Starts** working in 4 to 6 hours.
- **Lowers** blood sugar most in 8 to 20 hours.
- **Finishes** working in 24 to 28 hours.

*NPH and Regular insulin mixture*

Two types of insulins mixed together in one bottle.

- **Starts** working in 30 minutes.
- **Lowers** blood sugar most in 7 to 12 hours.
- **Finishes** working in 16 to 24 hours.

## Does insulin work the same all the time?

After a short time, you will get to know when your insulin starts to work, when it works its hardest to lower blood sugar, and when it finishes working.

You will learn to match your mealtimes and exercise times to the time when each insulin you take works in your body.

How quickly or slowly insulin works in your body depends on:

- Your own response.
- The place on your body where you inject insulin.
- The type and amount of exercise you do and the length of time between your shot and exercise.

### *Where on my body should I inject insulin?*

You can inject insulin into several places on your body. Insulin injected near the stomach works fastest. Insulin injected into the thigh works slowest. Insulin injected into the arm works at medium speed. Ask your doctor or diabetes teacher to show you the right way to take insulin and in which parts of the body to inject it.

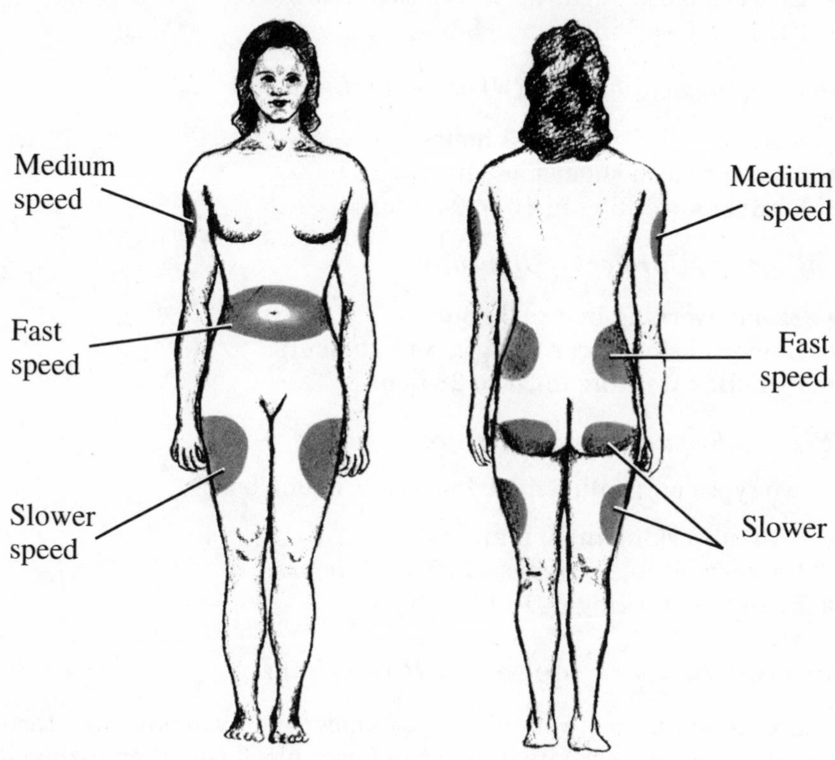


***Figure 34.6.*** *These are good places to give yourself insulin shots.*

### *How should I store insulin?*

- If you use a whole bottle of insulin within 30 days, keep that bottle of insulin at room temperature. On the label, write the date that is 30 days away. That is when you should throw out the bottle with any insulin left in it.

- If you do not use a whole bottle of insulin within 30 days, then store it in the refrigerator all the time.

- If insulin gets too hot or cold, it breaks down and does not work. So, do not keep insulin in very cold places such as the freezer, or in hot places, such as by a window or in the car's glove compartment during warm weather.

- Keep at least one extra bottle of each type of insulin you use in your house. Store extra insulin in the refrigerator.

## *Might I Take More Than One Diabetes Medicine at a Time?*

Yes. Your doctor may ask you to take more than one diabetes medicine at a time. Some diabetes medicines that lower blood sugar work well together. Here are examples.

### *Two Diabetes Pills*

If one type of pill alone does not control your blood sugar, then your doctor might ask you to take two kinds of pills. Each type of pill has its own way of acting to lower blood sugar. Here are pills used together:

- A sulfonylurea and metformin.
- A sulfonylurea and acarbose.
- Metformin and acarbose.

### *Diabetes Pills and Insulin*

Your doctor might ask you to take insulin and one of these diabetes pills:

- Insulin and a sulfonylurea.
- Insulin and metformin.
- Insulin and troglitazone.

## What Should I Know about Low Blood Sugar?

Sulfonylureas and insulin are the two diabetes medicines that can make blood sugar go too low. Low blood sugar can happen for many reasons:

- Delaying or skipping a meal.
- Eating too little food at a meal.
- Getting more exercise than usual.
- Taking too much diabetes medicine.
- Drinking alcohol.

You know your blood sugar may be low when you feel one or more of the following:

- Dizzy or light-headed.
- Hungry.
- Nervous and shaky.
- Sleepy or confused.
- Sweaty.

If you think your blood sugar is low, test it to see for sure. If your blood sugar is at or below 70 mg/dl, eat one of these items to get 15 grams of carbohydrate:

- 1/2 cup (4 oz.) of any fruit juice.
- 1 cup (8 oz.) of fat-free or low-fat milk.
- 4 teaspoons of granulated white sugar.
- 1/3 cup (3 oz.) regular soda.
- 6 to 7 small Lifesavers or 4 large Lifesavers.
- Glucose gel or tablets (take the amount noted on package to add up to 15 grams of carbohydrate).

Test your blood sugar again 15 minutes later. If it is still below 70 mg/dl, then eat another 15 grams of carbohydrate. Then test your blood sugar again in 15 minutes.

If you cannot test your blood sugar right away but you feel symptoms of low blood sugar, follow the steps above.

If your blood sugar is not low, but you will not eat your next meal for at least an hour, then have a snack with starch and protein. Here are some examples:

- Crackers and peanut butter or cheese.
- Half of a ham or turkey sandwich.
- A cup of milk and crackers or cereal.

## How Do I Know If My Diabetes Medicines Are Working?

Learn to test your blood sugar. Ask your doctor or diabetes teacher about the best testing tools for you and how often to test. After you test your blood sugar, write down your blood sugar test results. Then ask your doctor or diabetes teacher if your diabetes medicines are working. A good blood sugar reading before meals is between 70 and 140 mg/dl.

Ask your doctor or diabetes teacher about how low or how high your blood sugar should get before you take action. For many people, blood sugar is too low below 70 mg/dl and too high above 240 mg/dl.

One other number to know is the result of a blood test your doctor does called hemoglobin A1c (*HE-mah-glow-bin A-1-C*) or glycated hemoglobin (*GLY-kay-ted HE-mah-glow-bin*). It shows your blood sugar control during the last 2 to 3 months. For most people, a good hemoglobin A1c is 7 percent.

## How to Find More Help

**Diabetes Teachers** (nurses, dietitians, pharmacists, and other health professionals)

- To find a diabetes teacher near you, call the American Association of Diabetes Educators toll-free at 1-800-TEAMUP4 (1-800-832-6874).

**Recognized Diabetes Education Programs** (teaching programs approved by the American Diabetes Association)

- To find a program near you, call 1-800-DIABETES (1-800-342-2383) or look at its Internet home page <http://www.diabetes.org> and click on "Diabetes Info."

**Dietitians**

- To find a dietitian near you, call The American Dietetic Association's National Center for Nutrition and Dietetics at 1-800-366-1655 or look at its Internet home page <http://www.eatright.org> and click on "Find a Dietitian."

## Chapter 35

# All About Insulin

### What Is Insulin?

Inside the pancreas, beta cells make the protein insulin. With each meal, beta cells release insulin to help the body use or store the glucose it gets from food.

People with insulin-dependent (type 1) diabetes no longer make insulin. Their beta cells have been destroyed. They need insulin shots to use glucose from meals.

People with non-insulin-dependent (type 2) diabetes make insulin, but their bodies don't respond well to it. Some people with type 2 diabetes need diabetes pills or extra insulin in shots to help their bodies use their own insulin better.

If you have type 1 or type 2 diabetes and inject insulin, you have many questions about insulin. Insulin cannot be taken as a pill. Because it is a protein, it would be broken down during digestion just like the protein in food. It must be injected into the fat under your skin for insulin to get into your blood.

There are almost 30 types of insulin made by two companies in the United States. These insulins differ in how they are made, how they work in the body, and price. Today's insulins are very pure. Allergic reactions to insulin are rare.

Insulin comes from either animals or is made in labs by bacteria that have gene instructions to make human insulin. Human insulin does not come from humans. There are three broad types of insulin, based on:

- How soon the insulin starts working (onset).
- When it works the hardest (peak time).
- How long it lasts in your body (duration).

However, each person responds to insulin in his or her own way. That is why onset, peak time, and duration are given as ranges.

Short-acting (Regular) insulin usually reaches the blood within 30 minutes after injection. It peaks 2 to 4 hours later and stays in the blood for about 4 to 8 hours.

Intermediate-acting (NPH and Lente) insulins reach the blood 2 to 6 hours after injection. They peak 4 to 14 hours later and stay in the blood for about 14 to 24 hours.

Long-acting (Ultralente) insulin takes 6 to 14 hours to start working. It has no peak or a very small peak 14 to 24 hours after injection. It stays in the blood between 20 and 36 hours.

Some types of insulin come mixed together. For example, you can buy Regular and NPH insulins already mixed in one bottle. They make life easier if you need to inject two kinds of insulin at the same time. However, you can't adjust the amount of one insulin without also changing how much you get of the other insulin.

## Strength

Insulins come dissolved in liquids at different strengths. Most people use U-100 insulin. This means it has 100 units of insulin per millimeter of fluid. Be sure that the syringe you use matches the insulin strength. U-100 insulin needs a U-100 syringe. In Europe and Latin America, U-40 insulin is also used.

If you're outside the United States, be certain to match your insulin strength with the correct size syringe.

## Additives

All insulins have added ingredients to keep them fresh and help them work better. Intermediate- and long-acting insulins also have ingredients to make them act longer. The additives may vary among different brands of the same kind of insulin and may cause slight differences in the onset and duration times.

## Storage and Safety

Insulin makers advise storing insulin in the refrigerator, but using cold insulin can make the shot more painful. You can keep the bottle of insulin you are currently using at room temperature or warm the bottle by gently rolling it between your hands before you fill the syringe.

If you buy more than one bottle of insulin at a time, store the extra bottles in the refrigerator until you start to use them.

Never store insulin at very cold (under 36 degrees Fahrenheit) or very hot (over 86 degrees Fahrenheit) temperatures. Extreme temperatures destroy insulin. Do not put your insulin in the freezer or in direct sunlight.

Before using any insulin, check the expiration date. Insulin may lose potency slightly if the bottle has been used for more than 30 days. Look at the bottle closely to make sure the insulin looks normal. If you use Regular, it should be perfectly clear—no floating pieces or color.

If you use NPH or Lente, it should be cloudy, with no floating pieces or crystals on the bottle. If you find any problems, return the bottle of insulin for an exchange or refund.

## Insulin Therapy

With your health care team's help, you can find an insulin therapy routine that will control your blood glucose, help you feel good, and fit your lifestyle.

Conventional insulin therapy means taking the same shots at the same times each day—usually a shot in the morning and a shot in the evening.

For most people, conventional therapy prevents dangerously high or low blood glucose levels. But conventional therapy may leave blood glucose levels too high. These higher glucose levels increase the risk of problems with your eyes, kidneys, and nerves.

For that reason, many doctors now advise intensive insulin therapy. This therapy aims to keep your blood glucose as close to normal as possible. Intensive therapy means either taking three or four shots daily or using an insulin pump.

For good results, you must take a very active role in your diabetes care and test your blood glucose level often. Based on your blood glucose records, you and your health care team will fine-tune your treatment plan.

Intensive therapy takes more work but gives you more choices. You are not tied to certain eating or exercise times. However, because you are keeping your blood glucose levels lower, there is a chance of more low blood glucose reactions.

You may also gain some weight. Because you are matching insulin needs closely to glucose levels, your body is able to use and store more of the calories from glucose instead of losing them in the urine.

Talk with your health care team about whether the greater freedom and chance to avoid diabetes complications are worth the drawbacks of intensive therapy.

## Insulin Delivery

Most people who require insulin take shots. Another choice is an insulin pump. Insulin pumps are devices that give a steady dose of Regular insulin. In addition, you signal the pump to give extra Regular insulin to cover meals.

Insulin comes through a plastic tube called an infusion line. This tube is attached to a needle that is inserted into fat under the skin (usually in the abdomen) and taped into place. About the size of a beeper, an insulin pump can be attached to a belt loop or even worn in a shirt or skirt pocket.

## Fine-Tuning Control

Whether you are on conventional or intensive insulin therapy, many factors affect your blood glucose levels. These include:

- How much and when you exercise.
- Where you inject your insulin.
- When you take your injections.
- What you eat.
- Illness.
- Stress.

To feel your best, work with your health care team to learn how each of these factors can affect your glucose control. When you want to improve your insulin routine, consider the following.

## Self-monitoring

It is hard to improve your blood glucose control without testing your blood glucose. Writing down your results and looking over weeks or months of results can help you predict and avoid low or high blood glucose levels.

Tests show how exercise, an exciting event, or a special meal changed your glucose level. By knowing that, you can change your insulin to prevent problems.

## Site Rotation

The place on your body where you inject insulin affects blood glucose control. Insulin enters the blood at different speeds when injected at different sites. Insulin shots work fastest when given in the abdomen.

Insulin arrives in the blood a little more slowly from the upper arms and even more slowly from the thighs and buttocks.

Injecting insulin in the same general area (for example, your abdomen) will give you the best results from your insulin. This is because the insulin will reach the blood with about the same speed with each shot. Don't inject in exactly the same place each time but move around the same area.

If you take several shots a day, you may want to choose one site (perhaps the upper arm) for morning shots, another site for lunch shots, and a third site for evening shots.

If you inject near the same place each time, hard lumps or extra fatty deposits may develop. Both of these problems are unsightly and make the insulin action less reliable.

Any member of your health care team should be able to show you how to correctly rotate your injection sites.

## Timing

Good blood glucose control is all in the timing. The idea is to time your shots so that insulin goes to work when glucose from your food starts to enter your blood. To do this, you need to know how soon your insulin starts to lower your blood glucose. You can find this out by self-monitoring.

## Too Much or Not Enough Insulin?

High morning blood glucose levels before breakfast can be a puzzle. If you haven't eaten, why did your blood glucose level go up? There are two common reasons. If you have very low blood glucose while sleeping, your body releases glucose from the liver. This causes a high blood glucose level in the morning.

Morning nausea and headache may be signs that you've had low blood glucose while sleeping. You may need to eat a bedtime snack to avoid low blood glucose in early morning hours. To see whether this is the problem, set your alarm to self-monitor around 2 or 3 am for several nights.

The other reason for high fasting blood glucose levels on waking is the dawn phenomenon. Near dawn, the levels of certain hormones in your blood naturally increase.

These hormones cause blood glucose to rise, usually around 5 or 6 am. This usually means you need to take a bedtime injection of intermediate- or long-acting insulin that will go to work around dawn.

## Syringe Reuse

Some doctors believe that you can safely reuse your syringe. However, if you are ill, have open wounds on your hands, or have poor resistance to infection for any reason, you should not risk syringe reuse.

Syringe makers will not guarantee the sterility of syringes that are reused. Keeping them germ-free is up to you. Keep the needle clean by keeping it capped when you're not using it.

Don't try to clean it with alcohol. Alcohol wiping removes the coating that helps the needle slide into the skin easily.

Never let the needle touch anything but clean skin and the top of the insulin bottle. Most important, never let anyone use a syringe you've already used, and don't use anyone else's syringe, ever.

Reusing syringes may help you cut costs, avoid buying large supplies of syringes, and reduce waste. However, talk with your doctor or nurse before you begin reusing. They can help you decide whether reuse would be a wise choice for you.

## Syringe Disposal

It's time to dispose of a syringe when the needle is dull or bent or if it has come in contact with anything other than clean skin. Proper syringe disposal is important. Your syringe is medical waste.

If you can do it safely, clip the needles off the syringes. When you remove the needle, no one can use the syringe. It's best to buy a device that clips, catches, and contains the needle. Do not use scissors to clip off needles—the flying needle could hurt someone or become lost.

If you don't destroy your needles, recap them. Place the needle or entire syringe in an opaque (not clear) heavy-duty plastic bottle with a screw cap or a plastic or metal box that closes firmly. Do not use a container that will allow the needle to break through. Make sure your syringe container doesn't get recycled.

Your area may have special rules for getting rid of medical waste like used syringes. Ask your refuse company or city or county waste authority what method meets their rules. When traveling, bring your used syringes home. Pack them in a heavy-duty holder, such as a hard plastic pencil box, for transport.

# Chapter 36

# *Using Insulin Lispro*

### *What is insulin lispro, and how can it help control my blood sugar levels?*

Insulin lispro (brand name: Humalog) is the newest type of insulin on the market. It's a fast-acting insulin that starts working sooner than other insulins. It also reaches peak activity faster and goes away sooner. Insulin lispro helps keep your blood sugar levels from going too high after you eat. Studies show that insulin lispro may do this better than regular insulin. In fact, insulin lispro may replace regular insulin for many patients with diabetes mellitus.

The medicines your doctor has prescribed are very important in keeping your diabetes under control. To keep your blood sugar level steady, your doctor will probably prescribe either a longer-acting insulin or another drug for you to take each day in addition to the insulin lispro.

### *When and how do I take insulin lispro?*

Insulin lispro should be injected under the skin within 15 minutes before you eat. Your doctor will tell you how much insulin lispro to inject. Remember, you must eat 15 minutes after you take this insulin shot.

---

Insulin lispro is a little easier to take than regular insulin. If you've been using regular insulin, you've had to inject the insulin and then wait 30 to 45 minutes before eating. Many people find it hard to time regular insulin injections and mealtimes. Sometimes they end up eating too early or too late. Then they don't get the best blood sugar control. Since insulin lispro is taken so close to meals, it may help you get the best possible blood sugar control.

### *Can I mix insulin lispro with other insulins?*

It's best that you mix insulin lispro only with Humulin U or Humulin N, which are brand names for certain longer-acting insulins. Insulin lispro should always be drawn into the syringe first. This will keep the longer-acting insulin from getting into the insulin lispro bottle. After mixing insulin lispro in the same syringe with Humulin U or Humulin N, you must inject the mixture under your skin within 15 minutes. Remember to eat soon after the injection.

### *How do I prepare the correct dose?*

To prepare a dose of insulin lispro, follow these steps:

1. Wash your hands.
2. Take the plastic cover off the new insulin bottle and wipe the top of the bottle with a cotton swab that you have dipped in alcohol. It's best to allow the insulin to be at room temperature before you inject it.
3. Pull back the plunger of the syringe. This way, you can draw air into the syringe equal to the dose of insulin lispro that you are taking. Then put the syringe needle through the rubber top of the insulin bottle. Inject air into the bottle by pushing the syringe plunger forward. Then turn the bottle upside down.
4. Make sure that the tip of the needle is in the insulin. Pull back on the syringe plunger to draw the correct dose of insulin into the syringe. The dose of insulin is measured in units.
5. Make sure there are no air bubbles in the syringe before you take the needle out of the insulin bottle. Air bubbles can cut down the amount of insulin that you get in your injection. If air bubbles are present, hold the syringe and the bottle

straight up in one hand, tap the syringe with your other hand and let the air bubbles float to the top. Push on the plunger of the syringe to move the air bubbles back into the insulin bottle. Then withdraw the correct insulin dose by pulling back on the plunger.

## *Where do I inject the insulin lispro?*

Insulin lispro is injected just under the skin. Your doctor or office staff will show you how and where to give an insulin injection. First, clean your skin with cotton dipped in alcohol. Most people are able to grab a fold of skin and inject insulin at a 90-degree angle. If you're thin, you may need to pinch the skin and inject the insulin at a 45-degree angle. When the needle is in your skin, you don't need to draw back on the syringe plunger to check for blood.

The usual places to inject insulin are the upper arm, the front and side parts of the thighs and the abdomen (tummy area). Don't inject insulin closer than two inches to your navel (belly button).

To keep your skin from thickening, try not to inject the insulin in the same place over and over. Instead, change injection places. But if you usually inject insulin into your arm, just inject in different spots on your arm rather than switch to the thigh or abdomen. This works better because insulin is absorbed at different rates from your arm, your thigh and your abdomen.

## *What do I do if I have an "insulin reaction"?*

Hypoglycemia is the name for a condition in which the blood sugar level is too low. In people who take insulin, this condition is called an insulin reaction. Your blood sugar level can get too low if you exercise more than usual, if you don't eat enough or if you don't eat on time. If you have an insulin reaction, you may feel some or all of these symptoms: headache, nervousness, shakiness, heavy sweating, rapid heartbeat, hunger, confusion or dizziness. Most people who take insulin have insulin reactions at some time.

If you're going to be treated with insulin lispro, you need to be aware of insulin reactions and how to treat them. Insulin lispro will help you control your blood sugar level, but it does act quickly. While you and your doctor are working together to adjust your dose of this insulin, you may have some insulin reactions.

Just in case you have an insulin reaction, you should carry at least 15 grams of a fast-acting carbohydrate with you at all times. Here are examples of quick sources of energy that can relieve the symptoms of an insulin reaction:

- Nondiet sodas—one half to three fourths of a cup
- Fruit juices and fruits—one-half cup of juice or 2 tablespoons of raisins
- Candy—five Lifesavers
- Milk—one cup
- Glucose tablets—three tablets that are 5 grams each.

If you don't feel better 15 minutes after having a fast-acting carbohydrate or if monitoring shows that your blood sugar level is still too low, have another 15 grams of a fast-acting carbohydrate.

If your blood sugar level is too low and, because of some physical problem, you need help from another person, you should teach family members and friends how to give you a drug called glucagon. Glucagon comes in a powder and a liquid that must be mixed together. Then the mixture has to be injected. Be sure that you take the time to learn about using glucagon.

### *How can I keep my blood sugar level from becoming too high or too low?*

You need to check your blood sugar level regularly using a blood glucose monitor. Your doctor or the office staff can teach you how to use the monitor. You'll need to write each measurement down and show this record to your doctor, so your doctor can tell you how much insulin to take.

Blood sugar measurements are different depending on stress, exercise, how fast you absorb your food, and hormonal changes related to puberty, menstrual cycles, pregnancy, etc. Illness, traveling or a change in your routine may mean that you have to monitor your blood sugar level more often.

This information provides a general overview on using insulin lispro and may not apply to everyone. Talk to your family doctor to find out if this information applies to you and to get more information on this subject.

This data is provided to you by your family doctor and the American Academy of Family Physicians. Other health-related information is available from the AAFP on the World Wide Web (http://www.aafp.org/healthinfo). Information may also be obtained from HealthAnswers® ( http://www.healthanswers.com).

## Chapter 37

# *Insulin Delivery*

Syringes...pumps...jet injectors... pens...infusers... they all do the same thing—deliver insulin. These items carry insulin through the outermost layer of skin and into fatty tissue so it can be used by the body. This category also includes injection aids—products designed to make giving an injection easier.

### *Syringes*

Today's syringes are smaller and have finer points and special coatings that work to make injecting as easy and painless as possible. When insulin injections are done properly, most people discover they are relatively painless.

Check with your doctor or diabetes educator and test several brands before you buy. Your equipment should suit your needs.

#### *Questions to ask:*

- Does the syringe dose match your insulin strength? If you take U-100 insulin, use U-100 syringes. (Generally, this is not a problem in the United States because U-100 is standard here.

---

*Diabetes Forecast*, October 1997; © 1997 American Diabetes Association; reprinted with permission. "Insulin Delivery Methods Under Development" is excerpted from "Devices to Take Insulin," National Diabetes Information Clearinghouse, a service of the National Institute of Diabetes and Digestive and Kidney Diseases, March 17, 1998.

- Does your syringe match your insulin dosage? If you take 30 units or less of insulin, you may use the 3/10-cc syringe. The 1/2-cc syringe may be used by those taking 50 units or less, and the 1-cc syringe is designed for those needing up to 100 units of insulin. Using a syringe that more closely matches your dose may help you more accurately draw up your insulin. If you are changing the syringe you use, check dosage lines carefully. In some syringes, one line is equal to one unit of insulin, but in others, each line is equal to two units of insulin.

- Can you easily draw up your dosage in a particular syringe? Does the syringe barrel have the kind of markings you can read easily—or are they too close together? Does having a plunger that's a different color make it easier for you?

- Would a shorter needle be a better choice for you or your child with diabetes? Some syringes now have shorter needles which many people find to be more comfortable. However, the depth of the injection can change the absorption. Ask your doctor or diabetes educator to assess whether this would be a good alternative to your current syringe.

- Does this brand come packaged as you prefer?

Cost is another factor because many stores use insulin syringes as key sale items. Shop around for a good price, but ask yourself: Is giving up a good local pharmacist to save $2 at an out-of-the-way store worth the money?

You may be interested in reusing your syringes. Most manufacturers do not recommend this and there may be some increased risk to patients (i.e., needle dullness causing discomfort and possible infection). While this practice remains controversial, many patients reuse syringes without any problems. Once again, your health care team can advise you on the practice.

And please, always follow appropriate guidelines when disposing of your syringes and lancets. Some states have very specific laws governing disposal of such items, while others have no guidelines. Even if no guidelines exist, you should be considerate of those who could possibly come in contact with used syringes and lancets. They can be safely placed in a puncture-proof container that can be sealed shut before it is placed in the trash.

## *Pumps*

The insulin pump is not an artificial pancreas (because you still have to monitor your blood glucose level). But improved blood sugar control can be achieved, and many people prefer this continuous system of insulin delivery over injections.

Insulin pumps are computerized devices, about the size of a call-beeper, that you can wear on your belt or in your pocket. They deliver a steady, measured dose of insulin through a cannula (a flexible plastic tube) with a small needle that is inserted through the skin into the fatty tissue and taped in place. In the newer products, the needle is removed and a soft catheter remains in place. On your command, the pump releases a bolus (a surge) of insulin; this is usually done about half an hour before eating to blunt the rise in blood glucose after the meal. Of course, if you use Humalog, the new ultra-fast-acting insulin, the time of the bolus would be considerably closer to the meal.

Because the pump releases incredibly small doses of insulin continuously, this delivery system most closely mimics the body's normal release of insulin. Also, pumps deliver very precise insulin doses for different times of day, which in many instances are necessary to correct the dawn phenomenon, or the rise of blood sugar that occurs in the hours before and after waking.

Many people have chosen the insulin pump because they believe it enables them to enjoy a more flexible lifestyle. But insulin pumps are not for everyone. To use a pump, you must be willing to test your blood glucose at least four times a day and learn how to make adjustments in insulin, food, and exercise in response to those test results. Before you consider pump therapy, ask yourself: Am I willing to assume this level of responsibility for my diabetes care?

You'll want to check with your insurance carrier before you buy a pump and all the supplies. Although most carriers do cover these items, notable exceptions are Medicare and many HMOs.

If you are interested in buying a pump, talk to your health care team.

## *Injection Aids*

This category includes devices that make giving an injection easier as well as syringe alternatives.

Talk with your doctor or diabetes educator about these kinds of products. Oftentimes, they will make sample products available to you before you make a purchase. You'll want to look for an item that is easy for you to use and is durable. Some items require more skill and dexterity on the part of the user than others, so test several before you buy. Testing will help you choose the one that is easiest for you to use.

**Insertion aids.** These devices accelerate needle insertion into the skin. Some even aid in pushing down the plunger. Most are spring-loaded and hide the needle from view.

**Syringe alternatives.** At present, this category includes infusers, insulin pens, and jet injectors.

Infusers create "portals" into which you inject insulin. With an infuser, a needle is inserted into subcutaneous tissues and remains taped in place, usually on the abdomen, for 48-72 hours. The insulin is injected into it, rather than directly through the skin into the fatty tissue. Some people are prone to infections with this type of product, so be sure to discuss the necessary cleaning procedures with your health care team.

Carrying around an insulin pen is like having an old-fashioned cartridge pen in your pocket—only instead of a writing point, there's a needle, and instead of an ink cartridge, there's an insulin cartridge. There are even disposable insulin pens now available. The devices are convenient, accurate, and often used by people on a multi-dose regimen. Insulin cartridges may come in limited total capacities of Regular, NPH, lispro, or 70/30 premixed insulin. They are particularly useful for people whose coordination is impaired, or for people who are on the go.

Jet injectors release a tiny jet stream of insulin, which is forced through the skin with pressure, not a puncture. These devices have no needles. However, they can sometimes cause bruising. You will need to work with your health care team to ensure good blood glucose control as you adjust to one of these devices.

You'll want to ask manufacturers about training on the use of a jet injector, as well as how to clean it and how to troubleshoot. If jet injectors interest you, discuss their use with your health care team. Before buying, check to be sure your insurance covers jet injectors.

## Aids for People with Visual Impairments

There are several products designed to make injections easier for people who are visually impaired. Some products handle more than one task.

**Non-visual insulin measurement.** Helps you measure an accurate dose of insulin. Some click at each 2-unit increment of insulin.

**Needle guides and vial stabilizers.** Help you insert the needle into the correct insulin vial for drawing up an injection.

**Syringe magnifiers.** Enlarge the measure marks on a syringe barrel.

It is important to note that certain of these aids fit only with specific brands of syringes, so check to be sure the product you want works with your syringe.

## Insulin Delivery Methods Under Development

**Implantable insulin pumps.** Implantable insulin pumps are surgically implanted, usually on the left side of the abdomen. The pump is disk shaped and weighs about 6 to 8 ounces. The pump delivers a basal dose of insulin continuously throughout the day. Users deliver bolus insulin doses with a handheld telemetry unit that instructs the pump to give the specified amount of insulin.

An advantage of this method is that, like insulin produced naturally from the pancreas, the insulin from the pump goes directly to the liver to prevent excess sugar production there.

**Insulin patch.** The insulin patch, placed on the skin, gives a continuous low dose of insulin. To adjust insulin doses before meals, users can pull off a tab on the patch to release insulin. The problem with the patch is that insulin does not get through the skin easily.

The U.S. Government does not endorse or favor any specific commercial product or company. Trade, proprietary, or company names appearing in this summary are used only because they are considered essential in the context of the information provided herein.

## Additional Information on Alternative Methods of Insulin Delivery

The National Diabetes Information Clearinghouse collects resource information on diabetes for Combined Health Information Database (CHID). CHID is a database produced by health-related agencies of the Federal Government. This database provides titles, abstracts, and availability information for health information and health education resources.

To provide you with the most up-to-date resources, information specialists at the clearinghouse created an automatic search of CHID. To obtain this information you may view the results of the automatic search on Alternative Methods of Insulin Delivery available on line at http://chid.aerie.com.

Or, if you wish to perform your own search of the database, you may access the CHID Online web site and search CHID yourself at http://chid.nih.gov.

This information is provided by the National Diabetes Information Clearinghouse, a service of the National Institute of Diabetes and Digestive and Kidney Diseases.

# Chapter 38

# *New Diabetes Drugs: Pathways to Better Control*

In the past year and a half, some remarkable new drugs have hit the market, giving you and your doctor the means to manage your diabetes better than ever before. You may have heard about some of these new drugs, and your doctor may already have suggested a change in your medicine. These new drugs work, and they work well, but the same treatment may not be right for each individual. Everybody's diabetes is different, and a "cookie cutter" approach to diabetes management doesn't work. This chapter will explain what these new medicines do, how they can improve diabetes control, and which might be right for you.

Until recently we've had only two types of medicine to help control diabetes when diet and exercise are not enough: oral sulfonylurea tablets and injections of insulin. Now, in less than two years, the Food and Drug Administration (FDA) has approved two new kinds of oral medicine as well as new sulfonylureas and a new type of insulin, and soon we'll have another type of oral medicine and even more kinds of new insulins. With all these choices, selecting the right treatment for each person becomes a real challenge.

To understand how these new drugs work, it would help to review some of the changes that occur in your body that lead to blood glucose being elevated.

---

## Type I Basics

If you have Type I (insulin-dependent) diabetes, you probably have this down cold. But to understand the impact of some of these new drugs, it's important to have a firm grasp of the major problem in Type I diabetes. In Type I diabetes, the cells in the pancreas that are responsible for producing insulin have been damaged. Over a relatively short period of time, these cells (called the beta cells) can no longer produce and secrete any insulin. And without insulin, the body can't regulate the storage, delivery, and use of glucose. Any treatment of Type I diabetes therefore has to revolve around replacing insulin.

Until medical science learns how to introduce healthy beta cells into the body or to make an artificial pancreas, new developments in Type I treatment depend on improving the ability to deliver insulin in a way that matches food intake. Doing this just right is hard, but the basic idea is simple: Replace the missing insulin.

## Type II Basics

Type II (non-insulin-dependent) diabetes is more complicated. Multiple factors contribute to the development of high blood sugar levels, and these different factors may be more or less important in any one person.

Resistance to insulin. Resistance to the action of insulin is present in most people with Type II diabetes. This means the body's tissues are less sensitive to insulin and higher levels of insulin are needed to move glucose into the cells. So one type of medicine that will help treat diabetes is one that makes tissues more sensitive to insulin. Weight loss and exercise decrease insulin resistance, and even with the advent of powerful new drugs, diet and exercise remain mainstays of effective Type II management.

Shortage of insulin. Even with insulin resistance, diabetes won't develop unless the beta cells aren't able to increase their production of insulin. In Type II diabetes, insulin is present but there isn't enough. Therefore, a medicine that increases the ability of the beta cells to produce insulin will also help control blood sugar levels.

Too much glucose from the liver. When you're not eating, your body is still able to maintain enough glucose in the blood to continue to function. The liver does this by producing glucose from stored fuels. One of the functions of insulin is to keep the liver from pumping out too much glucose, but that's exactly what the liver does when there isn't enough insulin around. Another way to help control diabetes, then, is to control this overproduction of glucose by the liver.

## The Old Treatments

### *Sulfonylureas*

For people with Type II diabetes, oral sulfonylureas have been the standard initial treatment for many years. There is a long history of experience with them, and they've been well tolerated, safe, and effective. For these reasons, these drugs will continue to be widely used.

Sulfonylureas work by stimulating the pancreas to produce more insulin. They're effective for most people when diet and exercise alone are no longer able to control blood sugar. In fact, when sulfonylureas aren't effective early in the course of treatment, it may be because the problem is really late-onset Type I diabetes, which can look a lot like Type II.

Another reason sulfonylureas may not work at first is that glucose toxicity can get in the way. Glucose toxicity occurs when blood glucose levels are so high that the high sugar itself makes the pancreas less able to produce insulin and makes insulin resistance worse. When this happens, insulin injections may be necessary at first to get the blood sugar down. Once better control is established, a sulfonylurea may work.

The most commonly used sulfonylureas today are glyburide (sold under the names Micronase, DiaBeta, and Glynase) and glipizide (brand name Glucotrol). These preparations, referred to as second-generation sulfonylureas, are quite effective in reducing blood sugar and have few unwanted effects. However, the peak action of these drugs occurs within hours of being taken, so to get the best results and to avoid low blood sugars, it is important to take them at the right time. Often, they have to be taken twice a day to be fully effective. A small amount of weight gain is common at the time treatment with sulfonylureas is started. This occurs at least partly because previously high blood sugar is used more efficiently and much of it gets stored as fat.

All sulfonylurea medicines work basically the same way, so if one becomes less effective over time, changing to another sulfonylurea is unlikely to work better.

### *Insulin*

A few words are necessary here about the terms Type I (insulin-dependent) and Type II (non-insulin-dependent). These terms refer to the underlying cause of the diabetes, not to the type of treatment used. People with Type I diabetes need insulin to live. Without it, they will develop a metabolic imbalance called ketoacidosis and soon die.

A person with Type II diabetes, on the other hand, may need insulin to control blood sugar and prevent complications of diabetes but is not dependent on insulin for survival. So when a person with Type II diabetes starts taking insulin injections, the diabetes is still Type II and does not change to Type I, or insulin-dependent, diabetes. In fact, many people with Type II diabetes need insulin treatment at some time—either temporarily, such as at the time of surgery, or as the main treatment after many years of diabetes.

Until recently, insulin has only been available as a short-acting preparation (Regular insulin), in longer-acting forms (NPH and Lente insulins), as a very long-acting type, used less often, called Ultralente, and as premixed combinations: 70/30 (70% NPH and 30% Regular) and 50/50 (50% NPH and 50% Regular). The premixed insulins are most helpful for those who have stable insulin needs. Trying to get the timing of insulin action to match food intake can be a challenge, and it tends to be more difficult for people with Type I diabetes because their only source of insulin is by injection.

## The New Stuff

Four new oral treatments and one new insulin have recently arrived in pharmacies. Of the oral drugs, two are new sulfonylurea preparations, and two are new agents that have been tested extensively elsewhere in the world and are now available in the United States. The new insulin offers several advantages over previously available insulins.

### New Sulfonylureas

The biggest news in sulfonylurea treatment is the development of new forms of these drugs that give a steady blood glucose level throughout the day. They are just as effective as the old preparations but can be given in a single daily dose, and probably with less risk of low blood sugar. The two forms of sulfonylureas that give more even blood glucose levels with a single daily dose are an extended-release form of glipizide (brand name Glucotrol XL) and a medicine just released called glimepiride (marketed as Amaryl).

If you're currently taking a different sulfonylurea and it's working well, there's probably no reason to change to a newer preparation. But we think the new long-acting preparations are a safer and more convenient way to begin treatment with a sulfonylurea.

You get most of the effect of sulfonylurea medicines with relatively low doses. This is especially true with the new long-acting preparations;

you get practically the full effect with a single 5-milligram capsule of extended-release glipizide or one 4-milligram glimepiride pill. If the dose is increased progressively without bringing improvement in control, further increases aren't likely to give additional benefit and it's probably time to add a second treatment. This "secondary failure" seems to be part of the natural progression of Type II diabetes. After 5 to 7 years, sulfonylureas are often not enough to control blood glucose levels; at that point the need to add another treatment is common. This is when some of the newer drugs should be considered.

## *Metformin*

You may already be familiar with this new drug. It was approved by the FDA almost two years ago. Its brand name is Glucophage. Metformin probably works mainly by keeping your liver from overproducing glucose. It's a highly effective oral medicine that can be used alone as the first medicine given for Type II diabetes. It can also be used in combination with sulfonylureas. Depending on your individual needs, the dose can range from 500 milligrams once daily to 850 milligrams three times a day. At maximal doses, metformin has about the same glucose-lowering power as the sulfonylureas. Since metformin works by a different mechanism than the sulfonylurea drugs, both drugs can be used in combination and the effect of each drug is additive to the other, producing a powerful glucose-lowering effect.

There are some significant advantages to metformin. Metformin doesn't cause low blood sugar, as sometimes occurs with sulfonylurea therapy. People don't gain weight when they take metformin for their diabetes, and they sometimes see their cholesterol and triglyceride levels decline. Metformin also doesn't increase insulin levels in the blood; this may be beneficial since some experts worry that high insulin levels could increase the risk of heart problems.

On the other hand, side effects such as nausea, abdominal discomfort, or diarrhea may occur; these symptoms are usually mild and often lessen or disappear with time. Side effects are also less common if metformin is taken with food and if the dose is increased gradually (Metformin is usually taken in divided doses, two to three times a day with meals). Finally, in rare circumstances, a dangerous buildup of lactic acid in the blood may occur. This serious side effect can be avoided by not using this medicine if you have kidney or liver disease, use alcohol heavily, or are seriously ill with other conditions.

### Acarbose

This drug was approved by the FDA for the treatment of Type II diabetes late last year; its commercial name is Precose. It works by blocking the enzymes that break down dietary starches so they can be absorbed in the small intestine. Blocking the enzymes helps decrease the rapid rise in blood sugar that would normally occur right after a meal. None of the other oral drugs for diabetes has as great an effect on after-meal rises in blood sugar, so acarbose is particularly useful for people who have their most significant blood sugar elevations after meals.

Acarbose has been approved for use alone or in combination with sulfonylureas, but it has also been used with metformin and with insulin, and it adds to the blood glucose lowering effect of each of these medicines.

Although it has only been formally approved for use in Type II diabetes, acarbose can also produce a benefit in Type I diabetes. In Type I diabetes, insulin often doesn't get absorbed quickly enough to help prevent a large rise in blood sugar after a meal, and acarbose can delay the absorption of carbohydrate so the insulin and food intake are better matched.

Acarbose isn't as powerful as sulfonylureas or metformin. Its blood glucose lowering effect is about half of what can usually be achieved with sulfonylureas or metformin, so it's not likely to be helpful if blood sugar levels are very high. Like metformin, acarbose by itself doesn't cause low blood sugar. It also doesn't cause weight gain. It's probably most useful early in the course of Type II diabetes, or as an addition to other drugs. Its greatest limitation comes from its gastrointestinal side effects: gas, bloating, and abdominal discomfort. These side effects can be minimized by starting with a very low dose and gradually increasing the amount taken. The side effects tend to decrease with time as the intestines adapt.

To be effective, this drug must be taken at the start of the meal. Treatment usually starts with half of a 50-milligram tablet just once a day. A dose of 50 milligrams three times a day gives maximal effect for most people.

If you take acarbose along with insulin or a sulfonylurea and you experience a low blood sugar reaction, you will have to use glucose to treat it instead of table sugar or fruit juice. The reason for this is that the main sugar in table sugar, fruit juice, and most other foods is sucrose, and acarbose blocks the absorption of this sugar.

### Lispro

This very-fast-acting insulin analog, sold under the brand name Humalog, was approved by the FDA in June of this year for treating both Type I and Type II diabetes. An insulin analog is an insulin that has been modified to change its effect. In the case of lispro, an insulin was created that starts working within 5 minutes of injection and peaks in one hour. Regular insulin, which was the only short-acting insulin available before the introduction of lispro, starts to work in 30-60 minutes and peaks in 2-4 hours. This is slower than food is absorbed, even when Regular insulin is injected 30 minutes before eating, as is customary. The faster onset and peak action of lispro allow a much better match between food intake and insulin action. Lispro can be taken right as you start eating a meal, eliminating the risk of having an insulin reaction if you have already taken your insulin and your meal is delayed.

Lispro will bring the most benefit to people with Type I diabetes who take short-acting insulin before meals combined with a longer-acting insulin once or twice a day. People who monitor their blood sugar frequently and make dose decisions based on the results can use lispro to help them mimic the way the pancreas secretes insulin in nondiabetic individuals. Lispro starts working quickly and clears the body quickly, so it is important that a longer-acting insulin be included in the treatment regimen to prevent the liver from overproducing glucose between meals.

## Combining Treatments

### Oral Combinations

The different oral medicines work in different ways, so you might expect them to be more powerful when used together. This turns out to be true—at least for the medicines we have at present. Sulfonylureas, acarbose, and metformin have been used in various combinations, and in all combinations studied they're more effective together than alone. Therefore, adding a second medicine when the first one no longer controls your blood sugar makes sense. Most of the time, this means adding metformin when a sulfonylurea is not enough. For instance, if you initially responded well to a sulfonylurea but now your blood sugar levels are no longer well controlled, adding metformin might be a good next step. Metformin is more likely to control your blood sugar if it's added to the sulfonylurea, not substituted for it. The reverse is also true; if metformin works at first but your blood sugars start climbing, adding a sulfonylurea is likely to bring your sugar level down again.

Another reason to combine two medications is to get the same glucose-lowering effect with smaller side effects. For instance, acarbose used with sulfonylureas may reduce the tendency to gain weight.

### *Oral Medicine with Insulin*

When combinations of oral treatments are no longer effective in controlling blood sugar in Type II diabetes, it's time to start insulin. One way to make this change is to stop the oral medicine and start two injections of insulin daily—one before breakfast and one before the evening meal.

Another method that works for many people is to combine oral treatment with one injection of insulin per day. Here's how that works: One or more oral medicines are continued, sometimes at a lower dose, during the day. An insulin injection is then added either before dinner or at bedtime, and the insulin dose is increased until the morning blood sugar reading is satisfactory. This is a safe and easy way to make the transition to taking insulin, and it may keep on working well for several years. But when the morning blood sugar is controlled and the afternoon blood sugar rises, it's time to start taking two injections a day.

## On the Horizon

### *Troglitazone*

Within the next year, we're likely to have another exciting drug to use for Type II diabetes. Troglitazone is expected to be the first of a group of drugs called thiazolidinediones. These drugs have been referred to as "insulin sensitizers." They work by reducing the resistance to insulin that is found in most people with Type II diabetes. This is good news, because some researchers worry that high levels of insulin in the blood may increase the risk of circulatory problems. Obviously, a treatment that lowers insulin resistance allows control of blood sugars with less insulin (either insulin your own body makes or insulin you take by injection).

So far, the known side effects of troglitazone are few, but more experience is accumulating to further document its safety. Researchers do know that troglitazone doesn't cause low blood sugars and that it tends to improve blood pressure and perhaps cholesterol and triglyceride levels.

The early studies of troglitazone showed that some people respond dramatically to the drug while others may not respond at all. Studies are currently being conducted to try to determine in advance who will benefit from this new drug.

Another important question being studied is whether using troglitazone could prevent the development of Type II diabetes in people who don't yet have diabetes but are at high risk. Women who have had diabetes during a pregnancy are one group that might benefit from this approach. Both troglitazone and metformin are being included in a large, new, government-sponsored study called the Diabetes Prevention Program. In this study, researchers will use different drugs and combinations of diet and exercise to see if Type II diabetes can be delayed or prevented.

### *Insulin Analogs*

Several new insulin analogs are currently under development. Like the insulins available now, these newer insulins are given by injection. The main differences among insulins are how fast they work and how long they continue to have an effect. The newest insulin available, lispro, starts working very quickly and clears out of the system very quickly.

One insulin currently being developed may give a more steady basal effect than current insulins can achieve. Insulin does more than just lower the blood-sugar rise that follows a meal; it also prevents the liver from releasing too much glucose into the bloodstream between meals. Consequently, the body needs a constant low level of circulating insulin; this is basal insulin. We'll learn more about this insulin as further studies are conducted.

## So Many Choices

So there's good news and bad news. The good news is that there's now a treatment for nearly every kind of diabetes. The bad news is that treatment is getting more complicated. As the number of available drugs grows larger, the number of possible combinations increases even faster.

Which treatments are right for you? That depends. Not all diabetes is the same; that's especially true for Type II diabetes. Obviously, the correct treatment for Type I diabetes is insulin, but which kind and in which combinations? Using the available insulins to best match your food intake requires attention to your individual needs.

In Type II diabetes, there are even more options because not everyone with Type II diabetes responds best to the same treatment. There's no way to predict which drug will work for you. Fortunately, however, you can tell how well your treatment is working by monitoring your blood glucose levels frequently and having your doctor check your hemoglobin $A_{1C}$ regularly. Your treatment can then be changed if your blood sugar levels are not being controlled. Because Type II diabetes is a progressive disorder, it usually takes a series of changes in treatment strategy over time to keep control of blood sugar levels.

All this can mean a lot of work for you. It's for a good cause, though. This kind of stepwise treatment, using new medicines alone and in combinations, should keep your diabetes in better control than was possible in the past. And controlling your blood sugar is the most important step you can take to prevent complications.

*—by Diane M. Karl, M.D., and Matthew C. Riddle, M.D.*

Dr. Karl is Medical Codirector of the Diabetes Treatment Center of Providence Portland Medical Center and Clinical Assistant Professor of Medicine at Oregon Health Sciences University, in Portland, Oregon. Dr. Riddle is Professor of Medicine and Head of the Section of Diabetes at Oregon Health Sciences University.

## Chapter 39

# *Diabetes Drugs of the 1990s*

Several new diabetes medications have entered the marketplace recently. And according to the Pharmaceutical Research and Manufacturers of America, 21 more diabetes-related medications are coming down the pipeline, from research and clinical testing to the FDA approval process. Two drugs, metformin and troglitazone, are being tested in NIH/CDC's Diabetes Prevention Program to see if they can actually prevent diabetes.

At-risk groups such as Hispanic/Latinos, African Americans, and obese and hypertensive individuals are being included in clinical trials. Amaryl and Glyset were tested among substantial populations of Hispanics and African Americans, for instance.

Cost comparisons of new diabetes drugs are difficult, especially since doctors and patients are trying out new regimens. Most of the new diabetes drugs are roughly similar in price to many of the older treatments. First-generation sulfonylureas, for instance, averaged $30 per 100 tablets of 500-mg tablets, and $61 per 100 250-mg tablets, an average of $45 per 100 tablets. Rezulin, the most expensive of the new drugs, ranges between $96 and $193 per 100 tablets, depending on the dose. Rezulin, however, offers an entirely new biological mechanism and may save other costs, so dollar-for-dollar comparison is impossible. Rezulin prices have fallen 11 to 33 percent as the drug's market share has increased.

---

*Diabetes Dateline*, Winter 1998, National Institute of Diabetes and Digestive and Kidney Diseases.

Following are brief descriptions of recently approved diabetes pills and the first insulin analogue in 14 years. These summaries cannot be interpreted as endorsements of any kind by the National Institute of Diabetes and Digestive and Kidney Diseases (NIDDK); they include some but not all characteristics of the drugs, which may differ under varying circumstances.

## Drug Class: Sulfonylureas

These oral hypoglycemic medications for type 2 diabetes work by stimulating the beta cells in the pancreas to release more insulin.

- **Mechanism of action:** All sulfonylureas work by stimulating insulin production by pancreatic beta cells.
- **Side effects:** Over extensive periods, the drugs may exhaust beta cells' activity. These medicines can cause hypoglycemia. Excessive insulin production from these medications may cause weight gain or atherosclerosis.
- **New sulfonylurea drugs:** Most may be taken alone or with other diabetes drugs, with appropriate diabetes meal planning and exercise. These drugs can be taken at reduced frequency than older drugs in the class.

### *Glucotrol XL (Generic: glipizide)*

Pfizer Inc. FDA approval: 1994. Same mechanism of action and side effects as above.

- **Usage:** Taken once daily or more.
- **Advantages:** Reduced frequency of dosage can make adherence easier.

### *Glynase PresTabs (Generic: glyburide)*

Pharmacia & Upjohn. FDA approval: April 1992. Same side effects as above.

- **Mechanism of action:** In addition to pancreatic stimulation, some extra-pancreatic mechanisms may be involved.
- **Advantages:** Reduced frequency of dosage can make adherence easier. Blood glucose lowering effect may persist despite gradual decline in insulin secretory response to the drug.

***Amaryl (Generic: glimepiride)***
Hoechst Marion Roussel. FDA approval: December 1995.

- **Mechanism of action:** Binds to different sulfonylurea receptor site than other drugs in this class. Amaryl may stimulate less insulin secretion than others.
- **Usage:** Once daily alone or with other diabetes medications.
- **Advantages:** Reduced frequency of dosage can improve adherence. Increases insulin sensitivity and may cut insulin dose in half. Does not elevate insulin levels as much as other sulfonylureas.

## Drug Class: Biguanides

In the liver, biguanides suppress glucose production and lower insulin resistance.

***Glucophage (Generic: metformin)***
Bristol-Myers Squibb. FDA approval: June 1994.

- **Mechanism of action:** Helps the body use insulin more efficiently. Decreases glucose production in liver and increases cellular glucose uptake, increasing muscle utilization of glucose.
- **Side effects:** Rarely, accumulates and causes severe lactic acidosis, which can be fatal. The acidosis usually occurs in patients who use alcohol (even low or moderate amounts), have renal dysfunction, or have liver impairments. May cause loss of appetite, stomach ache, or nausea.
- **Advantages:** May cause small weight loss when therapy begins and improves blood lipid profiles. Does not cause hypoglycemia or weight gain when used alone. Does not stress pancreas through insulin overproduction.

## Drug Class: Alpha-glucosidase Inhibitors

These drugs work in the small intestine and inhibit enzymes that digest carbohydrates, delaying carbohydrate absorption and lowering postmeal glucose levels. New alpha-glucosidase inhibitor drugs:

***Precose (Generic: acarbose)***
Bayer Corporation. FDA approval: September 1995.

- **Mechanism of action:** Delays carbohydrate absorption in the small intestine and lowers glucose levels after meals.

- **Usage:** May be taken alone or with diabetes drugs, along with appropriate diabetes meal planning and exercise.
- **Side effects:** Does not cause hypoglycemia or weight gain when used alone. Frequently may cause diarrhea, cramping, abdominal pain, or gas, headaches, and hyperglycemia at first. Symptoms may be alleviated by starting at a lower dose and gradually increasing to therapeutic level.
- **Advantages:** Lowers postmeal blood glucose levels. Does not stress the pancreas by stimulating excess insulin production.

### *Glyset (Generic: miglitol)*

Bayer Corporation. FDA approval: December 1996.

- **Mechanism of action:** Inhibits enzymes that control glucose absorption in the small intestine and lowers glucose levels after meals.
- **Usage:** May be taken alone or with sulfonylureas.
- **Side effects:** Early, temporary digestive complaints including flatulence, soft stools or diarrhea, or abdominal pain. Can cause serious side effects in patients with chronic intestinal diseases, inflammatory bowel disease, colonic ulceration, or partial intestinal obstruction.
- **Advantages:** Shown to be effective in Hispanic and African-American patients with type 2 diabetes. Does not cause hypoglycemia, excessive insulin levels, or weight gain.

## *Drug Class: Thiazolidinediones*

New class for insulin-requiring patients with type 2 diabetes. Acts in muscles, sensitizes cells to insulin action, and reduces glucose production by the liver.

### *Rezulin (Generic: troglitazone)*

Parke-Davis, a division of Warner-Lambert Company. FDA approval: January 1997 and August 1997 for combination therapy.

- **Mechanism of action:** The drug lowers insulin resistance to injected or natural insulin and enhances insulin action in muscle fat and liver. Now approved for broad range of people with type 2 diabetes.

- **Usage:** Alone or in combination with sulfonylureas or insulin, once daily with meal.
- **Side effects:** In general use, insulin doses may need to be lowered to prevent hypoglycemia. Labeling now includes warning that patients with severe heart failure or liver disease may be poor Rezulin candidates. They may experience reversible but rarely complete liver failure. The warning recommends a schedule of liver function tests for patients taking Rezulin. Patients taking oral contraceptives may have lowered birth control protection on this drug. Rezulin may also alter the action of cholestyramine. Patients on or considering the use of both these medications should discuss their options carefully before starting Rezulin. Patients may also experience pain.
- **Advantages:** Does not strain the pancreas by excessive insulin production or stimulating weight gain. Reduces peripheral insulin resistance. Insulin injections may be reduced or eliminated. Reduces glucose production by the liver, improves blood lipid levels, and reduces need for antihypertensive and dyslipidemic medications. No weight gain. No known drug interactions.

## *Drug Class: Insulins*

Insulin is released from the pancreas and enables cells to metabolize glucose. Several animal- and human-DNA analogues are available to augment the natural supply.

### ***Humalog (Generic: insulin lispro)***

Eli Lilly and Company. FDA approval: June 1996.

- **Mechanism of action:** This insulin differs from regular insulin in two ways: its rapid onset of action and shorter duration. Its onset is 5 to 15 minutes and its peak of activity comes within an hour. Its peak activity is over within 2 to 4 hours.
- **Usage:** Just before meals. Those with type 1 diabetes use the insulin analogue in conjunction with an intermediate or long-acting insulin. An "insulin cocktail" is evolving, with some people also using regular insulin.
- **Side effects:** Best used by people accustomed to frequent blood glucose monitoring and multiple daily injections.

- **Advantages:** Closest action to body's timing of insulin production response after eating a meal. Prevents high postmeal blood glucose. May reduce insulin requirements in those with type 2 diabetes, without stimulating insulin secretion or weight gain.

# Chapter 40

# Rezulin Update

## Updated News About Rezulin

Earlier this year, a new oral medication for type 2 diabetes, Rezulin, was cleared for marketing by the Food and Drug Administration (FDA). It was originally approved in patients treating type 2 diabetes with insulin injections. Now, the FDA has approved two new "indications," or uses, for Rezulin in the treatment of type 2 diabetes. Rezulin may be added to a patient's treatment regimen that either: 1) involves only diet and exercise, or 2) involves a combination of diet, exercise, and an oral medication from the sulfonylurea class. The American Diabetes Association has prepared this question-and-answer sheet to provide you with more information about this medication for people with type 2 diabetes.

### *Rezulin has been around for awhile. What's new about this drug?*

You may have heard or read news reports about a new oral medication used to treat type 2 diabetes called Rezulin (generic name, troglitazone). Earlier in 1997, it received clearance for marketing as an "add-on" medication for patients treating type 2 diabetes with insulin. Now, two new indications, or uses, for Rezulin have been approved by the FDA.

---

"Updated News about Rezulin ®" ©1997 American Diabetes Association, reprinted with permission; and U.S. Food and Drug Administration (FDA) Talk Paper, T97-55, November 3, 1997.

### What does Rezulin do?

Rezulin helps control "hyperglycemia," a condition in which blood sugar (blood glucose) levels are too high. Rezulin works primarily to reduce insulin resistance, a condition in which the body does not respond properly to the amounts of insulin it produces. Insulin resistance is found almost always in people with type 2 diabetes, and is thought to be one of the underlying causes of the disease.

### How does the use of Rezulin fit with the other types of treatment available for people with type 2 diabetes?

Type 2 diabetes is a serious, complex disease, and there is no single, correct way to treat it. A health care team, led by a physician, should determine an individualized treatment plan with each person.

Treatment for people with type 2 diabetes usually begins with meal planning and regular daily exercise. These measures alone help some patients effectively manage their diabetes. If diet and exercise alone fail to bring a patient's blood glucose level close to his/her treatment goals, a doctor may add an oral medication to the diet and exercise plan. When the oral medication no longer works effectively, insulin may be added or substituted as a means to reduce a patient's blood glucose level. Rezulin gives health care providers another treatment option for their patients with type 2 diabetes.

### How does this new drug differ from other type 2 oral medications already available?

There are now four different classes of oral medications, along with insulin, for treating type 2 diabetes. (NOTE: All four classes of drugs can treat high blood sugar levels effectively when prescribed and used as indicated, either alone or in combination. However, since no two people with diabetes are exactly alike, different drugs or combinations may work more effectively in some individuals.)

The first class of medications is called the "sulfonylurea" (súl-fa-nul-úr-ee-ah) class. These medications work primarily to stimulate insulin production in the pancreas. There are a number of these drugs on the market, some of which are: Orinase®, Tolinase®, Glucotrol XL®, and Diabeta®.

The second class of medications used to treat type 2 diabetes is the "biguanide" (bi-gwan-ide) class. There is one drug approved and on the market in this class: Glucophage® (metformin). Glucophage works by primarily decreasing the amount of sugar secreted by the liver, thereby reducing a person's glucose levels. It also works to improve insulin sensitivity. It does not stimulate the pancreas to produce more insulin.

The third class of medications used to treat type 2 diabetes is called the "alpha glucosidase (glue-kos-a-dace) inhibitor" class. There is one drug approved in the class: Precose® (acarbose). Precose interferes with the digestive process, slowing down the digestion of starchy foods in the small intestine. Hence, the absorption of sugar into the blood is delayed, helping to prevent the sudden surges of glucose that occur after a meal.

The fourth class of medications for treating type 2 diabetes is called the "thiazolidinediones" (thee-ah-zah-la-deen-dye-owns) class. There is one drug approved in this class: Rezulin® (troglitazone). Called an "insulin resistance reducer," it works very differently than drugs in other classes.

People with type 2 diabetes almost always have a condition called insulin resistance, when insulin produced by the body is much less effective in lowering blood glucose levels. Over time, blood sugar and insulin levels rise. But even these levels of insulin are ineffective. To compensate, patients may need additional insulin to overcome the resistance. They may be prescribed an oral medication to help the pancreas produce more insulin and/or take insulin injections to lower blood sugar levels.

Rezulin works by decreasing insulin resistance, thereby improving blood glucose control. This therapy may reduce the need for some people with type 2 diabetes to rely on insulin injections to manage their diabetes.

### *What should I do if I'm interested in trying Rezulin?*

Rezulin is now approved for use as an addition to a treatment plan consisting of diet and exercise, or diet, exercise and a sulfonylurea drug. (NOTE: Rezulin is not indicated to be used in combination with Glucophage or Precose.) Consult your health care professional when considering Rezulin as a treatment option.

### *I treat my type 2 diabetes with insulin and I've heard that Rezulin can dramatically reduce a patient's daily insulin requirements. Does this mean that I may no longer require insulin injections if I use Rezulin?*

While 15% of those who completed clinical studies no longer required insulin injections to control glucose levels, the long term effectiveness of Rezulin was not determined. You should consult your health care provider as to whether or not Rezulin can help you meet your treatment goals.

### *I've recently heard news reports about a major side effect regarding Rezulin. What are they about?*

Parke-Davis, along with the Food and Drug Administration, announced a labeling change due to post marketing reports of cases of liver injury. Of the 650,000 Americans with diabetes currently on Rezulin, only 35 people were reported to have some form of liver problem. Two of those cases resulted in serious liver disease. Both the manufacturer and the FDA point out that Rezulin's role in these cases is unclear. [The text of an FDA "Talk Paper" discussing the labeling change for Rezulin can be found at the end of this chapter.]

### *I'm taking Rezulin now. Should I stop taking it?*

People with diabetes should never alter their diabetes treatment without the advice of their health care provider. However, should you experience severe symptoms (e.g. nausea, vomiting, abdominal pain, fatigue, anorexia, dark urine), we encourage you to see your physician immediately.

### *What can my doctor do?*

Your physician has received information regarding this new labeling change and warnings. If you have questions about your current treatment, you should talk to your doctor. Or, call the Parke-Davis Medical Affairs hotline at 1-800-223-0432 for more information.

### *Is there anyone who should not take Rezulin?*

Patients with severe heart disease or liver disease should use Rezulin with caution. Rezulin is not indicated for children or women during pregnancy.

### *I have type 1 diabetes. Can Rezulin become a component of my treatment regimen?*

Rezulin has not been indicated for the management of type 1 diabetes, which requires insulin for blood sugar control.

***What can I do to get in better control of my diabetes?***

Making regular visits with members of a team of health care professionals (including a doctor, nurse, and dietitian) is the best thing you can do to learn how to better control your diabetes. Of course, you should always eat right, exercise and take your medication and/or insulin as prescribed.

***Does the American Diabetes Association have other information available about diabetes?***

Yes. The American Diabetes Association publishes many different books, newsletters and brochures for people with diabetes and the health care professionals who care for them. We publish a monthly lifestyle magazine called *Diabetes Forecast* which hundreds of thousands of people with diabetes find useful in helping them take charge of their diabetes, as well as a bimonthly publication called *The Diabetes Advisor*. You can subscribe to *Diabetes Forecast* online, or call 1-800-806-7801. To subscribe to *The Diabetes Advisor*, call 1-800-806-7802. You can order books and other publications online or call 1-800-ADA-ORDER (1-800-232-6733). [The American Diabetes Association can be found online at www.diabetes.org.]

## From the U.S. Food and Drug Administration: Rezulin Labeling Changes

The manufacturer of the diabetes drug Rezulin (troglitazone) is changing prescribing information for the product and adding new warning information to the labeling, in response to reports of liver injury associated with use of the drug.

Rezulin is used in combination with insulin or sulfonylurea in patients with type II diabetes (adult-onset diabetes mellitus) whose blood glucose levels are not adequately controlled by these other therapies alone.

About 500,000 patients in the United States have been treated with Rezulin since it came on the market in January 1997; of those, approximately 85,000 have been taking the drug for six months or more. As of October 21, 1997, 35 post-marketing reports of liver injury of various degrees have been received. These reports ranged from mildly elevated blood levels of the liver transaminase enzymes to liver failure leading to one liver transplant and one death. Whether the drug was solely responsible for all of these reports of liver injury is as yet unknown, due to confounding medical factors in some of the reported cases.

Based on these reports, FDA and the manufacturer are recommending that serum transaminase levels in patients be checked routinely within the first one to two months of Rezulin therapy, every three months thereafter during the first year of treatment, and periodically thereafter. In addition, liver function tests should be performed on any patient on Rezulin who develops symptoms of liver dysfunction, such as nausea, vomiting, abdominal pain, fatigue, loss of appetite, or dark urine. Patients on Rezulin who develop jaundice or whose laboratory results indicate liver injury should stop taking the drug.

Based on clinical trials, approximately two percent of patients on Rezulin can be expected to have to stop taking the drug because of elevated liver enzymes. Few, if any, of these patients will go on to develop permanent liver damage if the drug is stopped.

The new prescribing information and labeling warning are designed to give health care providers and patients the latest available information about possible risks associated with Rezulin and recommendations for safer use of the drug.

Health care providers are urged to report any Rezulin-related adverse events, especially those suggestive of possible liver injury, to the manufacturer, Parke Davis, at 1-800-223-0432, or FDA MedWatch at (phone) 1-800-FDA-1088, (fax) 1-800-FDA 1078, (modem) 1-800-FDA-7737 or (mail) FDA, HF-2, 5600 Fishers Lane, Rockville, MD 20857.

Food and Drug Administration
U.S. Department of Health and Human Services
Public Health Service
5600 Fishers Lane
Rockville, Maryland 20857

FDA Talk Papers are prepared by the Press Office to guide personnel in responding with consistency and accuracy to questions from the public on subjects of current interest. Talk Papers are subject to change as more information becomes available. Talk Papers are not intended for general distribution outside FDA, but all information in them is public, and full texts are releasable upon request.

Consumer Hotline: (800) 532-4440

# Chapter 41

# *Watch Out for Drug Interactions*

The more you know about drugs and their effects, the better you will be able to manage your diabetes.

Emergency-room doctors in a major city hospital knew just what to do when a man with diabetes in his 60s came to them nearly unconscious, sweating, and with his heart racing. The man, who treated his diabetes with the oral medication Diabinese, was having classic symptoms of hypoglycemia (low blood sugar). The doctors gave him glucose intravenously, waited for his symptoms to disappear, and sent him on his way.

But when he returned two hours later and then again a third time, the doctors realized that more was going on than met the eye. After questioning him further, they learned that his doctor had prescribed an antibiotic medication called Septra the day before. This drug can cause a drop in blood sugar when taken with Diabinese.

This time, the doctors kept the man in the hospital to carefully control his blood sugar until the effects of his medications wore off. Meanwhile, they explained the problem to the man's personal physician, who changed the prescription to one that wouldn't interfere with the diabetes medication. Only then was the man rid of his symptoms and the emergency room rid of a steady customer.

A variety of conditions can affect the actions of drugs in your system. You may, for example, have an allergy to a specific drug, or it

---

Campbell, R. Keith, John R. White, Jr., and Philip D. Hansten "The Ins and Outs," *Diabetes Forecast*. February 1992 

may produce a side effect that makes it necessary to stop using the drug. In addition, two or more drugs taken at the same time might act together in an unwanted way, in a process called a drug interaction.

Other factors that can affect how a drug acts in your body include any diseases you may have, how much you exercise, and habits such as smoking or drinking. Talk with your doctor and pharmacist before you start taking any new medication. You have a special responsibility to know what a particular drug will do inside your body. On their own, many medications can raise or lower your blood sugar levels.

This chapter lists the major drugs known to affect diabetes control. But it cannot say how you will react to any of them. These medications will disturb diabetes control for some people, yet affect others slightly or not at all.

Also, even if a medication listed here affects your blood sugar level, you can probably still take it if you really need it. Your physician and pharmacist should be able to help you work the medication into your overall diabetes-management plan.

In the following lists, the *generic* (or general) name of a drug or class of drugs is given first, followed in parentheses by one or more of the popular brand names. Drugs written in ***boldface italics*** can raise or lower blood sugar severely. If you use diabetes pills, take special note of the drugs marked by an asterisk (*). When these drugs and diabetes pills are both used, the diabetes medicines can cause blood sugar to rise or fall even more drastically. (When "diabetes pills" or "oral diabetes medicines" are mentioned here, they refer to drugs of the *sulfonylurea* type.)

## Over-the-Counter and Under-the-Table Drugs

Like prescription drugs, over-the-counter and "recreational" drugs can have unwanted effects, and they can sometimes interact with each other or with prescription drugs. Because you can buy these drugs without a prescription, you must take extra care to use them wisely.

Always read the label on packages of non-prescription drugs for general warnings and warnings for people with diabetes. But be aware that not all substances that can affect your blood sugar come with warnings. The following are drugs that can affect blood sugar control:

- *Alcohol*. Like other drugs, alcohol can do different things to different people. Its main danger to people with diabetes concerns its tendency to cause a severe, possibly fatal fall in blood sugar levels when taken on an empty stomach. Alcohol's effects tend to be stronger for people with insulin-dependent diabetes and those who take oral diabetes medicine than in people whose diabetes is controlled by diet.

- Ironically, alcohol can have exactly the opposite effect—that of increasing blood sugar—in individuals who drink large amounts over a long period of time. The increase is probably caused by liver damage.

- *Aspirin*. The amount of aspirin you would typically take for a headache or temporary fever is no great cause for concern. However, the amount you might take to control chronic pain may lower your blood sugar, especially if you take oral diabetes medicine. If you need to take a large amount of aspirin, your doctor may have to adjust the dose of your diabetes medication.

- *Caffeine*. Found in coffee, tea, and many soft drinks, it is also the main ingredient of over-the-counter "pep" pills (Vivarin) and diuretics (Odrinil). Taken in large quantities, it can raise your blood sugar. Caffeine can also give you the "shakes" and may make you feel as if you are having an insulin reaction when you are not.

- *Cold Remedies and Diet Pills*. Many of these medications, including Sudafed, CoTylenol, Dexatrim, and Dietac, contain epinephrine-like compounds (including ephedrine, pseudoephedrine, phenylpropanolamine, phenylephedrine, and epinephrine). These substances can increase blood sugar (and also blood pressure) in some people with diabetes.

- *Marijuana*. This drug does not raise blood sugar directly, but it does cause a craving for sweets in many of those who use it. Giving in to this craving can cause blood sugar to skyrocket.

- *Sugary Medicines*. Most cough syrups and lozenges are made of sugar. What's worse, they are often taken during an illness, when blood sugar levels tend to be high already.

- Consult your doctor or pharmacist before using any medication containing sugar. Your pharmacist may be able to find a sugarless version of the medication you need, but be aware that drug manufacturers can add sugar to a product at any time, without prior notice. If you are not sure about a drug's sugar content, write the manufacturer.

- *Tobacco*. Smoking, according to some researchers, can raise blood sugar, but more studies are needed. Of course, such risks pale in comparison to other risks of smoking—such as heart disease and lung cancer—but they are still important.

## Drugs That Increase Blood Glucose Levels

- ***Corticosteroids.*** (prednisone, Decadron, Kenalog, cortisone, and others).* Most commonly used to relieve inflammation, redness, irritation, and swelling. Doctors prescribe corticosteroids for a variety of illnesses, including asthma, arthritis, multiple sclerosis, and myasthenia gravis.

- ***Diazoxide.*** (Hyperstat, Proglycem).* A powerful hyperglycemic (blood sugar-raising) agent used, under the name Proglycem, to treat low blood sugar caused by insulin-producing pancreatic tumors. Under the name Hyperstat, the drug is used to treat high blood pressure. Some doctors, however, may not realize that Hyperstat and Proglycem are different names for the same drug.

- ***Diuretics.**** A broad class of drugs that relieve water buildup by increasing the amount of water passed through the urine. They are most often used to treat high blood pressure and congestive heart failure. The thiazide diuretics (Diuril, HydroDIURIL, Esidrix) generally have the strongest effect on blood sugar, but other kinds (including Diamox, Hygroton, Edecrin, and Lasix) can also raise blood sugar significantly.

- ***Epinephrine*** and Epinephrine-like compounds, ***Adrenaline*** (Adrenalin).* Often used as a life-saving drug to help start the heart after it has stopped beating. It is also used to treat asthma and allergic reactions (for example, to bee stings). Similar compounds are used as decongestants in cold remedies and as appetite suppressants in diet pills.

- *Estrogens, Birth Control Pills* (sold under several brand names). Used to prevent pregnancy and also to lessen the effects of menopause.

- Lithium Carbonate.* (Eskalith, Lithane). Used in treating manic-depressive illness.

- *Nicoiitiic Acid, Niacin.* In large doses, sometimes used to treat high cholesterol levels. Since it is a B vitamin, niacin is also sold over the counter as a nutrition supplement. Large doses can raise blood sugar.

- *Phenobarbital.* * Used as a sedative or sleeping pill and sometimes for treating epilepsy. It raises blood sugar only in people who use diabetes pills.

- ***Phenytoin*** (Dilantin).* Often used in treating epilepsy and other nervous-system disorders. It does not raise blood sugar in all people with diabetes but can have strong effects in some.

- ***Propanolol*** (Inderal) and other beta-blocker drugs. In most people with diabetes, this drug lowers blood sugar levels (see below), but in a few people it can have the opposite effect.

- *Rifampin* (Rifadin). * Used in treating tuberculosis. It raises blood sugar levels only in people who use diabetes pills, especially among those taking tolbutamide (Orinase).

- *Thyroid Preparations*, including Desiccated Thyroid. Used by people not producing thyroid hormones or who have had their thyroid gland removed. Excessive doses of these preparations may increase insulin requirements in people taking insulin.

## Drugs That Decrease Blood Glucose

- *Anabolic Steroids* (Dianabol). While steroids have some important medical uses, they are often used to merely increase muscle mass.

- *Chloramphenicol* (Chloromycetin).* A potent antibiotic used in treating serious infections, it has a number of side effects that limit its use. It lowers blood sugar levels only in people who use diabetes pills.

- *Coumarin Anticoagulants* (Dicumarol).* Used to thin the blood to prevent clotting, most often for heart attack patients. It lowers blood sugar only in people who use diabetes pills.

- *Fenfluramine* (Pondimin). An appetite suppressant used for weight control in some people.

- ***Methyldopa*** (Aldomet). * Used for treating high blood pressure. It lowers blood sugar only in people who use diabetes pills, particularly tolbutamide (Orinase).

- *Monoamine Oxidase Inhibitors, MAO Inhibitors* (Parnate, Nardil, Eutonyl).* Used to combat severe depression. They are seldom prescribed because of many possible side effects. In addition to lowering blood sugar levels, these drugs interact strongly with aged foods, including certain wines and cheeses.

- ***Phenylbutazone*** (Butazolidin).* An anti-inflammatory, used in treating arthritis. It lowers blood sugar only in people who use diabetes pills, particularly chlorpropamide (Diabinese).

- ***Propanolol*** (Inderal), and other beta-blocking drugs. Used in treating angina (chest pain from heart ailments), high blood pressure, unsteady heartbeats, and overactive thyroid glands. Not only can it lower blood sugar levels, it can also block the symptoms, including sweating and shakiness, that ordinarily let insulin users know their blood sugar is too low. Similar drugs, such as metoprolol and timolol, are now being introduced in the United States and appear to be safer for people with diabetes.

- ***Sulfa Drugs*** (Gantrisin, Septra, Bactrim).* Antibiotics used for treating infections. They do not lower blood sugar levels on their own, but they are chemically similar to the sulfonylureas (oral diabetes medicines). When taken together with the sulfonylureas, they can cause a significant fall in blood sugar level.

## Staying One Step Ahead of Drug Problems

By all means, follow the instructions of your doctor and pharmacist when using a drug. But don't rely entirely on others to keep you safe from drug problems. The better you understand the medications you take, the safer you'll be.

Always heed the instructions and warnings on drug packages. If you are seeing more than one doctor, make sure that each knows what the other has prescribed to avoid receiving the same drug twice or receiving drugs that interfere with each other. (If possible, use a single pharmacy, so that all your prescriptions will be listed in a single record.)

Don't leave the doctor's office before you know the generic names of your drugs, the dose to take, the times of day to take the medications, precautions (such as other drugs or foods that you should not take together with the drugs), and any side effects.

One important way to monitor a drug's actions in your body is to test your own blood or urine for glucose. You should be aware, however, that many drugs that affect the accuracy of urine tests do not affect blood testing, so home blood testing is preferred over urine testing. In either case, always read the package insert for both blood and urine tests for drugs that can cause false readings.

By educating yourself about the medications you use, you can help make sure that the drugs you use are your allies—not your enemies—in preserving good health.

*—by R. Keith Campbell, John R. White, Jr., and Philip D. Hansten*

John R. White, Jr., PharmD, is assistant professor of pharmacy practice and R. Keith Campbell, RPh. CDE, MPH, is professor of pharmacy practice and associate dean at the College of Pharmacy of Washington State University in Spokane. Philip D. Hansten, RPh, is professor of pharmacy at the University of Washington in Seattle.

## Layperson's Guides to Drugs

A convenient way to learn about drugs is to read a good book on medications and their effects. Most guides list drugs by both brand names and generic names. Several inexpensive guides are available in paperback form in many bookstores.

"About Your Medicines" (U.S. Pharmacopeial Convention, Inc., 12601 Twinbrook Parkway, Rockville, MD 20852, call toll-free: (800) 227-8772).

"The People's Pharmacy," (by Joe Graedon and Teresa Graedon, St. Martin's Press, 1985.

"Prescription Drugs" (by Editors of *Consumer Guide*, Publications International, Ltd., 1991.

# *Part Six*

# *Complications of Diabetes*

# Chapter 42

# Diabetic Neuropathy

## What Is Diabetic Neuropathy?

Diabetic neuropathy is a nerve disorder caused by diabetes. Symptoms of neuropathy include numbness and sometimes pain in the hands, feet, or legs. Nerve damage caused by diabetes can also lead to problems with internal organs such as the digestive tract, heart, and sexual organs causing indigestion, diarrhea or constipation, dizziness, bladder infections, and impotence. In some cases, neuropathy can flare up suddenly, causing weakness and weight loss. Depression may follow. While some treatments are available, a great deal of research is still needed to understand how diabetes affects the nerves and to find more effective treatments for this complication.

## How Common Is Diabetic Neuropathy?

People with diabetes can develop nerve problems at any time. Significant clinical neuropathy can develop within the first 10 years after diagnosis of diabetes and the risk of developing neuropathy increases the longer a person has diabetes. Some recent studies have reported that:

- 60 percent of patients with diabetes have some form of neuropathy, but in most cases (30 to 40 percent), there are no symptoms.

---

National Institute of Diabetes and Digestive and Kidney Diseases (NIDDK), NIH Pub. No. 97-3185, July 1995.

- 30 to 40 percent of patients with diabetes have symptoms suggesting neuropathy, compared with 10 percent of people without diabetes.

Diabetic neuropathy appears to be more common in smokers, people over 40 years of age, and those who have had problems controlling their blood glucose levels.

## DCCT: Can Diabetic Neuropathy Be Prevented?

A 10-year clinical study that involved 1,441 volunteers with insulin-dependent diabetes (IDDM) was recently completed by the National Institute of Diabetes and Digestive and Kidney Diseases. The study proved that keeping blood sugar levels as close to the normal range as possible slows the onset and progression of nerve disease caused by diabetes. The Diabetes Control and Complications Trial (DCCT) studied two groups of volunteers: those who followed a standard diabetes management routine and those who intensively managed their diabetes. Persons in the intensive management group took multiple injections of insulin daily or used an insulin pump and monitored their blood glucose at least four times a day to try to lower their blood glucose levels to the normal range. After 5 years, tests of neurological function showed that the risk of nerve damage was reduced by 60 percent in the intensively managed group. People in the standard treatment group, whose average blood glucose levels were higher, had higher rates of neuropathy. Although the DCCT included only patients with IDDM, researchers believe that people with noninsulin-dependent diabetes would also benefit from maintaining lower levels of blood glucose.

## What Causes Diabetic Neuropathy?

Scientists do not know what causes diabetic neuropathy, but several factors are likely to contribute to the disorder. High blood glucose, a condition associated with diabetes, causes chemical changes in nerves. These changes impair the nerves' ability to transmit signals. High blood glucose also damages blood vessels that carry oxygen and nutrients to the nerves. In addition, inherited factors probably unrelated to diabetes may make some people more susceptible to nerve disease than others.

How high blood glucose leads to nerve damage is a subject of intense research. The precise mechanism is not known. Researchers have discovered that high glucose levels affect many metabolic pathways in the nerves, leading to an accumulation of a sugar called sorbitol and depletion of a substance called myoinositol. However, studies in humans have not shown convincingly that these changes are the mechanism that causes nerve damage.

More recently, researchers have focused on the effects of excessive glucose metabolism on the amount of nitrous oxide in nerves. Nitrous oxide dilates blood vessels. In a person with diabetes, low levels of nitrous oxide may lead to constriction of blood vessels supplying the nerve, contributing to nerve damage. Another promising area of research centers on the effect of high glucose attaching to proteins, altering the structure and function of the proteins and affecting vascular function.

Scientists are studying how these changes occur, how they are connected, how they cause nerve damage, and how to prevent and treat damage.

## *What Are the Symptoms of Diabetic Neuropathy?*

The symptoms of diabetic neuropathy vary. Numbness and tingling in feet are often the first sign. Some people notice no symptoms, while others are severely disabled. Neuropathy may cause both pain and insensitivity to pain in the same person. Often, symptoms are slight at first, and since most nerve damage occurs over a period of years, mild cases may go unnoticed for a long time. In some people, mainly those afflicted by focal neuropathy (see Focal Neuropathy section below), the onset of pain may be sudden and severe.

## *Diabetic Neuropathy Can Affect Virtually Every Part of the Body*

**Diffuse (Peripheral) Neuropathy**

- Legs
- Feet
- Arms
- Hands

**Diffuse (Autonomic) Neuropathy**

- Heart
- Digestive System
- Sexual organs
- Urinary tract
- Sweat glands

**Focal Neuropathy**

- Eyes
- Facial muscles
- Hearing
- Pelvis and lower back
- Thigh
- Abdomen

## What Are the Major Types of Neuropathy?

The symptoms of neuropathy also depend on which nerves and what part of the body is affected. Neuropathy may be diffuse, affecting many parts of the body, or focal, affecting a single, specific nerve and part of the body.

### Diffuse Neuropathy

The two categories of diffuse neuropathy are peripheral neuropathy affecting the feet and hands and autonomic neuropathy affecting the internal organs.

*Peripheral Neuropathy*

The most common type of peripheral neuropathy damages the nerves of the limbs, especially the feet. Nerves on both sides of the body are affected. Common symptoms of this kind of neuropathy are:

- Numbness or insensitivity to pain or temperature
- Tingling, burning, or prickling
- Sharp pains or cramps
- Extreme sensitivity to touch, even light touch
- Loss of balance and coordination.

These symptoms are often worse at night.

The damage to nerves often results in loss of reflexes and muscle weakness. The foot often becomes wider and shorter, the gait changes, and foot ulcers appear as pressure is put on parts of the foot that are less protected. Because of the loss of sensation, injuries may go unnoticed and often become infected. If ulcers or foot injuries are not treated in time, the infection may involve the bone and require amputation. However, problems caused by minor injuries can usually be controlled if they are caught in time. Avoiding foot injury by wearing well-fitted shoes and examining the feet daily can help prevent amputations.

*Autonomic Neuropathy (also called visceral neuropathy)*

Autonomic neuropathy is another form of diffuse neuropathy. It affects the nerves that serve the heart and internal organs and produces changes in many processes and systems.

**Urination and sexual response.** Autonomic neuropathy most often affects the organs that control urination and sexual function. Nerve damage can prevent the bladder from emptying completely, so bacteria grow more easily in the urinary tract (bladder and kidneys). When the nerves of the bladder are damaged, a person may have difficulty knowing when the bladder is full or controlling it, resulting in urinary incontinence.

The nerve damage and circulatory problems of diabetes can also lead to a gradual loss of sexual response in both men and women, although sex drive is unchanged. A man may be unable to have erections or may reach sexual climax without ejaculating normally.

**Digestion.** Autonomic neuropathy can affect digestion. Nerve damage can cause the stomach to empty too slowly, a disorder called gastric stasis. When the condition is severe (gastroparesis), a person can have persistent nausea and vomiting, bloating, and loss of appetite. Blood glucose levels tend to fluctuate greatly with this condition.

If nerves in the esophagus are involved, swallowing may be difficult. Nerve damage to the bowels can cause constipation or frequent diarrhea, especially at night. Problems with the digestive system often lead to weight loss.

**Cardiovascular system.** Autonomic neuropathy can affect the cardiovascular system, which controls the circulation of blood throughout the body. Damage to this system interferes with the nerve impulses from various parts of the body that signal the need for blood and regulate blood pressure and heart rate. As a result, blood pressure may drop sharply after sitting or standing, causing a person to feel dizzy or light-headed, or even to faint (orthostatic hypotension).

Neuropathy that affects the cardiovascular system may also affect the perception of pain from heart disease. People may not experience angina as a warning sign of heart disease or may suffer painless heart attacks. It may also raise the risk of a heart attack during general anesthesia.

**Hypoglycemia.** Autonomic neuropathy can hinder the body's normal response to low blood sugar or hypoglycemia, which makes it difficult to recognize and treat an insulin reaction.

**Sweating.** Autonomic neuropathy can affect the nerves that control sweating. Sometimes, nerve damage interferes with the activity of the sweat glands, making it difficult for the body to regulate its temperature. Other times, the result can be profuse sweating at night or while eating (gustatory sweating).

### *Focal Neuropathy (including multiplex neuropathy)*

Occasionally, diabetic neuropathy appears suddenly and affects specific nerves, most often in the torso, leg, or head. Focal neuropathy may cause:

- Pain in the front of a thigh
- Severe pain in the lower back or pelvis
- Pain in the chest, stomach, or flank
- Chest or abdominal pain sometimes mistaken for angina, heart attack, or appendicitis
- Aching behind an eye
- Inability to focus the eye
- Double vision
- Paralysis on one side of the face (Bell's palsy)
- Problems with hearing.

This kind of neuropathy is unpredictable and occurs most often in older people who have mild diabetes. Although focal neuropathy can be painful, it tends to improve by itself after a period of weeks or months without causing long-term damage.

People with diabetes are also prone to developing compression neuropathies. The most common form of compression neuropathy is carpal tunnel syndrome. Asymptomatic carpal tunnel syndrome occurs in 20 to 30 percent of people with diabetes, and symptomatic carpal tunnel syndrome occurs in 6 to 11 percent. Numbness and tingling of the hand are the most common symptoms. Muscle weakness may also develop.

## How Do Doctors Diagnose Diabetic Neuropathy?

A doctor diagnoses neuropathy based on symptoms and a physical exam. During the exam, the doctor may check muscle strength, reflexes, and sensitivity to position, vibration, temperature, and light touch. Sometimes special tests are also used to help determine the cause of symptoms and to suggest treatment.

A simple **screening test** to check point sensation in the feet can be done in the doctor's office. The test uses a nylon filament mounted on a small wand. The filament delivers a standardized 10-gram force when touched to areas of the foot. Patients who cannot sense pressure from the filament have lost protective sensation and are at risk for developing neuropathic foot ulcers. Physicians may order the filament (with instructions for use) free from the Gillis W. Long Hansen's Disease Center, LEAP Program, 5445 Point Clair Road, Carville, Louisiana 70721; telephone (504) 642-4714.

**Nerve conduction studies** check the flow of electrical current through a nerve. With this test, an image of the nerve impulse is projected on a screen as it transmits an electrical signal. Impulses that seem slower or weaker than usual indicate possible damage to the nerve. This test allows the doctor to assess the condition of all the nerves in the arms and legs.

**Electromyography (EMG)** is used to see how well muscles respond to electrical impulses transmitted by nearby nerves. The electrical activity of the muscle is displayed on a screen. A response that is slower or weaker than usual suggests damage to the nerve or muscle. This test is often done at the same time as nerve conduction studies.

**Ultrasound** employs sound waves. The sound waves are too high to hear, but they produce an image showing how well the bladder and other parts of the urinary tract are functioning.

**Nerve biopsy** involves removing a sample of nerve tissue for examination. This test is most often used in research settings.

If your doctor suspects autonomic neuropathy, you may also be referred to a physician who specializes in digestive disorders (gastroenterologist) for additional tests.

## How Is Diabetic Neuropathy Usually Treated?

Treatment aims to relieve discomfort and prevent further tissue damage. The first step is to bring blood sugar under control by diet and oral drugs or insulin injections, if needed, and by careful monitoring of blood sugar levels. Although symptoms can sometimes worsen at first as blood sugar is brought under control, maintaining lower blood sugar levels helps reverse the pain or loss of sensation that neuropathy can cause. Good control of blood sugar may also help prevent or delay the onset of further problems.

Another important part of treatment involves special care of the feet, which are prone to problems. (See the section on foot care below.)

A number of medications and other approaches are used to relieve the symptoms of diabetic neuropathy.

### Relief of Pain

For relief of pain, burning, tingling, or numbness, the doctor may suggest an analgesic such as aspirin or acetaminophen or anti-inflammatory drugs containing ibuprofen. Nonsteroidal anti-inflammatory drugs should be used with caution in people with renal disease. Antidepressant medications such as amitriptyline (sometimes used with fluphenazine) or nerve medications such as carbamazepine or phenytoin sodium may be helpful. Codeine is sometimes prescribed for short-term use to relieve severe pain. In addition, a topical cream, capsaicin, is now available to help relieve the pain of neuropathy.

The doctor may also prescribe a therapy known as transcutaneous electronic nerve stimulations (TENS). In this treatment, small amounts of electricity block pain signals as they pass through a patient's skin. Other treatments include hypnosis, relaxation training, biofeedback, and acupuncture. Some people find that walking regularly or using elastic stockings helps relieve leg pain. Warm (not hot) baths, massage, or an analgesic ointment such as Ben Gay® may also help.

### Gastrointestinal Problems

Indigestion, belching, nausea or vomiting are symptoms of gastroparesis. For patients with mild symptoms of slow stomach emptying, doctors suggest eating small, frequent meals and avoiding fats. Eating less fiber may also relieve symptoms. For patients with severe gastroparesis, the doctor may prescribe metoclopramide, which speeds digestion and helps relieve nausea. Other drugs that help regulate digestion or reduce stomach acid secretion may also be used or erythromycine may be prescribed. In each case, the potential benefits of these drugs need to be weighed against their side effects.

To relieve diarrhea or other bowel problems, antibiotics or clonidine HC1, a drug used to treat high blood pressure, are sometimes prescribed. The antibiotic tetracycline may be prescribed. A wheat-free diet may also bring relief since the gluten in flour sometimes causes diarrhea.

Neurological problems affecting the urinary tract can result in infections or incontinence. The doctor may prescribe an antibiotic to clear up an infection and suggest drinking more fluids to prevent further infections. If incontinence is a problem, patients may be advised to urinate at regular times (every 3 hours, for example) since they may not be able to tell when the bladder is full.

### *Dizziness, Weakness*

Sitting or standing slowly may help prevent light-headedness, dizziness, or fainting, which are symptoms that may be associated with some forms of autonomic neuropathy. Raising the head of the bed and wearing elastic stockings may also help. Increased salt in the diet and treatment with salt-retaining hormones such as fludrocortisone are other possible approaches. In certain patients, drugs used to treat hypertension can instead raise blood pressure, although predicting which patients will have this paradoxical reaction is difficult.

Muscle weakness or loss of coordination caused by diabetic neuropathy can often be helped by physical therapy.

### *Urinary and Sexual Problems*

Nerve and circulatory problems of diabetes can disrupt normal male sexual function, resulting in impotence. After ruling out a hormonal cause of impotence, the doctor can provide information about methods available to treat impotence caused by neuropathy. Short-term solutions involve using a mechanical vacuum device or injecting a drug called a vasodilator into the penis before sex. Both methods raise blood flow to the penis, making it easier to have and maintain an erection. Surgical procedures, in which an inflatable or semirigid device is implanted in the penis, offer a more permanent solution. For some people, counseling may help relieve the stress caused by neuropathy and thereby help restore sexual function.

In women who feel their sexual life is not satisfactory, the role of diabetic neuropathy is less clear. Illness, vaginal or urinary tract infections, and anxiety about pregnancy complicated by diabetes can interfere with a woman's ability to enjoy intimacy. Infections can be reduced by good blood glucose control. Counseling may also help a woman identify and cope with sexual concerns.

## Why Is Good Foot Care Important for People with Diabetic Neuropathy?

People with diabetes need to take special care of their feet. Neuropathy and blood vessel disease both increase the risk of foot ulcers. The nerves to the feet are the longest in the body, and are most often affected by neuropathy. Because of the loss of sensation caused by neuropathy, sores or injuries to the feet may not be noticed and may become ulcerated.

At least 15 percent of all people with diabetes eventually have a foot ulcer, and 6 out of every 1,000 people with diabetes have an amputation. However, doctors estimate that nearly three quarters of all amputations caused by neuropathy and poor circulation could be prevented with careful foot care.

To prevent foot problems from developing, people with diabetes should follow these rules for foot care:

- Check your feet and toes daily for any cuts, sores, bruises, bumps, or infections—using a mirror if necessary.
- Wash your feet daily, using warm (not hot) water and a mild soap. If you have neuropathy, you should test the water temperature with your wrist before putting your feet in the water. Doctors do not advise soaking your feet for long periods, since you may lose protective calluses. Dry your feet carefully with a soft towel, especially between the toes.
- Cover your feet (except for the skin between the toes) with petroleum jelly, a lotion containing lanolin, or cold cream before putting on shoes and socks. In people with diabetes, the feet tend to sweat less than normal. Using a moisturizer helps prevent dry, cracked skin.
- Wear thick, soft socks and avoid wearing slippery stockings, mended stockings, or stockings with seams.
- Wear shoes that fit your feet well and allow your toes to move. Break in new shoes gradually, wearing them for only an hour at a time at first. After years of neuropathy, as reflexes are lost, the feet are likely to become wider and flatter. If you have difficulty finding shoes that fit, ask your doctor to refer you to a specialist, called a pedorthist, who can provide you with corrective shoes or inserts.

- Examine your shoes before putting them on to make sure they have no tears, sharp edges, or objects in them that might injure your feet.
- Never go barefoot, especially on the beach, hot sand, or rocks.
- Cut your toenails straight across, but be careful not to leave any sharp corners that could cut the next toe.
- Use an emery board or pumice stone to file away dead skin, but do not remove calluses, which act as protective padding. Do not try to cut off any growths yourself, and avoid using harsh chemicals such as wart remover on your feet.
- Test the water temperature with your elbow before stepping in a bath.
- If your feet are cold at night wear socks. (Do not use heating pads or hot water bottles.)
- Avoid sitting with your legs crossed. Crossing your legs can reduce the flow of blood to the feet.
- Ask your doctor to check your feet at every visit, and call your doctor if you notice that a sore is not healing well.
- If you are not able to take care of your own feet, ask your doctor to recommend a podiatrist (specialist in the care and treatment of feet) who can help.

## *Are There Any Experimental Treatments for Diabetic Neuropathy?*

Several new drugs under study may eventually prevent or reverse diabetic neuropathy. However, extensive testing is required by the U.S. Food and Drug Administration to establish the safety and efficacy of drugs before they are approved for widespread use.

Researchers are exploring treatment with a compound called myoinositol. Early findings have shown that nerves in diabetic animals and humans have less than normal amounts of this substance. Myoinositol supplements increase the levels of this substance in tissues of diabetic animals, but research is still needed to show any concrete lasting benefits from this treatment.

Another area of research concerns the drug aminoguanidine. In animals, this drug blocks cross-linking of proteins that occurs more quickly than normal in tissues exposed to high levels of glucose. Early clinical tests are under way to determine the effects of aminoguanidine in humans.

One approach that appeared promising involved the use of aldose reductase inhibitors (ARIs). ARIs are a class of drugs that block the formation of the sugar alcohol sorbitol, which is thought to damage nerves. Scientists hoped these drugs would prevent and might even repair nerve damage. But so far, clinical trials have shown that these drugs have major side effects and, consequently, they are not available for clinical use.

## Some General Hints

- Ask your doctor to suggest an exercise routine that is right for you. Many people who exercise regularly find the pain of neuropathy less severe. Aside from helping you reach and maintain a healthy weight, exercise also improves the body's use of insulin, helps improve circulation, and strengthens muscles. Check with your doctor before starting exercise that can be hard on your feet, such as running or aerobics.
- If you smoke, try to stop because smoking makes circulatory problems worse and increases the risk of neuropathy and heart disease.
- Reduce the amount of alcohol you drink. Recent research has indicated that as few as four drinks per week can worsen neuropathy.
- Take special care of your feet.

## What Resources Are Available for People with Diabetic Neuropathy?

**American Association of Diabetes Educators**
444 North Michigan Avenue
Suite 1240
Chicago, IL 60611
(800) 832-6874 or (312) 644-2233

A professional organization that can help individuals locate a diabetes educator in their community.

**American Diabetes Association National Service Center**
1660 Duke Street
Alexandria, VA 22314
(800) 232-3472 or (703) 549-1500

A private, voluntary organization that fosters public awareness of diabetes and supports and promotes diabetes research and education. The association has printed information on many aspects of diabetes, and local affiliates sponsor community programs. Local affiliates can be found in the telephone directory or through the national office.

**American Dietetic Association**
216 West Jackson Boulevard
Chicago, IL 60606-6995
(800) 877-1600 or (312) 899-0040

A professional organization that can help individuals locate a registered dietitian in their community.

**American Heart Association**
7320 Greenville Avenue
Dallas, TX 75231
(800) 242-1793

A private, voluntary organization that distributes literature on heart disease and how to prevent it. Local affiliates can be found in the telephone directory.

**Juvenile Diabetes Foundation International**
120 Wall Street
19th Floor
New York, NY 10005
(212) 785-9500 or (800) 223-1138

A private, voluntary organization that funds research on diabetes and promotes public awareness. Local chapters located across the country sponsor programs and fundraising activities. Information about local groups is available in telephone directories or from the national office.

**National Diabetes Information Clearinghouse**
1 Information Way
Bethesda, MD 20892-3560
(301) 654-3327

A program of the National Institute of Diabetes and Digestive and Kidney Diseases, the Federal Government's lead agency for diabetes research. The clearinghouse distributes a variety of publications to the public and to health professionals.

## Additional Reading

For more information about diabetic neuropathy and diabetes research:

Albert, L., Restraining pain: What's available for easing the pain of diabetic neuropathy, *Diabetes Forecast*, January 1988, pp. 39-41.

American Diabetes Association and the American Academy of Neurology, Report and recommendations of the San Antonio Conference on Diabetic Neuropathy, *Diabetes Care*, July/August 1988, pp. 592-597.

Bell, D. & Clements, R., Diabetes and the digestive system, *Diabetes Forecast*, December 1987, pp. 43-46.

Clark, C.M., & Lee, D.A., Prevention and treatment of the complications of diabetes mellitus, *The New England Journal of Medicine*, May 4, 1995, pp. 1210-1218.

Cohen, M. et al., Managing diabetes complications, *Patient Care*, December 15, 1988, pp. 28-39.

Dyck, P.J., Aldose reductase inhibitors and diabetic neuropathy, *Diabetes Forecast*, May 1989, pp. 41-43.

Dyck, P.J., Resolvable problems in diabetic neuropathy, *The Journal of NIH Research*, June 1990, pp. 57-62.

Dyck, P.J., Thomas, P.K., and Asbury, A.K., *Diabetic Neuropathy*, Saunders, W.B., Company, 1987.

Gerding, D. et al., Problems in diabetic foot care, *Patient Care*, August 15, 1988, pp. 102-118.

Greene, D., & Stevens, M., Diabetic peripheral neuropathy: New approaches to treatment, classification, and staging, *Diabetes Spectrum*, July/August 1993, pp. 223-257.

Haase, G. et al., Neuropathy: Diabetic? Nutritional?, *Patient Care*, May 15, 1990, pp. 112-134.

Jaspan, J. et al., GI complications of diabetes, *Patient Care*, January 15, 1990, pp. 108-128.

Mills, P., Drugs that block complications, *Diabetes Self-Management*, September/ October 1988, pp. 14-16.

National Institute of Diabetes and Digestive and Kidney Diseases. *Diabetes Special Report*, 1994 (NIH Publication No. 94-3422). Bethesda, MD.

Vinik, A., et al., Diabetic neuropathies, *Diabetes Care*, December 1992, pp. 1926-1975.

Wakelee-Lynch, J., Relieving pain with peppers, *Diabetes Forecast*, June 1992, pp. 34-37.

Weiss, R., Behind the pain: Causes and treatment of diabetic neuropathy, *Diabetes Interview*, November 1993, pp. 1, 12-13.

The following booklets developed by the National Institute of Diabetes and Digestive and Kidney Diseases provide general information about diabetes. Copies may be ordered from the National Diabetes Information Clearinghouse.

- *Insulin-Dependent Diabetes*
- *Noninsulin-Dependent Diabetes*
- *The Diabetes Dictionary*

Chapter 43

# Periodontal Disease and Diabetes

If you have diabetes, you know the disease can harm your eyes, nerves, kidneys, heart and other important systems in the body. Did you know it can also cause problems in your mouth? People with diabetes have a higher than normal risk of periodontal diseases.

Periodontal diseases are infections of the gum and bone that hold the teeth in place. In advanced stages, they lead to painful chewing problems and even tooth loss. Like any infection, gum disease can make it hard to keep your blood sugar under control.

## What is the Link Between Diabetes and Periodontal Disease?

**Diabetic Control.** Like other complications of diabetes, gum disease is linked to diabetic control. People with poor blood sugar control get gum disease more often and more severely, and they lose more teeth than do persons with good control. In fact, people whose diabetes is well controlled have no more periodontal disease than persons without diabetes. Children with IDDM (insulin-dependent diabetes mellitus) are also at risk for gum problems. Good diabetic control is the best protection against periodontal disease.

Studies show that controlling blood sugar levels lowers the risk of some complications of diabetes, such as eye and heart disease and

---

National Institute of Dental Research, NIH Publication No. 97-2946, January 1997.

nerve damage. Scientists believe many complications, including gum disease, can be prevented with good diabetic control.

**Blood Vessel Changes.** Thickening of blood vessels is a complication of diabetes that may increase risk for gum disease. Blood vessels deliver oxygen and nourishment to body tissues, including the mouth, and carry away the tissues' waste products. Diabetes causes blood vessels to thicken, which slows the flow of nutrients and the removal of harmful wastes. This can weaken the resistance of gum and bone tissue to infection.

**Bacteria.** Many kinds of bacteria (germs) thrive on sugars, including glucose—the sugar linked to diabetes. When diabetes is poorly controlled, high glucose levels in mouth fluids may help germs grow and set the stage for gum disease.

**Smoking.** The harmful effects of smoking, particularly heart disease and cancer, are well known. Studies show that smoking also increases the chances of developing gum disease. In fact, smokers are five times more likely than nonsmokers to have gum disease. For smokers with diabetes, the risk is even greater. *If you are a smoker with diabetes, age 45 or older, you are 20 times more likely than a person without these risk factors to get severe gum disease.*

## How Does Periodontal Disease Develop?

**Gingivitis.** Poor brushing and flossing habits allow dental plaque—a sticky film of germs—to build up on teeth. Some of these germs cause gum disease. The gums can become red and swollen and may bleed during toothbrushing or flossing. This is called gingivitis, the first stage of periodontal disease.

Gingivitis can usually be reversed with daily brushing and flossing and regular cleanings by the dentist. If it is not stopped, gingivitis could lead to a more serious type of gum disease called periodontitis.

**Periodontitis.** Periodontitis is an infection of the tissues that hold the teeth in place. In periodontitis, plaque builds and hardens under the gums. The gums pull away from the teeth, forming "pockets" of infection. The infection leads to loss of the bone that holds the tooth in its socket and might lead to tooth loss.

There are often no warning signs of early periodontitis. Pain, abscess, and loosening of the teeth do not occur until the disease is advanced.

Since periodontitis affects more than just the gums, it cannot be controlled with regular brushing and flossing. Periodontitis should be treated by a periodontist (a gum disease specialist) or by a general dentist who has special training in treating gum diseases.

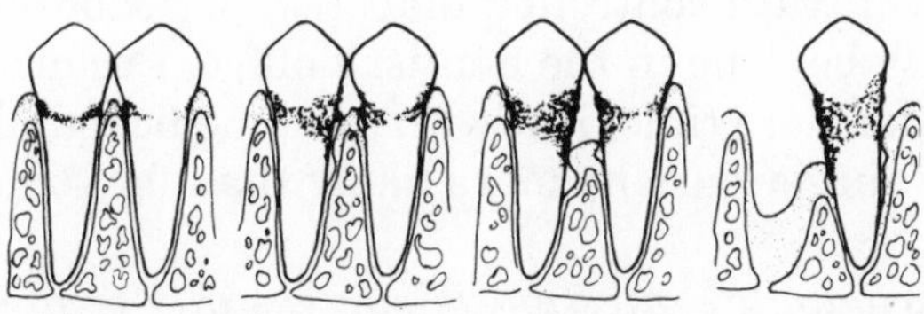

***Figure 43.1.*** *As plaque builds up, the gums become inflamed and, in time, affected teeth may loosen and could be lost.*

## How Is Periodontal Disease Treated?

**Plaque Removal.** Treatment of periodontitis depends on how much damage the disease has caused. In the early stages, the dentist or periodontist will use deep cleaning to remove hardened plaque and infected tissue under the gum and smooth the damaged root surfaces of teeth. This allows the gum to re-attach to the teeth. A special mouthrinse or an antibiotic might also be prescribed to help control the infection.

*Deep cleaning is successful only if the patient regularly brushes and flosses to keep the plaque from building up again.*

**Periodontal Surgery.** Gum surgery is needed when periodontitis is very advanced and tissues that hold a tooth in place are destroyed. The dentist or periodontist will clean out the infected area under the gum, then reshape or replace the damaged tooth-supporting tissues. These treatments increase the chances of saving the tooth.

## If You Have Diabetes

- It's important for you to know how well your diabetes is controlled and to tell your dentist this information at each visit.
- See your doctor before scheduling treatment for periodontal disease. Ask your doctor to talk to the dentist or periodontist about your overall medical condition before treatment begins.

- You may need to change your meal schedule and the timing and dosage of your insulin if oral surgery is planned.
- Postpone non-emergency dental procedures if your blood sugar is not in good control. However, acute infections, such as abscesses, should be treated right away.

For the person with controlled diabetes, periodontal or oral surgery can usually be done in the dentist's office. Because of diabetes, healing may take more time. But with good medical and dental care, problems after surgery are no more likely than for someone without diabetes.

*Once the periodontal infection is successfully treated, it is often easier to control blood sugar levels.*

## Are Other Oral Problems Linked to Diabetes?

**Dental Cavities.** Young people with IDDM have no more tooth decay than do nondiabetic children. In fact, youngsters with IDDM who are careful about their diet and take good care of their teeth often have fewer cavities than other children because they don't eat many foods that contain sugar.

**Thrush.** Thrush is an infection caused by a fungus that grows in the mouth. People with diabetes are at risk for thrush because the fungus thrives on high glucose levels in saliva. Smoking and wearing dentures (especially when they are worn constantly) can also lead to fungal infection. Medication is available to treat this infection. Good diabetic control, no smoking, and removing and cleaning dentures daily can help prevent thrush.

**Dry Mouth.** Dry mouth is often a symptom of undetected diabetes and can cause more than just an uncomfortable feeling in your mouth. Dry mouth can cause soreness, ulcers, infections, and tooth decay.

The dryness means that you don't have enough saliva, the mouth's natural protective fluid. Saliva helps control the growth of germs that cause tooth decay and other oral infections. Saliva washes away sticky foods that help form plaque and strengthens teeth with minerals.

One of the major causes of dry mouth is medication. More than 400 over-the-counter and prescription drugs, including medicines for colds, high blood pressure or depression, can cause dry mouth. If you are taking medications, tell your doctor or dentist if your mouth feels dry.

You may be able to try a different drug or use an "artificial saliva" to keep your mouth moist.

*Good blood glucose control can help prevent or relieve dry mouth caused by diabetes.*

## Keep Your Teeth

Serious periodontal disease not only can cause tooth loss, but can also cause changes in the shape of bone and gum tissue. The gum becomes uneven, and dentures may not fit well. People with diabetes often have sore gums from dentures.

If chewing with dentures is painful, you might choose foods that are easier to chew but not right for your diet. Eating the wrong foods can upset blood sugar control. The best way to avoid these problems is to keep your natural teeth and gums healthy.

## How Can You Protect Your Teeth and Gums?

Harmful germs attack the teeth and gums when plaque builds up. You can stop plaque build-up and prevent gum disease by brushing and flossing carefully every day.

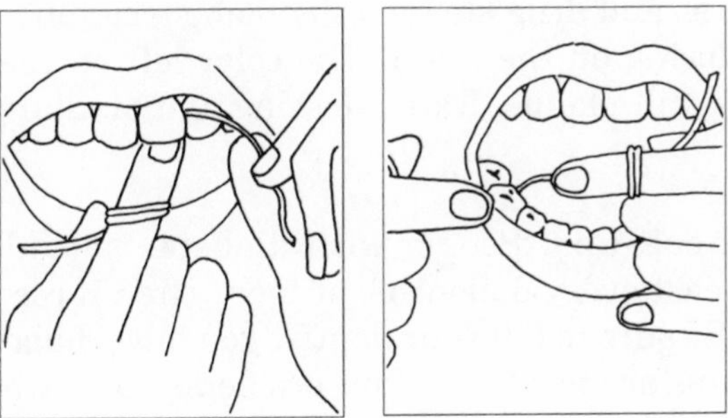

***Figure 43.2.*** *Floss carefully.*

- Use a piece of dental floss about 18 inches long.
- Using a sawing motion, gently bring the floss through the tight spaces between the teeth.
- Do not snap the floss against the gums.
- Curve the floss around each tooth and gently scrape from below the gum to the top of the tooth several times.
- Rinse your mouth after flossing.

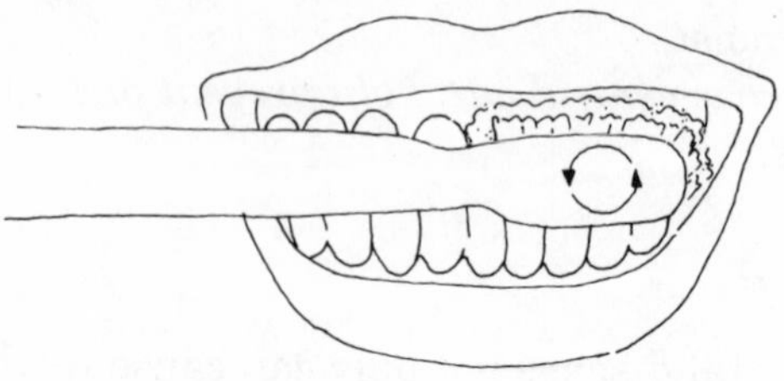

***Figure 43.3.*** *Brush carefully.*

- Gently brush teeth twice a day with a soft nylon brush with rounded ends on the bristles.
- Avoid hard back-and-forth scrubbing.
- Use small circle motions and short back-and-forth motions.
- Gently brush your tongue, which can trap germs.
- Use a fluoride toothpaste to protect teeth from decay.

**Check Your Work.** Dental plaque is hard to see unless it is stained. Plaque can be stained by chewing red "disclosing tablets" sold at grocery stores and drug stores or by using a cotton swab to smear green food coloring on the teeth. The color left on the teeth shows where there is still plaque. Extra flossing and brushing will remove this plaque.

**Dental Check-ups.** People with diabetes should have dental check-ups at least every 6 months, or more often if recommended by their dentist. Be sure to tell your dentist you have diabetes. Frequent dental check-ups are needed to find problems early when treatment is most effective. See your dentist as soon as possible if you have any problem with your teeth or mouth.

Preventing or controlling gum disease depends on teamwork. The best defense against this complication of diabetes is good blood sugar control, combined with daily brushing and flossing and regular dental check-ups.

# Chapter 44

# *Diabetic Retinopathy*

This chapter has been written to help people with diabetic retinopathy and their families better understand the disease. It describes the cause, symptoms, diagnosis, and treatment of diabetic retinopathy.

Diabetic retinopathy is a potentially blinding complication of diabetes that damages the eye's retina. It affects half of the 14 million Americans with diabetes.

At first, you may notice no changes in your vision. But don't let diabetic retinopathy fool you. It could get worse over the years and threaten your good vision. With timely treatment, 90 percent of those with advanced diabetic retinopathy can be saved from going blind.

The National Eye Institute (NEI) is the Federal government's lead agency for vision research. The NEI urges all people with diabetes to have an eye examination through dilated pupils at least once a year.

### *What is the retina?*

The retina is a light-sensitive tissue at the back of the eye. When light enters the eye, the retina changes the light into nerve signals. The retina then sends these signals along the optic nerve to the brain. Without a retina, the eye cannot communicate with the brain, making vision impossible.

---

National Eye Institute (NEI), NIH Pub. No. 95-3252, 1995.

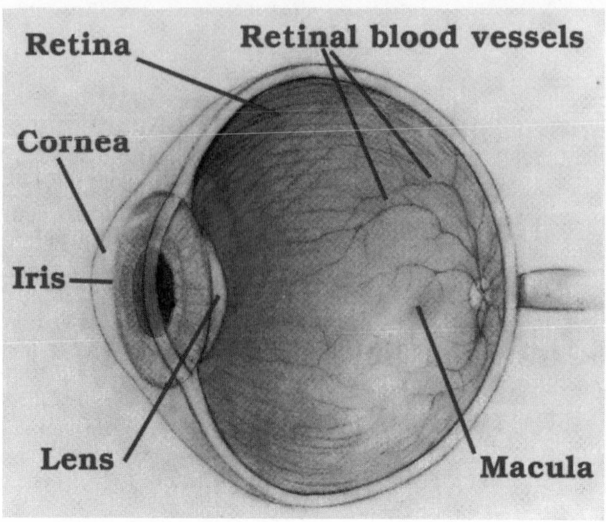


***Figure 44.1.*** *The Eye*

## *How does diabetic retinopathy damage the retina?*

Diabetic retinopathy occurs when diabetes damages the tiny blood vessels in the retina. At this point, most people do not notice any changes in their vision.

Some people develop a condition called **macular edema.** It occurs when the damaged blood vessels leak fluid and lipids onto the macula, the part of the retina that lets us see detail. The fluid makes the macula swell, blurring vision.

As the disease progresses, it enters its advanced, or **proliferative**, stage. Fragile, new blood vessels grow along the retina and in the clear, gel-like vitreous that fills the inside of the eye. Without timely treatment, these new blood vessels can bleed, cloud vision, and destroy the retina.

## *Who is at risk for this disease?*

All people with diabetes are at risk—those with Type I diabetes (juvenile onset) and those with Type II diabetes (adult onset).

During pregnancy, diabetic retinopathy may also be a problem for women with diabetes. It is recommended that all pregnant women with diabetes have dilated eye examinations each trimester to protect their vision.

### *What are its symptoms?*

Diabetic retinopathy often has no early warning signs. At some point, though, you may have macular edema. It blurs vision, making it hard to do things like read and drive. In some cases, your vision will get better or worse during the day.

As new blood vessels form at the back of the eye, they can bleed (hemorrhage) and blur vision. The first time this happens it may not be very severe. In most cases, it will leave just a few specks of blood, or spots, floating in your vision. They often go away after a few hours.

These spots are often followed within a few days or weeks by a much greater leakage of blood. The blood will blur your vision. In extreme cases, a person will only be able to tell light from dark in that eye. It may take the blood anywhere from a few days to months or even years to clear from inside of your eye. In some cases, the blood will not clear. You should be aware that large hemorrhages tend to happen more than once, often during sleep.

### *How is it detected?*

Diabetic retinopathy is detected during an eye examination that includes:

- **Visual acuity test:** This eye chart test measures how well you see at various distances.

- **Pupil dilation:** The eye care professional places drops into the eye to widen the pupil. This allows him or her to see more of the retina and look for signs of diabetic retinopathy. After the examination, close-up vision may remain blurred for several hours.

- **Ophthalmoscopy:** This is an examination of the retina in which the eye care professional: (1) looks through a device with a special magnifying lens that provides a narrow view of the retina, or (2) wearing a headset with a bright light, looks through a special magnifying glass and gains a wide view of the retina.

- **Tonometry:** A standard test that determines the fluid pressure inside the eye. Elevated pressure is a possible sign of glaucoma, another common eye problem in people with diabetes.

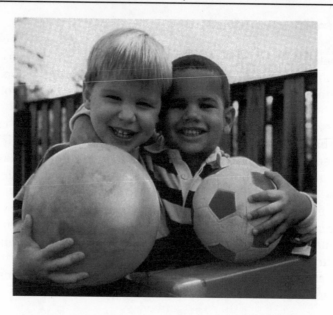

***Figure 44.2.*** *View of boys by person with normal vision.*

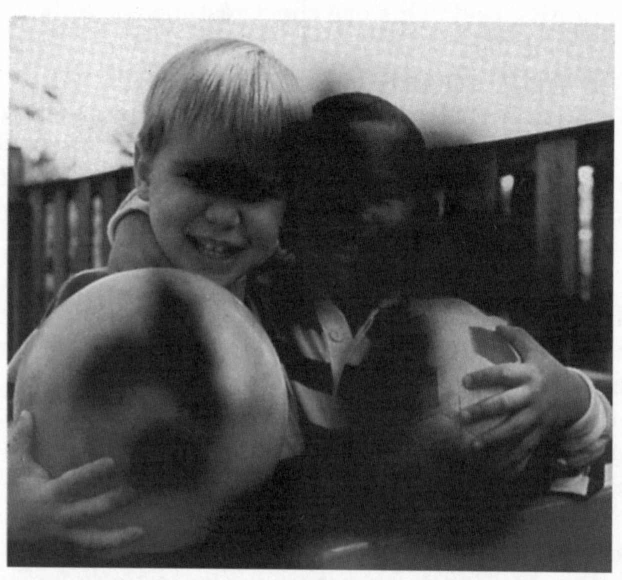

***Figure 44.3.*** *View of boys by person with diabetic retinopathy.*

Your eye care professional will look at your retina for early signs of the disease, such as: (1) leaking blood vessels, (2) retinal swelling, such as macular edema, (3) pale, fatty deposits on the retina—signs of leaking blood vessels, (4) damaged nerve tissue, and (5) any changes in the blood vessels.

Should your doctor suspect that you need treatment for macular edema, he or she may ask you to have a test called **fluorescein angiography**.

In this test, a special dye is injected into your arm. Pictures are then taken as the dye passes through the blood vessels in the retina. This test allows your doctor to find the leaking blood vessels.

### *How is it treated?*

There are two treatments for diabetic retinopathy. They are very effective in reducing vision loss from this disease. In fact, even people with advanced retinopathy have a 90 percent chance of keeping their vision when they get treatment before the retina is severely damaged. These treatments are:

**Laser Surgery:** Doctors will perform laser surgery to treat severe macular edema and proliferative retinopathy.

- **Macular Edema:** Timely laser surgery can reduce vision loss from macular edema by half. But you may need to have laser surgery more than once to control the leaking fluid.

  During the surgery, your doctor will aim a high-energy beam of light directly onto the damaged blood vessels. This is called **focal laser treatment**. This seals the vessels and stops them from leaking. Generally, laser surgery is used to stabilize vision, not necessarily to improve it.

- **Proliferative Retinopathy:** In treating advanced diabetic retinopathy, doctors use the laser to destroy the abnormal blood vessels that form at the back of the eye.

  Rather than focus the light on a single spot, your eye care professional will make hundreds of small laser burns away from the center of the retina. This is called **scatter laser treatment**. The treatment shrinks the abnormal blood vessels. You will lose some of your side vision after this surgery to save the rest of your sight. Laser surgery may also slightly reduce your color and night vision.

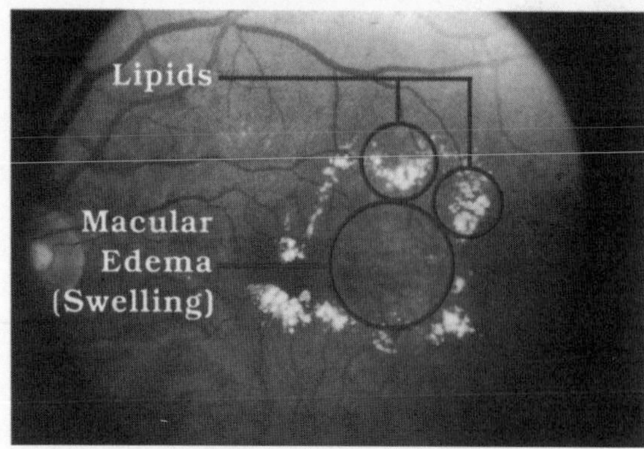


*Figure 44.4. The retina prior to focal laser treatment.*

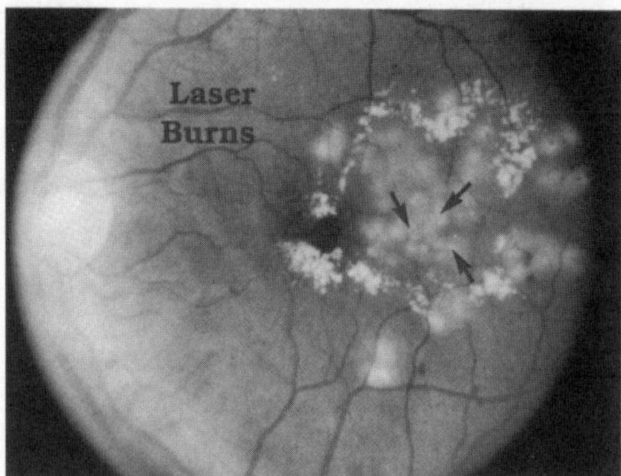


*Figure 44.5. The retina immediately after focal laser treatment.*

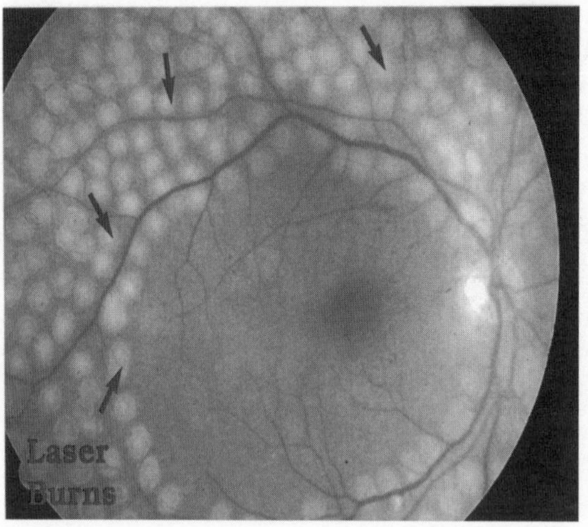


*Figure 44.6. Scatter laser treatment.*

Laser surgery is performed in a doctor's office or eye clinic. Before the surgery, your ophthalmologist will: (1) dilate your pupil and (2) apply drops to numb the eye. In some cases, the doctor also may numb the area behind the eye to prevent any discomfort.

The lights in the office will be dim. As you sit facing the laser machine, your doctor will hold a special lens to your eye. During the procedure, you may see flashes of bright green or red light. These flashes may eventually create a stinging sensation that makes you feel a little uncomfortable.

You may leave the office once the treatment is done, but you will need someone to drive you home. Because your pupils will remain dilated for a few hours, you also should bring a pair of sunglasses.

For the rest of the day, your vision will probably be a little blurry. Your eye may also hurt a bit. This is easily controlled with drugs that your eye care professional suggests.

**Vitrectomy:** If you have a lot of blood in the vitreous, you may need an eye operation called a **vitrectomy** to restore sight. It involves removing the cloudy vitreous and replacing it with a salt solution. Because the vitreous is mostly water, you will notice no change between the salt solution and the normal vitreous.

Studies show that people who have a vitrectomy soon after a large hemorrhage are more likely to protect their vision than someone who waits to have the operation. Early vitrectomy is especially effective in people with insulin-dependent diabetes, who may be at greater risk of blindness from a hemorrhage into the eye.

Vitrectomy is often done under local anesthesia (using drops to numb the eye). This means that you will be awake during the operation. The doctor makes a tiny incision in the sclera, or white of the eye. Next, a small instrument is placed into the eye. It removes the vitreous and inserts the salt solution into the eye.

You may be able to return home soon after the vitrectomy. Or, you may be asked to stay in the hospital overnight. Your eye will be red and sensitive. After the operation, you will need to wear an eyepatch for a few days or weeks to protect the eye. You will also need to use medicated eye drops to protect against infection.

Although laser surgery and vitrectomy are very successful, they do not cure diabetic retinopathy. Once you have proliferative retinopathy, you will always be at risk for new bleeding. This means you may need treatment more than once to protect your sight.

### *What research is being done?*

The NEI is currently supporting a number of research studies in both the laboratory and with patients to learn more about the cause of diabetic retinopathy. This research should provide better ways to detect, treat, and prevent vision loss in people with diabetes.

For example, it is likely that in the coming years researchers will develop drugs that turn off enzyme activity that has been shown to cause diabetic retinopathy. Some day, these drugs will help people to control the disease and reduce the need for laser surgery.

### *What can you do to protect your vision?*

The NEI urges all people with diabetes to have an eye examination through dilated pupils at least once a year. If you have more serious retinopathy, you may need to have a dilated eye examination more often.

A recent study, the Diabetes Control and Complications Trial (DCCT), showed that better control of blood sugar level slows the onset and progression of retinopathy and lessens the need for laser surgery for severe retinopathy.

The study found that the group that tried to keep their blood sugar levels as close to normal as possible, had much less eye, kidney, and nerve disease. This level of blood sugar control may not be best for everyone, including some elderly patients, children under 13, or people with heart disease. So ask your doctor if this program is right for you.

**For more information** about diabetic retinopathy or diabetes, you may wish to contact:

**American Academy of Ophthalmology**
655 Beach Street, P.O. Box 7424
San Francisco, CA 94109-7424
(415) 561-8500

**American Optometric Association**
243 Lindbergh Boulevard
St. Louis, MO 63141
(314) 991-4100

**American Diabetes Association**
1660 Duke Street
Alexandria, VA 22314
(703) 549-1500

**Juvenile Diabetes Foundation International**
432 Park Avenue South
New York, NY 10016
(212) 889-7575

**National Eye Institute**
2020 Vision Place
Bethesda, MD 20892-3655
(301) 496-5248

**National Diabetes Outreach Program**
**National Institute of Diabetes and Digestive and Kidney Diseases**
1 Diabetes Way
Bethesda, MD 20892-3560
1 -800-GET-LEVEL

# Chapter 45

# *Watching Out for Glaucoma*

As a person affected by diabetes, you have a greater chance of developing glaucoma than someone without diabetes. Glaucoma, in fact, is a very serious disease. But don't despair: There *are* steps you can take to treat it if you have glaucoma now.

Glaucoma is an eye disease that gradually causes a partial or complete loss of vision. Pressure inside the eye is the major factor in causing glaucoma. The eye is a ball filled with fluid. This fluid is constantly secreted by the eye and circulates inside the eye. The fluid exits through the front part of the eye to join the blood. This circulation process generates pressure within the eye and maintains it within certain limits. But disturbances in this cycle can lead to pressures higher than the eye can tolerate, thus causing glaucoma.

Although we don't know exactly why you are more prone to developing glaucoma than someone without diabetes, we do know that there are risk factors for glaucoma, such as age or a family history of glaucoma. Glaucoma is also associated with high blood pressure, diabetes, and hardening of the arteries (atherosclerosis). And Blacks are at a higher risk than members of other races.

In general, between 1 and 2 percent of the population older than 40 has glaucoma. But as a person with diabetes, *your* chances of being affected by glaucoma are higher than those of others, regardless of whether you have type I or type II diabetes.

---

## Types of Glaucoma

The most common type of glaucoma, usually called open-angle glaucoma, is a "silent" disease: It has no obvious physical symptoms. Open-angle glaucoma does not involve eye pain, headache, redness of the eye, or any other discomfort. The only way to detect it is through a complete eye examination, including checking eye pressure, the optic nerve, and field of vision. An optometrist may be able to do this type of exam, but I believe an ophthalmologist is better qualified to evaluate the importance of eye changes relative to the severity of diabetes, which is a disease affecting the whole body.

This type of glaucoma occurs more frequently in people with diabetes than in those without diabetes. Open-angle glaucoma develops slowly, so if it is detected early, treatment can prevent or slow loss of vision. People with open-angle glaucoma usually lose their side vision first, before losing their central vision. The field of vision gradually becomes narrower without central blurring. Eventually it becomes like "tunnel vision." And even that can be lost in the final stages.

The second, and less common, type of glaucoma is called narrow-angle glaucoma. Unlike open-angle glaucoma, narrow-angle glaucoma occurs as often in people with diabetes as in those without diabetes. Narrow-angle glaucoma, however, does involve symptoms, and they may appear suddenly. Eye pain, headaches of varying severity, redness of the eye, or blurring of vision may all occur. People with this kind of glaucoma have episodes of blurred vision, lasting from a few hours to a few days each time.

Again, a medical examination and treatment by an ophthalmologist may prevent irreversible eye damage and loss of vision. Because it may sometimes be difficult to tell the difference between periodic headaches and those due to narrow-angle glaucoma, a person with symptoms—especially someone with a family history of glaucoma—should have an eye examination designed to tell the two apart.

The third form of glaucoma is neovascular glaucoma. Neovascular glaucoma affects some people with diabetes and other people who suffer from a blockage of blood vessels in the eye or from chronic eye inflammation. The symptoms of this type of glaucoma are redness of the eye and a rapid rise in eye pressure. Neovascular glaucoma can cause pain and decreased vision. It tends to progress rapidly and can have devastating effects on vision.

The loss of vision from neovascular glaucoma is like open-angle glaucoma, but there is also underlying eye disease that may cause the vision to be lost suddenly, as with bleeding or inflammation. Sometimes, neovascular glaucoma responds favorably to laser treatment if detected early through an eye examination.

## What to Do about Glaucoma

Although glaucoma is not curable or preventable, it is almost always treatable. And when glaucoma is diagnosed early, it responds particularly well to treatment.

Since glaucoma is usually discovered by a routine eye examination, anyone who is younger than 30 years old and has had diabetes for five years should have a baseline eye exam, and annual eye exams thereafter. Anyone who develops diabetes after age 30 should have a baseline eye exam at diagnosis and annual examinations after that.

There are three forms of treatment for glaucoma that can be used either separately or in combination: eye drops with or without oral medication, laser surgery, or conventional surgery. All these approaches lower eye pressure.

When medications fail to control eye pressure, laser surgery is usually attempted. Laser treatment of the front part of the eye, a procedure done in a doctor's office, results in pressure control in about 70 percent of cases. Its beneficial effects last anywhere from a few months to several years.

If laser surgery is not successful, conventional surgery is available. This surgery, also called filtering surgery, consists of creating a new passage in the eye for fluids to flow, reducing pressure in the eye. It is usually done under local anesthesia and may be performed in an outpatient setting. This surgery generally has a success rate of 70 to 80 percent. The American Diabetes Association recommends that this surgery be performed by a retinal specialist or other ophthalmologist experienced in these procedures in people with diabetes.

## Some Treatment Side Effects

The treatments for glaucoma have several possible side effects or complications. Be sure to discuss any side effects you develop with your doctor. Eye drops may cause mild eye irritation, redness, or blurring of vision. Oral medications can cause fatigue, headaches, tingling sensations, and stomach aches. Oral glaucoma medications also may interfere with your body's fluid and potassium balance, if taken for prolonged periods of time or in conjunction with medication to lower elevated blood pressure.

Other side effects, arising in people who have particular medical conditions, have also been reported, though less frequently, following the use of certain glaucoma eye drops.

For example, complications may arise in people with heartbeat disturbances or heart failure, or in people who have breathing problems, such as asthma or emphysema. People with insulin-dependent (type I) diabetes should be careful when using certain glaucoma medications, such as beta-blockers, because these medications may mask some of the symptoms that indicate hypoglycemia (see “Beta Blockers and Diabetes,” *Diabetes Forecast*, May 1991).

If you have heart disease or elevated blood pressure, your glaucoma treatment should be closely supervised. Your ophthalmologist, with advice from your primary-care physician, can give you proper guidelines as to what medications you should or should not take.

As with other types of eye surgery, the risks of glaucoma surgery can be serious. They include blurring of vision, bleeding, cataract formation, and eye infection. But, in general, these are infrequent, and they are usually short-lived when they occur. And there is no risk to your general health, other than the usual risks of an anesthesia procedure itself.

Medical treatment of glaucoma, unfortunately, can be quite costly. Monthly expenses for medications range from as little as $10 to more than $100. Generic substitutes are not available for all glaucoma medicines. Regular follow-up, which is necessary for adequate glaucoma management, adds several hundred dollars per year to the cost. The cost of laser surgery is approximately $1,000 per eye, while that of filtering surgery ranges between $1,000 and $2,000.

If you have glaucoma, follow the instructions of your ophthalmologist for future care. If you need treatment for glaucoma, be sure you take any medications regularly, since delays can lead to irreversible vision loss. And inform other physicians who treat you about your glaucoma and the medications you take for it.

Most types of glaucoma can be controlled with some kind of medical or surgical treatment. With proper medical care and follow-up, losing all of your vision because of glaucoma should be the exception rather than the rule.

*—by Joseph G. Feghali, M.D.*

Joseph G. Feghali, M.D., is Assistant Professor and Director of the glaucoma service at West Virginia University in Morgantown, West Virginia.

## Chapter 46

# *Hypertension in Diabetes*

Lee was one of the lucky ones—through a routine checkup he found out early he had high blood pressure (hypertension). His doctor prescribed a program of weight loss, salt restriction, and medication, and Lee's blood pressure came down to normal. Lee was especially fortunate to have been diagnosed early, considering he has non-insulin-dependent (type II) diabetes. Uncontrolled high blood pressure can worsen complications of diabetes, including eye and kidney disease.

Unfortunately, many people with diabetes aren't as lucky as Lee was. They don't know they have high blood pressure or do know but don't have it controlled effectively. That is troubling, because people with diabetes are more likely to have hypertension than those who don't have diabetes.

Studies suggest that hypertension is about twice as common in people with diabetes as in those without.

High blood pressure so often escapes detection and treatment because it has no symptoms except in severe cases. High blood pressure lives up to its reputation as a silent killer: Many people realize they have it only when they suffer a complication like heart attack or stroke. That's good reason to break the silence about hypertension and diabetes.

---

## Understanding Blood Pressure

To understand what causes hypertension, it may help to look first at how normal pressures are created within the arteries. A certain level of pressure in arteries and smaller vessels is needed so nutrients in the blood can squeeze through tiny pores in the vessels and nourish the body's tissues.

With every heartbeat, blood is forced out of the heart and into the vessels. Blood first enters the aorta, the largest artery in the body. From there, it flows through smaller and smaller vessels. The narrower the vessel, the more it resists blood flow. It is the amount of blood that leaves the heart and the resistance it meets in the small vessels that creates pressure.

The level of pressure depends on three major factors: the volume of blood in the circulatory system, the speed and force with which the heart ejects the blood, and the diameter of the blood vessels into which the blood flows. Our body tries to keep the blood pressure at a normal level by tightly controlling these three major factors.

The volume of blood is controlled by adding or removing salt and water from it. The higher the volume, the greater the blood pressure. The lower the volume, the less the blood pressure will be. This volume depends on salt intake as well as a close interaction between the kidneys and the adrenal glands. Should the kidneys sense an overload of volume, they would simply respond by excreting excess water and salt into the urine. Conversely, if the kidneys' sensors perceive the volume of blood as being too low, they will send a signal to the adrenal glands. The adrenal glands respond by producing aldosterone, a hormone that aids the kidneys in limiting the amount of salt and water lost into the urine.

## Heart Function and Blood Vessel Resistance

The harder and faster the heart pumps, the higher the blood pressure tends to be. Likewise, the more constricted the blood vessels are, the higher the blood pressure will be.

To think about high blood pressure, imagine a hose with a nozzle attached. When the nozzle of the hose is fully opened, water freely drains out of it without much force. But when you partially tighten the nozzle, the pressure in the hose rises, causing water to spray out. In the same way the narrowed nozzle holds back water flow, small blood vessels hold back blood flow and cause pressure to build up.

The heart and blood vessels both are greatly influenced by the part of the nervous system called the autonomic nervous system (ANS). The ANS is that part of the nervous system that controls body processes that do not require conscious thought, such as digestion and sweating. The ANS originates in the brain and extends to our blood vessels and heart (as well as other organs).

The ANS releases two types of hormones, alpha hormones and beta hormones, that ultimately will fit into invisible biological keyholes or receptors contained within the heart and blood vessels.

Release of alpha hormones causes blood vessels to constrict, increases their resistance, and hence increases the blood pressure. The effect of beta hormones on blood vessels is to dilate them. When beta hormones fit into the beta receptors of the heart, it beats faster and harder, which tends to raise blood pressure. Under stressful circumstances, the autonomic nervous system will send a signal to the adrenal gland, causing it to release epinephrine. Epinephrine is different from the other hormone that the adrenal gland releases, aldosterone. It causes the heart to beat faster and stronger.

All of the above body systems—the heart, kidneys, adrenal glands, and autonomic nervous system—act together to regulate blood pressure. Here is a typical scenario: The body's control system senses a low blood pressure. As a result, the kidneys send signals to the adrenal glands, which send hormones to the kidneys, causing them to retain salt and water. Meanwhile, the ANS sends messages to the heart, causing it to beat faster and harder. At the same time, a message is sent to the blood vessels, telling them to constrict. If the body perceives, the situation as an emergency, the adrenal glands will also release epinephrine. All these responses are coordinated to raise blood pressure back to normal.

## *What Causes Hypertension?*

Sometimes, however, the delicately balanced mechanism for regulating blood pressure fails and hypertension develops. In some cases, hypertension can be linked to a specific problem such as kidney disease, a common complication in people who have type I diabetes. High blood pressure that is traceable to a medical problem is called secondary hypertension.

In about 95 percent of cases, however, no clear cause for hypertension is found. This is called essential, or primary, hypertension. Research suggests that essential high blood pressure might be partly due to insulin resistance—an inability by the body to respond normally to insulin. People with insulin resistance have raised levels of insulin in the blood. High insulin levels can make the ANS too active and cause the kidneys to hold on to salt and water. Both of these can lead to hypertension.

A single reading in a doctor's office is not enough to diagnose essential hypertension. Just the stress of seeing the doctor can raise blood pressure (a condition called "white coat hypertension"). Because stress can quickly raise blood pressure, a diagnosis of essential hypertension should be made only after several high readings on different occasions.

Aging seems to play a role in essential hypertension, particularly in people who have type II diabetes. In some people, aging causes stiffening, thickening, and narrowing of the blood vessels. The damaged blood vessels resist blood flow, and high blood pressure develops. Unfortunately, hypertension itself can further damage the walls of blood vessels, increasing resistance and blood pressure. High cholesterol and fatty deposits in the artery walls also contribute to this increased resistance to blood flow. High blood sugar, well known for its potentially damaging effects to blood vessels, also can add to the problem.

## What's the Harm?

If most patients with high blood pressure have no symptoms, can it really be that bad? The answer is an unequivocal yes.

Hypertension does most of its harm by damaging blood vessels. In the brain, blood vessel damage can block or even rupture an artery, causing a stroke.

Narrowing and blockage of the heart's blood supply can cause chest pain or a heart attack. Also, the strain of the heart pumping against a high resistance can cause the heart to weaken and lead to congestive heart failures and thickening of the heart's muscle wall.

Damage to the small blood vessels that supply the kidney can impair kidney function. In fact, hypertension commonly quickens the course to renal failure. Some experts of eye disease believe that hypertension can cause retinopathy (eye disease) to progress and increase the risk of bleeding into the eye and blindness.

## Behind the Numbers

Because hypertension can lead to such serious problems, it is important to have your blood pressure checked periodically.

Blood pressure is reported as two numbers—for example, 120 over 80. The higher number is called the systolic blood pressure. This is the blood pressure when the heart contracts. The lower number is called the diastolic blood pressure and represents the blood pressure when the heart is relaxed.

Normally, systolic blood pressures range from 90 to 130, and diastolic numbers range from 60 to 85. A diastolic pressure from 85 to 89 is called high normal blood pressure; 90 to 104, mild hypertension; 105 to 114, moderate hypertension; and 115 and above, severe hypertension.

Sometimes the systolic blood pressure is high even though the diastolic pressure remains less than 90. This is termed isolated systolic hypertension. Isolated systolic blood pressures higher than 160 should be considered as important as hypertension in which both pressures are high.

## Drug-Free Treatment

Before treating hypertension, your doctor will probably conduct a complete history and physical examination. In addition, he or she may choose to perform some basic diagnostic tests to help determine the cause of your hypertension and any complications as a result of it. These tests may include a chest X-ray to determine whether the heart is enlarged, a cardiogram to assess the condition of the heart, and blood work and urinalysis to check kidney function.

Generally speaking, unless blood pressure is seriously high, doctors first try to lower blood pressure without drugs. Some of the methods of reducing blood pressure without the use of medicines include:

- *Losing weight.* Being overweight can cause hypertension. So, weight loss can often reverse obesity-related hypertension. It is not always necessary to get to your ideal weight for blood pressure to come down. Often, a modest weight loss is enough to get blood pressure back to normal.

- *Restricting salt.* Reducing salt intake to less than 5 grams per day can reduce blood pressure in about one-third of those with high blood pressure. Avoiding processed foods containing salt and not adding salt to foods is enough to reduce blood pressure in some people whose high blood pressure is especially sensitive to salt intake.

- *Limiting alcohol.* Drinking more than 2 ounces of alcohol a day has been linked to hypertension. Your doctor may ask you to limit your alcohol intake to no more than 1 ounce daily. That's approximately one mixed drink, one glass of wine, or a can of beer.

- *Getting exercise.* Regular exercise can lower your blood pressure by helping you lose weight.
- *Quitting smoking.* Cigarette smoking may not directly raise blood pressure, but it does cause peripheral vascular disease and coronary artery disease—a risk for people who have diabetes and hypertension.

## Treatment with Medications

Most physicians will try to use nonpharmacological therapy for several weeks or even months before resorting to medications. However, sometimes lifestyle changes aren't enough to lower a person's blood pressure. Then, he or she needs to be treated with antihypertensive medications.

Understanding the factors that regulate blood pressure has led to the development of several different types of antihypertensive medications. These differ in the way they reduce blood pressure. Basically, blood pressure medications work in one of three ways: by reducing salt and water volume of the circulatory system, by decreasing the rate and force of the heart, and by decreasing the resistance to blood flow. A medication may have more than one mode of action.

- *Volume reducers.* This class of medications is called diuretics. They promote extra salt and water excretion by the kidneys. A smaller circulatory volume results in a lower blood pressure.
- *Heart force and rate reducers.* Heart force and heart rate are reduced by beta blockers, a class of drugs that blocks the effect of beta hormone stimulation on the heart. Beta blockers make the heart beat slower and less forcefully, and reduce blood pressure. Beta blockers probably have other blood-pressure-lowering mechanisms, but in most people their effect on the heart seems to be the major one.
- *Reducers of resistance.* There are several classes of drugs that lower resistance. They differ on how they dilate the blood vessels.

    *Vasodilators* directly dilate the blood vessels, lowering resistance.

*Inhibitors of autonomic nervous system alpha stimulation* decrease the autonomic nervous system's alpha stimulation of blood vessels. Alpha stimulation causes blood vessels to constrict. Some drugs, including clonidine and methyldopa, inhibit nerve impulses in the brain. Others block alpha hormones from interacting with blood vessels. A third class depletes alpha hormones from nerve endings. This last class of drugs is rarely used today because of side effects.

*Angiotensin-converting-enzyme (ACE) inhibitors* block the conversion of nonactive hormones (angiotensin I) into hormones that raise blood pressure (angiotensin II).

*Calcium channel blockers* cause blood vessels to dilate. They act by interfering with the action of calcium, a factor that causes blood vessels to constrict.

To reduce the side effects of a medication, manufacturers often combine two agents in one pill. For example, a diuretic that depletes potassium might be combined with another diuretic to conserve it. Combination pills are often used to increase effectiveness. For example, an ACE inhibitor might be combined with a diuretic.

Combination pills offer some treatment advantages, but they also have drawbacks. Although side effects are reduced, they are not eliminated. The side effects of a combination pill are the same as if two separate pills were taken. Combination pills also offer the doctor less flexibility in changing the dose of the two medications.

## The Right Medication for You

Ideally, a medication would reduce blood pressure without causing side effects or complications. Unfortunately, no drug is free from the potential of side effects.

To minimize side effects from antihypertensives, doctors use a careful strategy for prescribing medication. They first select a drug whose beneficial effects—a decrease in blood pressure and the risk of heart attack or stroke—outweigh the possible side effects.

Because side effects become more likely as the dose is increased, doctors first prescribe the minimum dose that is likely to be effective, then increase the dose if hypertension is still not controlled.

If the doctor feels that a higher dose of the drug would bring on side effects, he or she might try another antihypertensive or a combination of pills.

Special considerations are given to treating hypertension in people who have diabetes. Certain antihypertensive medications can worsen complications of diabetes. Some of the common problems encountered with antihypertensives in people with diabetes are:

- *Hyperglycemia*. Diuretics and beta blockers can inhibit the secretion of insulin, raising blood-sugar levels. This is generally only an issue with those who have non-insulin-dependent (type II) diabetes, since those who have insulin-dependent (type I) diabetes no longer produce insulin. Often, however, people with diabetes need to use diuretics and beta blockers. If so, the hyperglycemia is offset by adjusting a person's diabetes regimen.

- *Hypoglycemia*. Beta blockers tend to suppress the early warning signs (tremors, palpitations) of hypoglycemia. Therefore people who take insulin and use beta blockers may have to test their blood sugar more often to avoid hypoglycemia. In rare cases, beta blockers may prolong hypoglycemic reactions.

- *Impotence*. Impotence is a common complication in men who have diabetes. Several antihypertensive medications can either cause or worsen impotence. It is important that you discuss any problems with impotence before starting and during the time you are using antihypertensive medications.

- *Cholesterol and triglyceride levels*. People with diabetes have a greater incidence of increased triglyceride and cholesterol levels. Diuretics may cause a short-term rise in blood-cholesterol and triglyceride levels. Beta blockers may raise triglyceride levels and increase the ratio of LDL ("bad") cholesterol to HDL ("good") cholesterol.

- *Other metabolic problems*. Diuretics can cause low potassium or magnesium levels, which can lead to abnormal electrical and rhythm disturbances of the heart. Using potassium pills or a diuretic with potassium-sparing properties can often avoid this problem. ACE inhibitors can sometimes cause potassium levels to rise above normal in people with kidney disease.

- *Peripheral vascular disease*. The narrowing of both large and small arteries, which results in reduced blood flow to the extremities (such as the toes, is more common in people who have diabetes. In those people, who have severe peripheral. vascular disease, certain types of beta-blocking medications can cause the arteries to narrow and decrease blood flow.

- *Kidney disease.* Kidney disease and hypertension have several important links. Kidney disease can cause hypertension, and hypertension can worsen kidney disease. A special approach to hypertension is needed in patients with kidney disease.

- *Autonomic neuropathy.* Autonomic nerves play an important role in blood-pressure regulation. The autonomic nerves speed up the heart and increase resistance to blood flow in patients when blood pressure dips too low. These are important corrective mechanisms. Diabetes often impairs the ability of the autonomic nervous system to protect the body against hypotension (low blood pressure). Therefore, people with autonomic neuropathy should avoid medications that interfere with the alpha autonomic nervous system.

Your doctor can evaluate which drug will best control your blood pressure without causing excessive side effects or complications. Often, your physician may have to try several different medications before finding the most effective one that you can tolerate best. This may take several weeks. In general, I prefer to start treatment with calcium channel inhibitors, ACE inhibitors, or alpha blockers for people with diabetes. These drugs have few adverse effects on glucose control or levels of blood cholesterol, fats, or electrolytes, and they rarely cause impotence or worsen the symptoms of vascular disease. Of course, they still can cause side effects and any problems should be reported to your doctor. Even though diuretics and beta blockers have potential side effects, in most cases they are safe and effective.

In some people, high blood pressure is hard to control. Then the physician may want to either switch the medication or try a combination of medications. Sometimes as many as three or four medications must be combined to achieve blood-pressure control.

To avoid side effects, your physician will make changes in your antihypertensive medications slowly. Trying to find the right medication to control blood pressure takes time.

At the start of antihypertensive treatment, some people have minor side effects including headache, depression, unsteadiness, sleep disturbances, weak limbs, and fatigue. Often, these side effects are temporary and disappear after the first few days of therapy as the body adjusts to the medication. If symptoms persist, changes can be made in the medication. It is important to discuss any problems with your physician.

Hypertension is a chronic disease that often lasts a lifetime. You may be able to reduce the dose of your medication over time, however. Some people with mild hypertension have been able to stop treatment all together. Never stop taking the medications, however, without the advice of your physician.

If you haven't had your blood pressure checked, resolve to do it soon. Bringing down high blood pressure can slow down kidney disease and prevent the development of heart failure. If you have hypertension, be one of the lucky ones who have it detected and treated early.

*– by William A. Kaye, M.D., F.A.C.P.*

William A. Kaye, a practicing endocrinologist and nephrologist in West Palm Beach, Florida, is the Director of the Diabetes Center of the Palm Beaches and a Clinical Assistant Professor of Medicine at the University of Miami School of Medicine.

**Table 46.1.** Hypertension Drugs.

| Drug Name | Brand Name | Complications and Side Effects |
|---|---|---|
| 1. Diuretics | | Worsening in blood-glucose control in type II, transient rise in cholesterol, elevation of triglycerides, elevation of uric acid, gout, potassium and magnesium depletion, low blood pressure with standing, impotence, ineffective in renal failure |
| a. Thiazides and related diuretics | | |
| Bendroflumethiazide | Naturetin | |
| Benzthiazide | Aquatag, Exna, Marazide | |
| Chlorothiazide sodium | Diuril, Diachlor | |
| Chlorthalidone | Hygroton, Hylidone, Thalitone | |
| Cyclothiazide | Anhydron | |
| Hydrochlorothiazide | Esidrix, Hydrodiuril, Hydro-T, Oretic, Thiuretic | |
| Hydroflumethiazide | Diucardin, Saluron, Sonazide | |

(continued)

**Table 46.1.** Hypertension Drugs, continued.

| Drug Name | Brand Name | Complications and Side Effects |
|---|---|---|
| a. Thiazides and related diuretics, continued | | |
| Indapamide | Lozol | |
| Methyclothiazide | Aquatensen, Enduron, Ethon | |
| Metolazone | Diulo, Zaroxolyn | |
| Polythiazide | Renese | |
| Quinethazone | Hydromox | |
| Trichloromethiazide | Aquazide, Diurese, Metahydrin, Naqua, Niazide, Serpente, Triazide, Trichlorex | |
| b. Loop diuretics | | Same as above, possibly less impotence, effective in renal failure |
| Bumetanide | Bumex | |
| Ethracrynic acid | Edecrin | |
| Furosemide | Lasix | |
| c. Potassium-sparing agents | | Elevated potassium levels, impotence |
| Amiloride hydrochloride | Midamir | |
| Spironolactone | Aldactone, Aldostone, Dyrenium | |
| 2. Beta-adrenergic blockers | | Shortness of breath, masking of hypoglycemia, impotence, increased triglycerides, decreased HDL ("good") cholesterol, fatigue, depression, prolonged recovery from insulin reactions, worsening of blood-glucose control, aggravated vascular disease |
| Acebutolol hydrochloride | Sectral | |
| Atenolol | Tenormin | |
| Betaxolol | Kerlone | |
| Cartelol | Cartrol | |
| Metoprolol tartrate | Lopressor | |
| Nadolol | Corgard | |
| Oxprenolol hydrochloride | | |
| Penbutolol | Levatol | |

(continued)

**Table 46.1.** Hypertension Drugs, continued.

| Drug Name | Brand Name | Complications and Side Effects |
|---|---|---|
| 2. Beta-adrenergic blockers, continued | | |
| Pindolol | Visken | |
| Propranolol hydrochloride | Inderol, Ipran | |
| Propranolol long-acting (LA) | Inderol | |
| Timolol maleate | Blocadren | |
| 3. Central adrenergic inhibitors | | Dry mouth, drowsiness, dizziness, constipation, low blood pressure with standing, impotence |
| Clonidine hydrochloride | Catapres | |
| Guanabenz acetate | Wytensin | |
| Guanfacine | Tenex | |
| Methyldopa | Aldomet, Amodopa | |
| 4. Alpha-I blocker | | Fall of blood pressure with standing, especially with first dose |
| Doxazosin | Cardura | |
| Prazosin hydrochloride | Minipress | |
| Terazocin | Hytrin | |
| 5. Combined alpha and beta blocker | | Same as alpha- I blockers and nonselective beta blockers |
| Labetalol hydrochloride | Normodyne, Trandate | |
| 6. Vasodilators | | Headache, palpitation, nausea, fluid retention |
| Hydralazine hydrochloride | Apresoline, Alazine | |
| Minoxidil | Loniten | |

(continued)

**Table 46.1.** Hypertension Drugs, continued.

| Drug Name | Brand Name | Complications and Side Effects |
|---|---|---|
| 7. Angiotensin-converting enzyme inhibitors | | Cough, rash, loss of taste, elevated potassium levels, protein in urine |
| Benazepril | Lotensin | |
| Captopril | Capoten | |
| Cilazapril | Inhibace | |
| Enalapril maleate | Vasotec | |
| Fosinpril | Monopril | |
| Prinivil | Lisinopril, Zestril | |
| Ramipril | Altace | |
| Quinapril | | |
| 8. Calcium channel blocking agents | | Hypotension, flushing, headache, edema, constipation (verapamil) |
| Bepridil | Vascor | |
| Diltiazem hydrochloride | Cardizem | |
| Felodpine | Plendil | |
| Isadipine | Dynacirc | |
| Nicardipine | Cardene | |
| Nifedipine | Procardia, Adalat | |
| Verapamil hydrochloride | Calan, Isoptin | |
| Verapamil hydrochloride (LA) | Calan SR | |

# Chapter 47

# *Stroke in the Diabetic Patient*

A higher prevalence of stroke is found in the patient with both diagnosed and undiagnosed diabetes and glucose intolerance. Because of local cerebral acidosis caused by ischemia and hyperglycemia, morbidity and mortality from a stroke are increased. Most studies show that individuals with admission serum glucose > 120 mg/dl (6.7 mM) have a higher morbidity and mortality from a stroke. The prevalence of cerebral infarcts, especially lacunar infarcts, is increased and the prevalence of subarachnoid hemorrhage, cerebral hemorrhage, and transient ischemic attacks are decreased in the diabetic patient. Age, race, hypertension, and the presence of diabetic nephropathy and coronary and peripheral vascular disease are risk factors for stroke in the diabetic patient, whereas obesity, smoking, hyperlipidemia, and glycemic control are not. Investigation and treatment of the diabetic patient with a stroke is discussed.

Diabetes literature is replete with information on the microvascular complications of neuropathy, nephropathy, retinopathy, and the macrovascular complications of coronary artery disease and peripheral vascular disease (PVD), but little information is available on cerebrovascular disease in the diabetic patient. This is surprising because strokes are more common, and the mortality and morbidity resulting from strokes are increasing in the diabetic population.

---

Bell, David S. H. "Stroke in the Diabetic Patient" *Diabetes Care*, Vol. 17, No. 3. March 1994 © American Diabetes Association, reprinted with permission.

## Causes of Stroke in the Diabetic Patient

A stroke can be defined as a focal, neurological disorder with a sudden onset [1]. In the nondiabetic population, a stroke results from ischemic cerebral infarction in 80% of cases and cerebral hemorrhage in 20% of cases. Hemorrhage into the subarachnoid space occurs as the result of a rupture of a small berry aneurysm, whereas an intracerebral hemorrhage occurs as a result of the rupture of an aneurysmal dilatation of small penetrating arteries weakened by medial fibrinoid necrosis, which is associated with hypertension [1]. Studies in diabetic patients have shown a decreased prevalence of both intracerebral and subarachnoid hemorrhage when compared with the nondiabetic population [2,3].

An ischemic stroke results from an inadequate cerebral perfusion that deprives the brain of essential oxygen and glucose. This can be global and occur as a result of systemic hypotension or can be focal occurring as a result of an arterial embolism to, or occlusion of, intracerebral arteries. The source of the emboli can be cardiac, in which case 45% are associated with nonrheumatic atrial fibrillation and a thrombus in the left atrium, and 15% are associated with a mural thrombus after a myocardial infarct. In the diabetic patient with a myocardial infarct, it has been shown that the prevalence of cardioembolic stroke is higher than in the nondiabetic patient [4]. However, the major source of extracranial embolism causing an ischemic stroke is the extracranial portion of the internal carotid artery [5].

Whereas in the diabetic patient, the prevalence of classic cerebral infarction has been shown to be slightly increased in postmortem studies, the association with extracranial carotid disease is not as clear in the nondiabetic patient [6]. In the only prospective study of diabetic patients, a >50% carotid stenosis was seen in 8.2% of diabetic patients compared with 0.7% of age- and sex-matched control subjects. Overall, 20% of those with a significant carotid stenosis had an ischemic event compared with 2% of those without significant carotid stenosis. However, only 28% of the diabetic patients with an ischemic event had a significant carotid stenosis, and in those cases the infarction usually occurred on the side of the stenosis [7]. Thus, carotid disease would not seem to be the major cause of cerebral ischemia in the diabetic patient, and this has been confirmed in autopsy studies where most ischemic strokes have been shown to occur as a result of occlusion of the small paramedian penetrating arteries [2,6,8]. These arteries are >0.5 mm in size, do not communicate with collaterals, and their occlusion causes small infarcts within the white matter of the brain.

These infarcts do not result in glial scarring. They are cystic, which gives them the characteristic appearance described as a lacunar infarct [9].

The cause of the occlusion of the penetrating arteries is unclear and could be attributable to collapse, thrombus, embolus, microatheroma or spasm, or any combination of these factors [9]. Studies in diabetic patients have shown a failure to increase cerebral blood flow in response to a vasodilating stimuli such as 5% inhaled carbon dioxide [10]. This deficiency is thought to occur as a result of diabetic autonomic neuropathy and/or endothelial disease leading to a decrease in the release of endothelial vasodilating factors such as nitric oxide. This failure of vasodilation may be one explanation for the high prevalence of lacunar infarcts in the diabetic patient and also may explain the low prevalence of migraine headaches in the diabetic population [11].

## Increased Incidence of Stroke in the Diabetic Patient

Several large population studies have shown an increase in the prevalence of stroke in the known diabetic population, the undiagnosed diabetic population, and those with glucose intolerance. A summary of these studies is presented in Table 47.1 [12-22]. From these studies note the presence of an increased relative risk in the female diabetic population compared with the male diabetic population, and note that the greatest relative risk in both sexes is in the fifth and sixth decades with the relative risk decreasing dramatically at higher decades [25]. In addition, note a large geographic variation in the relative risk of stroke in the diabetic population with the highest relative risk being reported as 6-fold higher in diabetic males and 13-fold higher in diabetic females in Sweden [22]. In the U.S., the southeastern states are often referred to as the "stroke belt" and probably have the highest relative risk because of their large African-American population with their increased prevalence of hypertension [20].

Many patients presenting with a stroke have undiagnosed diabetes. This can be defined as an increased random serum glucose accompanied by an increased GHb. One study showed that of 200 patients presenting with strokes, 7% had previously undiagnosed diabetes [23]. Several other studies have confirmed this finding [24,25].

In the patient with insulin-dependent diabetes mellitus (IDDM), the frequency of stroke and death from stroke is less than in the patient with non-insulin-dependent diabetes mellitus (NIDDM). Krowelski et al. [26], studying mortality in a group of IDDM patients, reported only one death from a stroke (a cerebral hemorrhage). Deckert et al. [27], studying a group of patients who had had IDDM for more than 40

**Table 47.1.** Increased Prevalence of stroke in the diabetic population.

| Reference | Location | Relative risk in diabetic patient |
|---|---|---|
| 12 | Framingham, MA | Males × 4 in 5th and 6th decade, × 1 in 7th decade |
| | | Females × 1 in 5th decade, × 4 in 6th decade, × 3 in 7th decade |
| 13 | U.S. | × 4 45- to 64-year-olds |
| | | × 2.5 65- to 74-year-olds |
| 14 | Rochester, MN | × 1.4 in population with median age of 75 years |
| 15 | U.S. | Hospitalized patients × 1.4 aged 45–69 years |
| 16 | Monroe Co., NY | Hospitalized patients × 3.3 |
| 17 | Tilsburg, Holland | Hospitalized patients × 2.2 |
| 18 | Jerusalem, Israel | Hospitalized patients × 6 in 5th decade, × 3 in 6th decade, × 2 after age 60 |
| 19 | Chicago, IL | × 1.3 in elderly patients receiving financial assistance |
| 20 | Seal Beach, CA | × 1.7 males × 2.6 females |
| | Chicago, IL | |
| 20 | Birmingham, AL | × 3.3 males × 5.7 females |
| 21 | Hawaii | × 2.0 |
| | Japan | × 2.0 |
| 22 | Sweden | × 6 males |
| | | × 13 females |

years, reported a 10% incidence of stroke and a 7% mortality from stroke. Turnbridge [28], studying 448 patients with diabetes dying under the age of 50 in 1979 showed that 7% died of a stroke compared with 41% from ischemic heart disease, 19% from renal disease, 15% from diabetic ketoacidosis, and 4% from hypoglycemia.

The increased prevalence of stroke and the mortality from stroke in the patient with IDDM may be related to the development of diabetic nephropathy. When proteinuria develops, not only is there an increase in systolic and diastolic blood pressure but also an increase in Von Willebrand factor, fibrinogen, platelet adhesiveness and numbers, and a decrease occurs in basal and stimulated levels of tissue plasminogen activator and plasminogen activator inhibitor [29-31]. A report on the survival of IDDM patients who received a kidney transplant showed that after transplantation diabetic patients had significantly more cerebrovascular accidents (23 vs. 2%) compared with nondiabetic kidney transplant recipients [32].

In addition to the diabetic population, patients with glucose intolerance, that is, a normal fasting serum glucose and elevated levels of glucose on the glucose tolerance test performed before the stroke or 3 months after the stroke, also have a higher prevalence of stroke [25]. In the prospective Honolulu Heart Study, the prevalence of thromboembolic but not hemorrhagic stroke was increased in those with a serum glucose >120 mg/dl 1 h after a 50-g glucose load [21]. This was a threshold effect and was not linear, i.e., the prevalence was just as high in those with 1-h glucose levels between 120 and 150 mg/dl as in those with 1-h glucose levels > 190 mg/ dl.

Of nondiabetic patients who present with a stroke, 10% have high random serum glucose levels, normal GHb levels, and after recovery have normal glucose tolerance tests [33]. This phenomenon is termed stress hyperglycemia and is often associated with brain stem infarction and has been postulated to be a result of damage to the glucose regulating centers in the brain stem. Of significance, as discussed below, is that those patients with stress hyperglycemia have a much poorer prognosis than those patients who have normal glucose levels at the time of presentation with a stroke [34].

## *Risk Factors for Stroke in the Diabetic Patient*

Because patients with diabetes and particularly patients with NIDDM have multiple risk factors for ischemic heart disease, it would seem logical that these factors would also apply to cerebrovascular disease. However, many of these factors have not been shown to increase the risk of stroke in the diabetic patient.

## Demographic Factors

As in the nondiabetic patient, age is the biggest risk factor for a stroke in the diabetic population. Race also is a major factor in diabetic patients. In both the black and Japanese populations who have a high prevalence of stroke, the incidence is further increased in the diabetic population. A population-based study of African Americans showed that even though the frequency of diabetes and hypertension was increased in the group with strokes, this did not entirely account for the increased prevalence of stroke [35]. Previously, it has been hypothesized that the African-American population may be more susceptible to the damaging effects of growth factors, particularly angiotensin II, on small arteries [36]. This could be responsible for the increased incidence of cerebral hemorrhage and lacunar infarction in the black population. This pathological change, which is associated with hypertension, occurs even when hypertension has been adequately controlled in the black hypertensive patient. In addition, as mentioned above, the female with diabetes loses the protection of her sex; the prevalence of strokes is equally high in male and female diabetic patients.

## Hypertension

Undoubtedly, the major risk factor for stroke is hypertension. This association is stronger for systolic hypertension than for diastolic hypertension, but both are risk factors [37]. In spite of the 40% increased incidence of hypertension in the diabetic population, diabetes and glucose intolerance are still independent risk factors for strokes [38]. This could be because of an increased tendency toward atherosclerosis of the carotid arteries in these patients or because of an increased blood viscosity in the diabetic patient [39]. In addition, in several population studies, insulin resistance and hyperinsulinemia have been shown to be associated with both an increased prevalence of cardiovascular disease and hypertension [40].

## Diabetes Complications

Patients who have diabetes complications have a higher prevalence of stroke. Individuals with coronary artery disease or PVD have a higher prevalence of stroke [28,41,42]. The presence of diabetic nephropathy, which is associated with an increase in hypertension, hyperlipidemia, platelet aggregation, clotting factors, and arterial wall endothelial permeability, also is not surprisingly associated with an increased prevalence of stroke [37]. No evidence associates background diabetic retinopathy or proliferate retinopathy with an increased prevalence of stroke.

## Other Factors

Surprisingly, in the diabetic patient, cigarette smoking, obesity, glycemic control, and hyperlipidemia are not independent risk factors for stroke. In the Honolulu Heart Study, hyperglycemia was shown to be a risk factor only by comparing the group with a fasting serum glucose of < 120 mg/dl with those whose fasting serum glucose was >200 mg/dl [21]. In the same study and in a similar artificial way, hyperlipidemia was shown to be an independent risk factor only by comparing those with serum cholesterol levels of < 200 mg/dl with those whose serum cholesterol levels were >280 mg/dl [21].

## Increased Morbidity and Mortality from Stroke in the Diabetic Patient

Several studies have shown an increase in short- and long-term mortality in the diabetic patient who has had a stroke [24,34,43]. The most carefully matched of these studies was a Finnish study in which the survival of diabetic patients was compared with a group of randomly selected nondiabetic patients and a group of age- and sex-matched nondiabetic control subjects with a stroke [41]. After 5 years, 40% of the control groups were alive but only 20% of the diabetic group were alive. This compared with an expected survival in the general population of 80%. The increased mortality was related more to ischemic heart disease than to hypertension. Note that 20% of the diabetic patients who had a stroke were first diagnosed with diabetes when they presented with their stroke.

Several studies have shown an increase in morbidity after a stroke in patients with diabetes, glucose intolerance, and stress hyperglycemia. The increased morbidity seems not to be related to the predisposing metabolic status but to the admission glucose level. In most studies the cut-off point is a serum glucose of 120 mg/dl (6-6 mM) [44]. Berger [45] reported an increased likelihood of cerebral edema above this level. A study from England showed that only in those patients with a presenting blood glucose of < 120 mg/dl did complete recovery of the hemiparesis occur within 4 weeks, i.e., none of those with a presenting serum glucose > 120 mg/dl had complete recovery of the hemiplegia within that time [33]. In addition, Pulsinelli [43] showed in diabetic patients < 65 years of age a higher percentage (70 vs. 43%) of those with a random serum glucose < 120 mg/dl returned to work when compared with those with a glucose > 120 mg/dl.

The reason for the increased morbidity and mortality associated with hyperglycemia is not well understood. In animal studies, acute hyperglycemia preceding cerebral ischemia increases histological brain damage and leads to a worse outcome, whereas hypoglycemia has the opposite effect. On the other hand, when hyperglycemia is acutely induced after the acute ischemic event there is little effect on the size of the infarction or on the outcome. Few animal studies address the effects of chronic hyperglycemia on stroke damage. Overall, these studies have shown that chronic hyperglycemia worsens stroke damage [14,43,44,46-48]. Because in both a clinical setting and in animal studies there seems to be a relationship between stroke damage and hyperglycemia, knowledge of the mechanisms responsible for this would help in developing clinical and pharmacological methods to minimize stroke size.

There are three possible explanations for the worsening of stroke damage in the presence of hyperglycemia [46]. The first is that under the hypoxic conditions caused by a stroke, glucose is anaerobically metabolized to lactic acid, and the resultant cerebral intracellular and extracellular acidosis causes damage to neurons, glial tissue, and vascular tissue [47-49]. It is probable that the production of lactic acid in the ischemic area is helped by changes in the blood-brain barrier or at the cell membranes of neurons and glial cells that allow an increase in glucose delivery to the cell. In animal models, the effects of glycemia also may differ at different anatomical sites. In the center of an infarct, excess glucose will worsen damage, whereas in the surrounding ischemic area, an increase in glucose level may lessen damage. This is probably because in the ischemic area there is less hypoxia and therefore less lactic acid generation.

The second explanation is that during ischemia an increase occurs in the extracellular concentrations of the neurotransmitters glutamate and aspartate, which are both excitory and neurotoxic [50,51]. Under normal circumstances release of glutamate causes stimulation of a nerve at a postreceptor site and depolarization. Under conditions of hyperglycemia and hypoxia the extracellular concentration of these amino acids, which literally stimulate neurons to death, is increased because of excessive release combined with a failure of energy-dependent reuptake that would normally result in detoxification of glutamate and aspartate. This results in hyperstimulation of the postsynaptic neuron that eventually causes neuronal death but spares glial and vascular tissue.

A third theory is that with ischemia and hyperglycemia and with neuronal hyperstimulation an increase occurs in intracellular calcium, which may cause neuronal damage [(52)]. This is important because nimodipine, a calcium channel blocker, has been shown to mitigate the cerebral acidosis and possibly neuronal damage caused by ischemia and hyperglycemia [(53)].

## Clinical Presentation in Diabetic Patients

In general, the clinical features, diagnosis, investigation, and acute treatment of stoke in the diabetic patient do not differ from stroke occurring in the nondiabetic patient. However, an awareness of metabolic events that can clinically mimic a stroke in the diabetic patient is essential.

When faced with a diabetic patient with a cerebral event, it is most important to rule out hypoglycemia as a nonvascular cause of a neurological disorder with a sudden onset. In this regard, a history of oral hypoglycemic drug use or insulin use, food and alcohol intake, use of β-blockers, and recent activity levels is important. The time at which the event occurred and its relationship to the time of action of insulin or sulfonylurea also should be noted. The effects of exercise, alcohol, and oral hypoglycemic agents are prolonged and may need treatment with intravenous glucose for a prolonged period of time. It is therefore mandatory to immediately check the blood glucose in every diabetic patient presenting with a cerebral event. In addition, a hemiplegia may follow an epileptic seizure and last for 1-2 days (Todd's paralysis). Hypoglycemia may precipitate a grand mal seizure in either a predisposed diabetic patient or a diabetic patient with severe hypoglycemia. It is therefore important to seek a history suggestive of seizure, i.e., incontinence, tongue biting, or muscle pains from the patient or seek an eye witness account.

Focal neurological findings, such as seizures and hemiparesis, that disappear with correction of dehydration and hyperglycemia are features of hyperosmolar nonketotic diabetic coma. Thus, when a patient with diabetes and altered consciousness presents with a stroke-like syndrome, hypersomolar nonketotic diabetic coma becomes part of the differential diagnosis.

## Primary Prevention of Stroke in the Diabetic Patient

Prevention of stroke in the diabetic patient requires early recognition and treatment of hypertension. In the diabetic population, smoking, glycemic control, obesity, and hyperlipidemia have not been shown to be independent risk factors for stroke (see above), but because these are risk factors for atherosclerosis in general, it would seem prudent to treat these factors aggressively. In addition, the lack of association of smoking, obesity, hyperglycemia, hyperlipidemia, and insulin resistance with stroke in the diabetic patient is based on only a few studies; therefore, these risk factors could still be relevant. With the evidence that aspirin in small dosages can prevent myocardial infarct [(54)] and lower the risk of stroke in those patients with established cerebrovascular disease [(55)], and with the knowledge that cerebral hemorrhage has a lower incidence in the diabetic patient [(3)] and that diabetic patients have increased platelet aggregation [(56)], it would seem logical for the diabetic patient over 40 years of age to take at least one baby aspirin per day.

## Secondary Prevention of Stroke in the Diabetic Patient

Those patients nor receiving anticoagulation therapy should be treated with antiplatelet therapy. Several studies have now shown that in nondiabetic patients with transient ischemic attacks (TIAs) or a minor stroke, aspirin lowers the risk of infarction [(55)]. Recently, ticlopidine, another anti-platelet agent, has been shown to be more effective than aspirin, especially in diabetic patients [(57)]. However, with ticlopidine, serum cholesterol rises and a rare patient may develop neutropenia so that regular monitoring of the white cell count is required.

In the Physicians Health Study [(54)], using 325 mg of aspirin on alternate days, a significant reduction in the incidence of myocardial infarction occurred, but the incidence of hemorraghic stroke increased 15%, which was said to be statistically nonsignificant. A British study showed a similar increase in hemorrhagic strokes with a higher dose of aspirin but no decrease in the incidence of myocardial infarction [(58)]. Thus, with primary prevention, the benefit of aspirin relates more to the prevention of myocardial infarct than to the prevention of stroke, but in secondary prevention, the incidence of stroke is decreased at least in the nondiabetic population.

However, we know that platelet adhesiveness is increased in the diabetic population [(56)] and that cerebral hemorrhage is less common [(3)].

Therefore, the use of anti-platelet therapy should be both safer and more efficacious. Surprisingly, only one study has evaluated the effect of anti-platelet therapy in the diabetic population. The VA Cooperative Study [59], examined 231 veterans with recent gangrene and amputation and followed them for 6 years. The group created with aspirin (325 mg/day) and dipyridamole (75 mg three times a day) had a lower incidence of TIAs and strokes than the control group (8 vs. 19%) but a higher mortality. This result was impressive because before the study, the treatment group had had a higher incidence of strokes and TIAs (19 vs. 7%). The European Stroke Prevention Study [60] compared the effect of a combination of 75 mg dipyridamole [illegible] 330 mg of aspirin given three times a day with placebo given t[illegible] sons with a recent TIA or cerebral infarction. Diabetic patie[illegible] not show a statistically significant decrease in the occurrence of st[illegible] perhaps because of the small number of diabetic patients in [illegible] In addition, the reduction in recurrence of stroke was les[illegible] betic than the nondiabetic population (48 vs. 32%). O[illegible]-platelet therapy would seem to be indicated in diabetic pa[illegible]ho have had TIAs or strokes. No studies of primary preventio[illegible] the diabetic population exist.

The addition of carotid endarterectomy to aspirin therapy in the nondiabetic population is more effective than aspirin alone in preventing strokes in patients with TIAs or nondisabling strokes with an ipsilateral high grade stenosis (between 70 and 100%) [61]. No study has yet evaluated the effectiveness of carotid endarterectomy in preventing cerebral infarction in patients with asymptomatic carotid stenosis. However, 100,000 carotid endarterectomies are performed each year in the U.S., and the indications for this procedure have been questioned. Four major trials of carotid endarterectomy in the U.S. will report in 1993. The indications in the diabetic patient would at this time be the same as in the nondiabetic person, i.e., the presence of carotid stenosis of between 70 and 100% and/or the presence of carotid ulceration with evidence of ischemia in the distribution of that artery. Studies of patients undergoing carotid endarterectomies have shown that diabetic patients have a similar perioperative mortality but an increased mortality after surgery mainly because of myocardial infarction [62].

Early ambulation and active rehabilitation in the diabetic patient with a stroke is essential, especially when neuropathy that may impair rehabilitation is present. Psychological rehabilitation accompanied by speech therapy also is essential. The patient who has lost the ability to communicate in addition to the ability to ambulate loses dignity, and this may be further compounded if incontinence develops. As a result of this, a high proportion of stroke patients develop significant clinical depression. This should be prevented, if possible, and when it occurs, it should be diagnosed quickly and treated appropriately.

## Future Treatment

In the future, fibrinolytic agents as now used in patients with an acute myocardial infarction will be used routinely in the treatment of the patient with an ischemic stroke. Placebo-controlled preliminary studies in humans have suggested that recombinant tissue plasminogen activator given within 6 hours of the onset of cerebral ischemia results in an improved outcome [63].

Animal studies have shown that glutamate receptor blockers given soon after the onset of stroke ameliorate the effects of cerebral ischemia [64]. This could potentially negate the increased morbidity and mortality resulting from stroke in the diabetic patient.

*—by David S. H. Bell, MB*

## References


1. Gilman S: Advances in neurology (Part II). *N Engl J Med* 326:1671-76, 1992

2. Aronson SM: Intercranial vascular lesions in patients with diabetes mellitus. *J Neuropathol Exp Neurol* 23:183-96, 1973

3. Adams HP, Patman SF, Kassell NF, Torner JC: Prevalence of diabetes mellitus among patients with subarachnoid hemorrhage. *Arch Neurol* 41:1033-35, 1984

4 Pullicino PM, Xuereb M, Aquiliana J, Piedmonte MR: Stroke following acute myocardial infarction in diabetics. *J Intern Med* 231:287-93, 1992

5. Weinberger J, Biscarra V, Weisberg MK, Jacobson JH: Factors contributing to stroke in patients with atherosclerotic disease of the great vessels: the role of diabetes. *Stroke* 16:709-12, 1983

6. Alex M, Baron EK, Goldenberg S, Bumenthal HT: An autopsy of cerebrovascular accidents in diabetes mellitus. *Circulation* 25:663-73, 1962

7. Kuebler TW, Bendick PJ, Fineberg SE, Markand ON, Norton JA Jr, Vinicor FN, Clark CM Jr: Diabetes mellitus and cerebrovascular disease: prevalence of carotid artery occlusive disease and associated risk factors in 482 adult diabetic patients. *Diabetes Care* 6:274-78, 1983

8. Bell ET: A postmortem study of vascular disease in diabetes. *Arch Pathol* 53:444-55, 1952

9. Mohr JP, Lacunes in Barnett HJM, Stein BM, Mohr JP, Yatsu FM (Eds.): *Stroke Pathophysiology, Diagnosis, and Management*. Vol 2. New York, Churchill Livingstone. 1986, p. 475-96

10. Dandona P, James IM, Newburg PA, Wollard ML, Beckett AG: Cerebral blood flow in diabetes mellitus: evidence of abnormal cerebrovascular reactivity. *Br Med J* 2:325-26, 1978

11. Burn WK, Machin D, Waters WE: Prevalence of migraine in patients with diabetes. *Br Med J* 289:1579-80, 1984

12. Wolf PA, Kannel WB, Verter J: Current status of stroke risk factors. In *Neurologic Clinics*. Barnett HJM, Ed. Philadelphia, Saunders, 1983, p. 317-43

13. Hadden WC, Harris MI: Prevalence of diagnosed diabetes, undiagnosed diabetes, and impaired glucose tolerance in adults 20-74 years of age. In *Vital and Health Statistics—Series 11: Data From the National Health Survey*. National Center for Health Statistics, 1987, p. 1-55

14. Roehmhodt ME, Palumbo PJ, Whisnant JP, Elusback LR. Transient ischemic attack and stroke in a community-based diabetic cohort *Mayo Clin Proc* 58:56-58, 1983

15. Kuller L, Anderson H, Peterson D, Cassel J, Spiers P, Curry H, Paegel B, Saslaw M, Sisk C, Wilber J, Millward D, Winklestein W, Lilienfield A, Seltser R. Nationwide cerebrovascular disease morbidity study. *Stroke* 1:86-99, 1970

16. Barker WH, Feldt KS, Felbel JH: Community surveillance of stroke in persons under 70 years old. *Am J Public Health* 73:260-65, 1983

17. Herman B, Leyten ACM, Van Luijk JH, Frenken CWGM, Op DE, Coul AAW, Schulte BPM: An evaluation of risk factors for stroke in a Dutch community. *Stroke* 13:334-39, 1982

18. Loug S, Melamed E, Cahane E, Carmen A: Hypertension and diabetes as risk factors in stroke patients. *Stroke* 4:751-59, 1973

19. Ostfeld AM, Shekelle RB, Kiawans H, Tufo HM: Epidemiology of stroke in an elderly welfare population. *Am J Public Health* 64:450-58, 1974

20. Stallones R, Dyken M, Fang HCH: Epidemiology for stroke facilities planning. *Stroke* 3:360-71, 1972

21. Kagan A, Popper JS, Rhoads GG: Factors related to stroke incidence in Hawaii in Japanese men. *Stroke* 11:14-21, 1980

22. Lindegard B, Hillbom M: Associations between brain infarction, diabetes, and alcoholism: observations from the Gothenburg population cohort study. *Acta Neurol Scand* 75:195-200, 1987

23. Gray CS, French JM, Bates D, Cartlidge NE, Venables GS, James OF: increasing age, diabetes mellitus, and recovery from stroke. *Postgrad Med J* 65:720-24, 1989

24. Riddle MC, Hart J: Hyperglycemia recognized and unrecognized as a risk factor for stroke and transient ischemic attacks. *Stroke* 13:356-59, 1982

25. Lamk S, Ma JT, Woo E, Lam C, Yu YL: High prevalence of undiagnosed diabetes among Chinese patients with ischemic stroke. *Diabetes Res Clin Pract* 14:133-37, 1991

26. Krolewski AS, Kosinski EJ, Warram JH, Leland OS, Busick EJ, Asmal AC, Rand LI, Christlieb AR, Bradley RF, Kahn CR: Magnitude and determinants of coronary artery disease in juvenile-onset insulin-dependent diabetes mellitus. *Am J Cardiol* 59:750-55, 1987

27. Deckert T, Poulsen JE, Larsen M: Prognosis of diabetics with diabetes onset before age thirty-one. *Diabetologia* 14:363-70, 1976

28. Turnbridge WMG: Factors contributing to deaths of diabetics under fifty years of age. *Lancet* 2:569-72, 1981

29. Jensen T, Borch-Johnsen K, Kofoed-Enevoldsen A, Deckert T: Coronary heart disease in young type I (insulin-dependent)

diabetic patients with and without diabetic nephropathy: incidence and risk factors. *Diabetologia* 30:144-48, 1987

30. Jensen T, Stender S, Deckert T: Abnormalities in plasma concentrations of lipoproteins and fibrinogen in type I (insulin-dependent) diabetic patients with increased urinary albumin excretion. *Diabetologia* 31:142-45, 1988

31. Jones SL, Close CF, Matlock NM, Jarrett J, Kim H, Viberti GC: Plasma lipid and coagulation factor concentrations in insulin-dependent diabetic patients with microalbuminuria. *Br Med J,* 298:487-90, 1989

32. Rischen-Vos J, van der Woode FJ, Tegzess AM, Zwinderman AH, Goozen HC, van den Akker PJ, van Es LA: Increased morbidity and mortality in patients with diabetes mellitus after kidney transplantation as compared with nondiabetic patients. *Nephrol Dial Transplant* 7:433-37, 1992

33. Gray CS, Taylor R, French JM, Alberti KG, Venables GS, James OF, Shaw DA, Cartlidge NES, Bates D: The prognostic value of stress hyperglycemia and previously unrecognized diabetes in acute stroke. *Diabetic Med* 4:237-40, 1987

34. Cox NH, Lorains JW: The prognostic value of blood glucose and glycosylated estimation in persons with stroke. *Postgrad Med J* 62:7-10, 1986

35. Kittner SJ, White CR, Losonczy KG, Wolf PA, Hebel JR, Black-white differences in stroke incidence in a national sample: the contribution of hypertension and diabetes mellitus. *JAMA* 264:1267-70, 1990

36. Dustan HP: Growth factors and racial differences in severity of hypertension and renal disease. *Lancet* 339:1339-40, 1992

37. Abbot RD, Donahue RP, MacMahon SW, Reed DM, Yunko K: Diabetes and the risk of stroke: The Honolulu Heart Program. *JAMA* 257:949-52, 1987

38. Barret-Connor E, Khaw KT: Diabetes mellitus: an independent risk factor for stroke? *Am J Epidemiol* 128:116-23, 1988

39. Emara MK, Saadah AM, Tohfa YA, Guindi RT, Gupta RK, Senthilselvan A: The hematocrit value in diabetic patients with ischemic stroke. *Diabetes Res* 12:189-92, 1989

40. Stern MP, Haffner SM: Body fat distribution and hyperinsulinemia as risk factors for diabetes and cardiovascular disease. *Arteriosclerosis* 6:123-30, 1980

41. Webster P: The natural history of stroke in diabetic patients. *Acta Med Scand* 207:417-24, 1980

42. Palumbo PJ, Elveback LR, Whisnant JP: Neurological complications of diabetes mellitus: transient ischemic attack, stroke, and peripheral neuropathy. *Adv Neurol* 19:593-601, 1978

43. Pulsinelli WA, Levy PE, Sigsbee B, Scherer P, Plum F: Increased damage after ischemic attacks in patients with hyperglycemia with or without established diabetes mellitus. *Am J Med* 74:540-44,1983

44. Melamed E: Reactive hyperglycemia in patients with acute stroke. *J Neurol Sci* 29:267-75, 1976

45. Berger C, Hakim IM: The association of hyperglycemia with cerebral edema in stroke. *Stroke* 17:865-71, 1986

46. McCall AL: Perspectives in diabetes: the impact of diabetes on the CNS. *Diabetes* 41:557-70, 1992

47. Smith ML, Von Hanwehr R, Siesjo BK: Changes in extra and intracellular pH in the brain during and following ischemia in hyperglycemic and in moderately hypoglycemic rats. *J Cereb Blood Flow Metab* 6:574-83, 1986

48. Rehncrona S, Rosen I, Siesjo BK: Brain lactic acidosis and ischemic cell damage: biochemistry and neurophysiology. *J Cereb Blood Flow Metab* 1:297-311, 1981

49. Collins RC, Dobkin BH, Choi DW: Selective vulnerability of the brain: new insights into the pathophysiology of stroke. *Ann Intern Med* 110:992-1000, 1989

50. Olney JW, Labrayere J, Wang G, Wozniak DF, Price MT, Sesma MA: NMDA antagonist neurotoxicity's mechanism and prevention. *Science* 254:1515-18,1991

51. Rothman SM, Olney JW: Glutamate and the pathophysiology of hypoxic-ischemic brain damage. *Ann Neurol* 19:105-11, 1986

52. Siesjo BK, Bengtsson F: Calcium fluxes, calcium antagonists, and calcium-related pathology in brain ischemia, hypoglycemia, and spreading depression: a unifying hypothesis. *J Cereb Blood Flow Metab* 9:127-40, 1989

53. Berger L, Hakim AM: Nimodipine prevents hyperglycemia-induced cerebral acidosis in middle cerebral artery occluded rats. *J Cereb Blood Flow Metab* 9:58-64, 1986

54. The Steering Committee of the Physicians Health Study Research Group: Preliminary report findings from the aspirin component of the ongoing Physicians Health Study. *N Engl J Med* 318:262-64, 1988

55. Antiplatelet Trialists Collaboration: Secondary prevention of vascular disease by prolonged antiplatelet treatment. *Br Med J* 296:320-31, 1988

56. Sagel J, Colwell JA, Crook L, Lamina M: Increased platelet aggregation in early diabetes mellitus. *Ann lntern Med* 83:733-38, 1975

57. Grotta JC, Norris JW, Kumm B: the TASS Baseline and Angiographic Data Subgroup: Prevention of stroke with ticlopidine: who benefits most? *Neurology* 42:111-15,1992

58. Peto R, Gray R, Collins R: Randomized trial of prophylactic daily aspirin in British male doctors. *Br Med J* 1296:313-16, 1988

59. Colwell JA, Bingham SF, Abraira C, Anderson JW, Comstock JP, Kwaan HC, and The Cooperative Study Group: Veterans Administration Cooperative Study on antiplatelet agents in diabetic patients after amputation for gangrene, II: effects of aspirin and dipyridamole on atherosclerotic vascular disease rates. *Diabetes Care* 9:140-48, 1986

60. Sivenius T, Laako M, Riekkinen P Sr, Smets P, Lowanthal A: European Stroke Prevention Study Effectiveness of antiplatelet therapy in diabetic patients in secondary prevention of stroke. *Stroke* 23:851-54, 1992

61. North American Symptomatic Carotid Endarterectomy Trial Collaborators: Beneficial effect of carotid endarterectomy in

symptomatic patients with high grade stenosis. *N Engl J Med* 325:445-53, 1991

62. Campbell DR, Hoar CS, Wheelock FC, Jr: Carotid artery surgery in diabetic patients. *Arch Surg* 119:1405-407, 1984
63. Mori E, Yomeda Y, Ohksawa S: Double-blind placebo-controlled trial of recombinant tissue plasminogen activator (rt-PA) in acute carotid stroke. *Neurology* 41 (Suppl. 1):347, 1991
64. Steinberg GK, Saleh J, Kunis D, DeLaPaz R, Zarnegar SR: Protective effect of *N*-methyl-*D*-aspartate antagonists after focal cerebral ischemia in rabbits. *Stroke* 20:1247-52, 1989

## Chapter 48

# *Amputation*

David S. Barr of Bodfish, Calif., took an 80,000-mile motorcycle trip that spanned North and South America, Europe, Asia, and Africa.

"Only 70 people have ever done anything like it before," Barr said. "There've been more people in outer space than have made this trip."

What makes it more extraordinary is that Barr, 41, is a double amputee. Fighting in Angola in 1981, he lost one leg above the knee and the other below the knee. But that hasn't kept him from riding a two-wheel 1972 Harley Davidson and writing a book about his around-the-world motorcycle trip.

And that is not all. Barr is one of only a handful of double-amputee parachutists who jump with special prosthetics. And he walks 3 or 4 miles a day and mows his own grass.

Advances in prosthetics, and the example set by amputees such as Barr, have shown more and more people that an amputation does not always mean confinement to a wheelchair. At private companies and key centers such as Northwestern University in Chicago and the University of Utah at Salt Lake City, research that sounds like something out of "The Six Million Dollar Man" could give amputees even more control over artificial limbs.

Physical therapist Marie A. Schroeder, chief of the Food and Drug Administration's restorative devices branch, explains that FDA regulates prostheses, but manufacturers do not have to undergo a full review for each new device. Instead, they must register the products and keep a record of any complaints.

---

"Big Steps Forward for Amputees," *FDA Consumer*, March 1997.

"But if there's a significant change in the technology, we could get involved," Schroeder said.

For instance, she said, her branch has seen some interest in implantable electrodes for stimulating muscles in spinal cord injury cases. Such devices would require review by FDA.

Some innovators are also exploring ways to use computers to design and manufacture custom prostheses, to attach muscles directly to a prosthesis, to develop powered fingers with microelectronics, and even to use brain waves to power prostheses.

For thousands of years, inventors have tried to replicate what nature cannot replace. Prostheses have been used since at least 300 B.C., when crude devices consisting of metal plates hammered over a wooden core, were attached to an amputated limb.

Advances in the science of prosthetics burgeon during and immediately after wars, when large numbers of people need to be fitted with artificial limbs. The technology of modern prosthetics has changed little since shortly after World War II.

"There's a real need for revolution in design," said Giovani M. Ortega, research and development project manager at Sabolich Prosthetics & Research in Oklahoma City, Okla., a division of NovaCare. "The systems that we have, have been around for a long time, and at best there have been only improvements. As far along as we've come, we're still far behind many other industries in terms of implementing new technologies."

Estimates of the amputee population in the United States vary widely, from fewer than 400,000 to more than 1 million. About 9 out of 10 amputations involve the leg, from the foot to above the knee.

Three-quarters of all amputations are the result of disease, often cancer or peripheral vascular disease. The latter is a narrowing of the arteries in the extremities that is often associated with diabetes. Most other amputations are the result of workplace or automobile accidents. And a small fraction, perhaps 3 percent, are due to birth defects that constrict bone growth.

## Preventing Amputation

Because so many amputations result from disease, considerable attention has been paid to prevention. For example, the American Diabetes Association recommends people stop smoking, which can speed the progress of peripheral vascular disease. Patients with diabetes should monitor their blood glucose levels carefully, eat a healthy, balanced diet, see their doctors regularly, control their weight, and check their feet each day for small cuts or blisters.

Electric blankets and heating pads carry warning labels that say people with diabetes should not use them without talking to their doctors first. This is because people with diabetes may lose sensation in their limbs. Patients can be seriously burned by an electric blanket or heating pad because they cannot feel how hot it really is.

Patients are also advised to develop an exercise plan after consulting with their doctors. Regular exercise maintains strength, flexibility, and blood flow to damaged areas and can help control pain. However, it's important not to stress the legs, feet or joints. Some good exercises are bicycling or easy rowing on a rowing machine. Swimming and aqua aerobics are also good choices.

"We know of many things that can help people avoid amputation, but unfortunately, it's no fun to do daily foot care or wear only proper fitting, well-designed shoes," said Jennifer Mayfield, M.D., chairwoman of the association's Foot Care Council. "Everybody keeps waiting for a magic bullet, and that would be nice, but it's not coming anytime soon."

Richard J. Gusberg, M.D., chief of vascular surgery at Yale University, said one of the first signs of peripheral occlusive disease is claudication, an aching, tired feeling in the leg muscles when they are exercised.

"The vast majority of people with claudication remain stable, or nearly stable, for an indefinite period of time," Gusberg said. In most cases the progress of the disease can be slowed if people control the risk factors, which includes reducing blood pressure, controlling their diabetes through diet or insulin, and reducing cholesterol levels. Regular exercise has also proven effective because it can strengthen circulation, he said.

The drug Trental (pentoxifylline) is approved by FDA for people with peripheral artery disease. Its use can decrease the thickness and stickiness of blood, and can reduce the deformities of red blood cells, so the blood can get through the narrowed arteries, but it is not effective in all patients, Gusberg said. The use of other drugs in treating occlusive disease has largely been abandoned, he said.

If the disease progresses, the patient might develop gangrene, or ulcers in the leg, as blood flow is reduced.

"When people get to that stage, most of them need to be evaluated for a bypass operation," Gusberg said. Replacing the arteries in the lower leg is effective for five years or more in 70 to 80 percent of cases.

## Sensory Loss

Another danger with diabetes is a deadening of the nerves in the extremities. John F. Glass, a biologist with FDA's pacing and neurological devices branch, said there are now a variety of devices that measure sensory loss in the affected limbs. In a patient with diabetes, loss of sensation because of nerve damage signals a need for diligence. Even minor injuries, undetected because the feeling is gone and thus left untreated, can become infected easily and lead to gangrene.

"If you're aware of sensory loss, you want to keep a close watch on it," Glass said. "There's a range of measurement devices, from those that detect general loss of sensation, to those that assess the specific degree of sensory loss, or that can quantify sensitivity to pressure or temperature."

Many of the devices are easy-to-use mechanical implements with no significant health risk to patients. One of the simplest is a hand-held device that looks like an old typewriter eraser with thin wires attached to it. The wires are placed on the toes or fingertips to see if there is tactile sensitivity.

Such simple devices are typically not reviewed by FDA before they are made available to the public. They are intended for use by the patient for monitoring only, not self-diagnosis.

"Loss of sensation in an extremity could indicate a lot of other conditions or disorders, so we would encourage the patient to see a physician immediately for a complete physical examination," Glass said.

## Unavoidable Limb Loss

Precautions such as Glass advocates can often delay the progression of the disease. Sometimes, though, the loss of a limb is unavoidable. In those cases, physical therapy starts a day or two after surgery. Since more than 9 out of 10 amputations involve one or both legs, physical therapy usually involves the use of parallel bars, and later a walker or crutches. Part of the training involves how to fall and get up safely.

There are other adjustments as well. Barr said the loss of both legs, and covering the stumps with plastic, means his body has become much less effective at cooling itself, so he has to be on the lookout for hyperthermia. And he learned other tricks to cope, as well.

"I'm constantly on the move, never standing still, always readjusting my balance even when I'm staying in one place, because I don't want one particular area on the stump to get sore," Barr said.

Until recently, patients were not fitted with an artificial limb for four to eight weeks after surgery, but new techniques allow the use of a protective foam over a sterile bandage, and the prosthesis can be fit as soon as the day following surgery.

## New Prosthetic Materials

For centuries, wood and leather were the only materials for prostheses, but today's physical therapist has a much wider range available, including advanced plastics and carbon fiber, which are much stronger and lighter and more durable.

"The industry is really moving towards composite materials, because they're lighter in weight, easier to work with, and more durable," said Douglas McCormack, vice president of the Amputee Coalition of America.

Silicone-based compounds used to make prosthetic arms, for instance, give the appearance of real skin, unlike the rigid plastic or metal limbs of years ago, and they are more comfortable for the person wearing them. Women can get prosthetic feet with life-like toes for when they wear sandals; men can get legs with the appearance of hair.

But even materials that work out in one application might not work in another.

"We tested a silicone foot at one point. On a machine it was subjected to 300 pounds of stress for a million cycles, and it didn't have any problems. But an amputee broke it within a few minutes. It really surprised us. Torque and other stresses can fatigue the material quickly," said Sabolich's Ortega. "You'd be amazed at the toll that a human body puts on even the strongest material."

New computer programs better determine where and what the forces are. But it's not just a question of choosing a material that will withstand those forces.

"With some of the new materials being developed, we could make a foot to take any of the pressures that the human body will give it," Ortega said. "The problem is it might not have any springiness. You give up flexibility for strength. You have to balance all the considerations in a prosthetic."

Prostheses are typically sold as components, so that someone who has an above-the-knee amputation would be able to choose leg, knee and foot units, often from different manufacturers, depending on their individual needs.

Most of the units are adjustable. Shock absorbers in knees, for instance, can be made more flexible as a person gains controls over the artificial leg. Ankles can be adjusted to the weight and activity level of the patient.

Arm amputees today can choose between prostheses that are powered by a harness and cable attached to the residual limb, or externally powered devices. Powered arms can be controlled by switches mounted inside or outside the socket, that the patient can activate by flexing certain muscle groups.

## Energy Requirements

Some prosthetics research is aimed at providing active devices, which do part of the work of the amputated limb, as opposed to passive devices that are controlled by the residual limb. An amputee with prostheses expends two to three times more energy than a nondisabled person to perform even the simplest activities, such as walking across a room or climbing stairs.

"A semi-active system, in which the limb itself performs part of the function, could reduce that energy requirement significantly," said Sabolich's Ortega. "And there would also be a psychological benefit, because the prosthesis would no longer be just a dead limb, but something that is helping."

Ortega said one area Sabolich is researching would provide sensory feedback from the prosthesis to the remaining limb. For instance, in an artificial leg, pressure sensors in the foot would send a mild electrical signal to the thigh muscles when there is pressure on the back, front or sides of the foot.

That kind of feedback would be similar to what they would get with the pressure of the ground against a natural foot, which would make their adjustment to the prostheses go more quickly, Ortega said.

Ortega said prosthetic designs are limited only by how large a power pack the amputee can carry.

"The crucial issue when it comes to trying to introduce any new prosthesis is the energy requirements," said Ortega. "Our muscles are so efficient, in terms of the power that they produce versus the fuel that they use, that we have a difficult time matching it."

Scientists are also working to build a better socket—the part of the prosthesis that attaches to the residual limb.

Dudley S. Childress, Ph.D., of Northwestern University's Rehabilitation Engineering Program, is working on applying the industrial practice known as rapid prototyping to socket production.

Sockets are now produced largely by hand. A cast is made of the residual limb, and plaster is poured into the cast to make a positive mold. The mold is then used to create a plastic or laminated polyester socket that fits over the residual limb.

Childress employs a computer-aided design program to measure the residual limb and design a socket. Then, using a modified "plastic deposition technology" called squirt shaping, a computer lays down small amounts of polypropylene to produce the desired shape, to very tight tolerances. In industry, the technology is used to quickly produce prototypes of everything from car parts to military weapons, to test them before starting mass production.

"Essentially, every socket is a prototype, and there are potentially some significant advantages to applying these techniques to prosthesis manufacture," Childress said. "We can make a socket in about 50 minutes, which isn't bad, but as people continue to work with the technology, it may be possible to get that down even faster."

The process would also allow manufacturers to make sockets out of different types of material than have been used in the past, or alter the thickness or characteristics of the material very quickly.

Another innovation being explored at Northwestern is powered prosthetic fingers. That might be difficult if you were going to match real fingers, he acknowledged, but most of the time that's unnecessary. Picking up a spoon and holding a book don't require much power, just control. Small motor technology and power storage capability have both improved vastly in recent years.

"If you want to do something like squeeze orange juice, you need force," Childress said. "But even for people without a prosthesis, that's tiresome, so we have all kinds of devices to do those jobs for us. So the intent of the powered fingers would be to provide prehensile [wraparound] force."

Childress said his laboratory is also looking at devices that would improve the "feel" of prostheses over current devices. It would be comparable, he said, to the way power steering reduces the muscle power needed to steer a car, but you can still "feel" the road through the wheel.

Cables in artificial fingers and hands would connect to the muscles of the forearm, either through holes in the muscle that are surgically lined with skin, or tendons could be taken outside the residual limb and covered with skin. Either option would give the muscle the sense of how hard it is working and how fast it is moving.

## Mundane, But Important, Needs

Joan E. Edelstein, Ph.D., director of Columbia University's physical therapy program, stresses the need for prosthetics research to focus not just on high-technology improvements, but to the more mundane but critical things such as fit, to make them as comfortable as possible, particularly among the elderly, whose needs may not be fully considered.

"Most patients are older people who have lost a limb because of diabetes, and the assumption is that they're going to be relatively undemanding of their prosthesis," Edelstein said.

Better prostheses for the elderly might prevent skin breakdown and infections, yet hardly any research dollars are being spent in that area, she said, explaining that, "It's not as glamorous as developing better prostheses for sport, or for children, and they are very difficult problems to overcome."

Research often proceeds along several courses at once, she noted, and you can never know which might yield the next major breakthrough.

*—by Robert A. Hamilton*

Robert A. Hamilton is a writer in Franklin, Conn.

# Chapter 49

# *Pancreas Transplantation*

Pancreas transplantation has been performed in thousands of patients with diabetes mellitus and has become accepted therapy in certain types of patients. Successful pancreas transplantation has been shown to eliminate the need for exogenous insulin, an outcome greatly desired by patients with type 1 diabetes. However, several significant issues surround the indications for pancreas transplantation and its respective benefits and risks.

This position statement presents the recommendations of the American Diabetes Association on pancreas transplantation in patients with type 1 diabetes. The recommendations are based on the American Diabetes Association's technical review on "Pancreas Transplantation for Patients With Diabetes Mellitus," which should be consulted for further information [(1)].

## *Recommendations*

1. Successful pancreas transplantation has been demonstrated to improve significantly the quality of life of people with diabetes, primarily by eliminating the need for exogenous insulin, frequent daily blood glucose measurements, and many of the dietary restrictions imposed by the disorder. Transplantation also can eliminate the acute complications commonly experienced by patients with type 1 diabetes (e.g., hypoglycemia).

---

Position Statement, *Diabetes Care* Supplement, Volume 21 Supplement 1, 

However, there is little evidence that pancreas transplantation can prevent or retard the development and/or progression of the long-term complications of diabetes. Nor is there evidence that pancreas transplantation can prolong the life of patients with diabetes mellitus.

2. Pancreas transplantation should be considered an acceptable therapeutic alternative to continued insulin therapy in diabetic patients with end-stage renal disease who have had or plan to have a kidney transplant. Such patients also must 1) meet the medical indications and criteria for kidney transplantation, 2) have significant clinical problems with exogenous insulin therapy, and 3) not have excessive surgical risk for the dual transplant procedure. Medicare and other third-party payors of medical care should include coverage for pancreas transplant procedures meeting these criteria. The pancreas transplant may be done simultaneously with, or subsequent to, a kidney transplant.

3. Pancreas-only transplants require lifelong immunosuppression to prevent rejection of the graft and recurrence of the autoimmune process that would again destroy the pancreatic islet cells. Immunosuppressive regimens used in transplant patients have side effects whose frequency and severity restrict their use in patients who would not survive without the transplant (e.g., patients with end-stage renal disease) or whose quality of life is unacceptable. Also, pancreas transplantation is a major surgical procedure. In addition to the side effects of lifelong immunosuppression, the procedure itself carries a small, but not negligible, risk of morbidity and mortality. Therefore, in the absence of renal failure, transplantation should be considered a therapeutic alternative to insulin therapy only in those few unusual patients who exhibit 1) a history of frequent acute severe metabolic complications requiring medical attention, 2) clinical and emotional problems with exogenous insulin therapy that are so severe as to be incapacitating, and 3) consistent failure of other therapeutic approaches to ameliorate the situation. Institutional guidelines for assuring an objective multidisciplinary evaluation of the patient's condition and eligibility for transplantation should be established and followed. Third-party payor coverage is appropriate only where such guidelines and procedures exist.

4. Institutions that perform pancreas transplantations should be tertiary care centers that have an active kidney transplant program and are equipped to adequately handle the complex medical and psychosocial needs of transplant patients.

5. Pancreatic islet cell transplants hold significant potential advantages over whole-gland transplants. However, at this time, islet cell transplantation is an experimental procedure.

## References

1. Porte D Jr, Baker L, Bollinger RR, Genuth S, Scharp DW, Sutherland DER: Pancreas transplantation for patients with diabetes mellitus (Technical Review). *Diabetes Care* 15:1668-1672, 1992

Approved June 1992. Revised 1997. The recommendations in this paper are based on the evidence reviewed in the following publication: Pancreas transplantation for patients with diabetes mellitus (Technical Review). *Diabetes Care* 15:1668-1672, 1992. **Currently, there is a committee considering a major revision of this position statement.**

# Chapter 50

# *Islet Cell Transplantation*

The treatment of Type I (insulin-dependent) diabetes has come a long way since the discovery of insulin, but a cure has remained elusive. That may change in the not-so-distant future. In the quest to end diabetes, researchers have looked for ways to restore normal pancreatic functioning. Scientists hope that pancreatic tissue transplants will become an effective and practical way to help the body produce its own insulin and thus avoid the complications of Type I diabetes.

## *Whole Pancreas Transplants*

Pancreas transplantation has long held promise as a cure for people with diabetes. A properly functioning transplanted pancreas can make insulin injections unnecessary, and it can offer a degree of precision in glycemic control that is impossible to mimic with insulin injections. Doctors have been transplanting whole pancreases into people with diabetes since 1966, and studies have shown that transplants can normalize blood glucose levels and may help prevent long-term diabetic complications.

Unfortunately, there's a catch. Transplanting a whole adult pancreas is a major, technically complex operation with many obstacles. For starters, it requires the use of immunosuppressive drugs to prevent organ rejection, and these drugs often have harmful side effects.

---

Because of these hazards and the fact that whole pancreas transplantation is not a lifesaving procedure, it is usually performed only in people who also require a kidney transplant because of kidney failure, which is life-threatening.

Another pressing issue is the relative shortage of adult pancreases available. Even as whole pancreas transplantations are being performed on an increasing number of people, it is clear that there are not enough adult pancreases for everyone who might benefit from one. If transplantation were ever to become completely safe and effective, then the estimated one million Americans with Type I diabetes (and 40 million people worldwide) would theoretically be candidates for surgery. Yet, only 1,000 to 1,500 adult pancreases are available for transplantation in the United States each year.

The problems inherent in whole pancreas transplantation have caused surgeons to explore other types of transplantation, such as transplanting only the insulin-producing islet cells from adult human or animal pancreases, transplanting pancreatic tissue from human fetuses, and implanting genetically engineered beta cells. Each of these therapies holds great promise for the future, but remember, it will probably be at least several years before their use becomes widespread.

## Human Islet Cells

Since only the islet cells of the pancreas, the cells that manufacture and secrete insulin, are necessary to correct Type I diabetes, one approach has been to transplant just these cells. These transplants were made possible when, in the 1960's, researchers at Washington University in St. Louis, Missouri, discovered a way to isolate islet cells using enzymes that digest the surrounding tissue. One of the benefits of islet cell transplantation is that it doesn't require major surgery. The islet cells can be injected into a vein, through which they move on to the liver, or they can be placed under the skin, in the abdominal cavity, or in other locations.

Islet cell transplants are plagued by some of the same problems as whole pancreas transplantation, particularly the need for immunosuppression, but scientists are exploring better ways to prevent the immune system from rejecting transplanted islet cells. For example, researchers are constantly searching for better immunosuppressive drugs to specifically block islet cell rejection without severely hampering the entire immune system. Cyclosporine is currently the most effective immunosuppressant, but researchers are also studying other agents, such as FK506 and rapamycin, alone or in combination with cyclosporine, to try to prevent rejection with few side effects. Another possibility is to treat the transplanted cells so that they will not trigger an immune response. One promising method for treating the transplanted islet cells is to expose them to radiation, an approach that has been used successfully in mice and rats.

One of the most promising approaches to preventing islet cell rejection is a technology called immunoisolation. This involves shielding the islets with a selectively permeable membrane. This membrane lets glucose, oxygen, and insulin pass in and out of the blood stream, but keeps out the antibodies and T cells of the immune system, which would otherwise destroy the islets.

Researchers are currently experimenting with the best way to use these special membranes in transplantation. One approach uses a perfusion device, a capsule that is grafted to an artery where it makes direct contact with the body's circulating blood; in this way, the device can draw nutrients from the blood and release insulin to circulate throughout the body. However, because this approach requires major surgery, researchers are also exploring less traumatic methods, such as coating small groups of islet cells (macroencapsulation) or individual islet cells (microencapsulation) and implanting them inside the abdominal cavity. While these devices would have limited contact with the circulation, nutrients and insulin would be exchanged by way of the body fluids permeating the tissues in which they are implanted.

Human islet transplantation has been tried experimentally in humans with some success. In 1993, surgeons at the Islet Transplant Center at St. Vincent's Medical Center in Los Angeles successfully transplanted microencapsulated islets into two people with diabetes. The two people were candidates for the procedure because they had already had kidney transplants and were on immunosuppressants. After the procedure, both people drastically reduced their insulin dosages, and their diabetic complications actually improved.

However, like whole pancreas transplantation, the feasibility of adult islet cell transplantation is hindered by a shortage problem; again, only 1,000 to 1,500 whole pancreases become available each year. If only the islets are used, three to four adult pancreases are needed per procedure, narrowing the number of potential recipients to only 250 to 500.

## Fetal Tissue

The shortage of adult human pancreases has led researchers to explore other sources of pancreatic tissue. One partial solution to this problem might be found in the highly controversial use of fetal pancreatic tissue. Studies have shown that human fetal pancreas tissue is easy to culture and that it can grow and mature once it is transplanted. It has also been shown that the tissue can be frozen and will function again once it is thawed. These factors could help to make such transplants available to a greater number of people.

There are roughly 1.5 million induced abortions in the United States each year although only a very small percentage of them yield usable tissue. Yet, if only 10% of these pancreases were available, using 10 to 20 fetal pancreases to treat each person, fetal tissue could potentially cure 7,500 to 15,000 people with diabetes. While this number still falls dramatically short of the number of people who could benefit from transplants, it could offer one more source of pancreatic tissue.

Work with fetal pancreas transplants began in the late 1970's when researchers in Los Angeles and Melbourne, Australia, grafted bits of fetal rat pancreas into diabetic rats of the same species. The implants not only survived, but grew and matured. After 3 to 12 weeks, they were able to normalize blood glucose levels and halt the early stages of retinopathy and kidney disease. Clinical transplantation of fetal tissue has also been reported in small studies in China, Europe, Russia, and the United States. In each case, fetal tissue transplantation lowered insulin requirements, but did not completely reverse diabetes. And, as with other types of pancreatic transplantation, the success was short-lived and the grafts were eventually rejected.

Research into this area was slowed considerably in 1988, when the Reagan Administration banned federal funding for research using tissue obtained from induced abortions. In 1993, the Clinton Administration lifted the ban, and research into this area is expected to continue.

## Animal Islet Cells

Islet cell transplants from pig pancreases may become another solution to the shortage problem. Pig insulin is very similar to human insulin, differing only by one molecule. In fact, before the advent of artificially produced human insulin, pork insulin was the insulin of choice. Since nearly 100 million pigs are used for food every year in the United States, slaughterhouses could easily supply enough pancreas tissue for everyone who wanted a transplant.

But again, there is the problem of immune system rejection. In addition to the immune response seen with human islet cells, other immune mechanisms guard against tissue from other species. However, this problem may be overcome by one of the immune isolation techniques now being developed. In fact, some biotechnology firms are banking on it.

BioHybrid Technologies, a biotechnology company in Lexington, Massachusetts, has been working on various versions of a bioartificial pancreas, a device containing pig islets that may some day be mass produced and implanted into people with diabetes. In 1991, in a paper in the journal *Science*, researchers from BioHybrid, in conjunction with surgeons at New England Deaconess Hospital and Harvard Medical School, reported successfully implanting bioartificial pancreases containing canine islets into diabetic dogs. The devices, which were roughly the size of hockey pucks, succeeded in maintaining near-normal fasting blood glucose levels in some of the dogs. Some of these devices continued to produce insulin for up to 3 1/2 years.

Over the last few years, these devices have evolved into microreactors, that is, small, resilient structures containing a small number of islets, which can be injected with a syringe. In dogs given low doses of immunosuppressants, implanted islets from the same species have survived and functioned for up to 5 1/2 months, and preliminary results with cross-species transplants also look promising. By the end of this year, BioHybrid researchers plan to seek approval from the Food and Drug Administration for clinical trials, and they may actually start those clinical trials by the end of 1996.

Another biotechnology firm, Neocrin Company, is developing a way to make a bioartificial pancreas that can be maintained by the body. Neocrin covers encapsulated islet cells with a membrane that not only blocks out the immune attack, but also allows new blood vessels to grow right up to its surface. This means that blood can feed the islet cells within the capsule, transport the insulin the cells produce, and cart away their waste products. Neocrin researchers have completed several years of studies in small animals and are now testing larger devices in large animals. Researchers at Neocrin have approached the Food and Drug Administration for approval to begin clinical trials and hope to begin human studies soon.

## Artificial Beta Cells

Yet another approach to solving the shortage problem is to create artificial beta cells that could be mass produced and used in an artificial pancreas. Researchers all over the country are pursuing this goal. While the individual approaches vary widely, they share a basic thread: All involve inserting new genes into naturally occurring cells. Some groups have already made significant strides in this line of research.

For example, in a study published in the January 15, 1992 issue of *Proceedings of the National Academy of Sciences*, researchers at the University of Dallas Southwestern Medical Center reported that they had created artificial beta cells using laboratory-grown cells from the University of California at San Francisco. The cells, originally derived from the pituitary glands of mice, were genetically altered so that they not only produced insulin, but could also respond to the rise and fall of blood glucose, just as normal pancreatic beta cells do. They did not implant them into animals or humans, however, because they still had to tackle the problem of rejection by the immune system.

Researchers at Albert Einstein College of Medicine in Bronx, New York, are also working on ways to mass produce genetically engineered beta cells that won't provoke rejection by the immune system. To solve the problem of immune rejection, these researchers are trying to camouflage the beta cells from the immune system. They hope to accomplish this by changing certain molecules on the beta cell surface that are normally red flags for an immune attack.

These are just two approaches among many for creating artificial beta cells, an experimental avenue that is still in its infancy. Meanwhile, the field of pancreatic tissue transplantation is growing rapidly. As researchers continue to develop ways to safely bypass the body's immune system, other approaches to pancreatic tissue transplantation may only be a few years away. And that means that, eventually, researchers may find a way to halt the progression of diabetes.

*—by Robert S. Dinsmoor*

Robert Dinsmoor is a freelance writer living in the Boston area. He is a Contributing Editor of *Diabetes Self-Management.*

# Chapter 51

# *Kidney Disease*

Each year in the United States, more than 50,000 people are diagnosed with end-stage renal disease (ESRD), a serious condition in which the kidneys fail to rid the body of wastes. ESRD is the final stage of a slow deterioration of the kidneys, a process known as nephropathy.

Diabetes is the most common cause of ESRD, resulting in about one-third of new ESRD cases (see Figure 51.1). Even when drugs and diet are able to control diabetes, the disease can lead to nephropathy and ESRD. Most people with diabetes do not develop nephropathy that is severe enough to cause ESRD. About 15 million people in the United States have diabetes, and about 50,000 people have ESRD as a result of diabetes.

ESRD patients undergo either dialysis, which substitutes for some of the filtering functions of the kidneys, or transplantation to receive a healthy donor kidney. Most U.S. citizens who develop ESRD are eligible for federally funded care. In 1994, the Federal Government spent about $9.3 billion on care for patients with ESRD.

African Americans and Native Americans develop diabetes, nephropathy, and ESRD at rates higher than average. Scientists have not been able to explain these higher rates. Nor can they explain fully the interplay of factors leading to diabetic nephropathy—factors including heredity, diet, and other medical conditions, such as high blood pressure. They have found that high blood pressure and high levels

---

National Institute of Diabetes and Digestive and Kidney Disorders (NIDDK), NIH Pub. No. 97-3925, July 1995.

of blood sugar increase the risk that a person with diabetes will progress to ESRD.

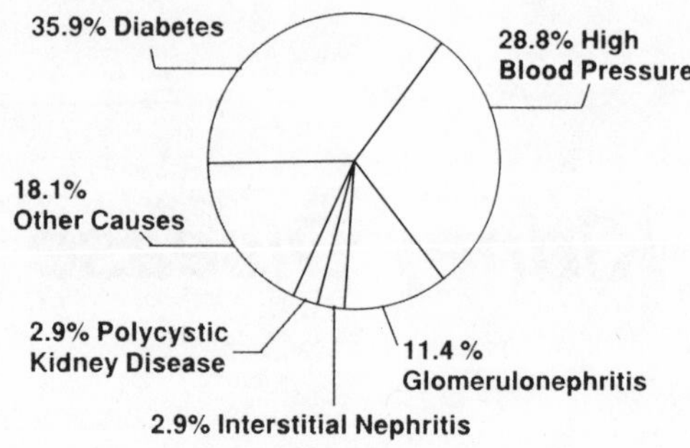


***Figure 51.1.** Primary Diagnoses (Causes) for ESRD (1991)*

## Two Types of Diabetes

In diabetes—also called diabetes mellitus, or DM—the body does not properly process and use certain foods, especially carbohydrates. The human body normally converts carbohydrates to glucose, the simple sugar that is the main source of energy for the body's cells. To enter cells, glucose needs the help of insulin, a hormone produced by the pancreas. When a person does not make enough insulin, or the body is unable to use the insulin that is present, the body cannot process glucose, and it builds up in the bloodstream. High levels of glucose in the blood or urine lead to a diagnosis of diabetes.

### NIDDM

Most people with diabetes have a form known as noninsulin-dependent diabetes (NIDDM), or Type II diabetes. Many people with NIDDM do not respond normally to their own or to injected insulin—a condition called insulin resistance. NIDDM occurs more often in people over the age of 40, and many people with NIDDM are overweight. Many also are not aware that they have the disease. Some people with NIDDM control their blood sugar with diet and an exercise program leading to weight loss. Others must take pills that stimulate production of insulin; still others require injections of insulin.

### IDDM

A less common form of diabetes, known as insulin-dependent diabetes (IDDM), or Type I diabetes, tends to occur in young adults and children. In cases of IDDM, the body produces little or no insulin. People with IDDM must receive daily insulin injections.

NIDDM accounts for about 95 percent of all cases of diabetes; IDDM accounts for about 5 percent. Both types of diabetes can lead to kidney disease. IDDM is more likely to lead to ESRD. About 40 percent of people with IDDM develop severe kidney disease and ESRD by the age of 50. Some develop ESRD before the age of 30. NIDDM causes 80 percent of the ESRD in African Americans and Native Americans.

## The Course of Kidney Disease

The deterioration that characterizes kidney disease of diabetes takes place in and around the glomeruli, the blood-filtering units of the kidneys. Early in the disease, the filtering efficiency diminishes, and important proteins in the blood are lost to the urine. Medical professionals gauge the presence and extent of early kidney disease by measuring protein in the urine. Later in the disease, the kidneys lose their ability to remove waste products, such as creatinine and urea, from the blood.

Symptoms related to kidney failure usually occur only in late stages of the disease, when kidney function has diminished to less than 25 percent of normal capacity. For many years before that point, kidney disease of diabetes exists as a silent process.

### Five Stages

Scientists have described five stages in the progression to ESRD in people with diabetes. They are as follows:

**Stage I.** The flow of blood through the kidneys, and therefore through the glomeruli, increases—this is called hyperfiltration—and the kidneys are larger than normal. Some people remain in stage I indefinitely; others advance to stage II after many years.

**Stage II.** The rate of filtration remains elevated or at near-normal levels, and the glomeruli begin to show damage. Small amounts of a blood protein known as albumin leak into the urine—a condition known as microalbuminuria. In its earliest stages, microalbuminuria may come and go. But as the rate of albumin loss increases from 20 to 200 micrograms per minute, microalbuminuria becomes more constant. (Normal losses of albumin are less than 5 micrograms per minute.) A special test is required to detect microalbuminuria. People with NIDDM and IDDM may remain in stage II for many years, especially if they have normal blood pressure and good control of their blood sugar levels.

**Stage III.** The loss of albumin and other proteins in the urine exceeds 200 micrograms per minute. It now can be detected during routine urine tests. Because such tests often involve dipping indicator strips into the urine, they are referred to as "dipstick methods." Stage III sometimes is referred to as "dipstick-positive proteinuria" (or "clinical albuminuria" or "overt diabetic nephropathy"). Some patients develop high blood pressure. The glomeruli suffer increased damage. The kidneys progressively lose the ability to filter waste, and blood levels of creatinine and urea-nitrogen rise. People with IDDM and NIDDM may remain at stage III for many years.

**Stage IV.** This is referred to as "advanced clinical nephropathy." The glomerular filtration rate decreases to less than 75 milliliters per minute, large amounts of protein pass into the urine, and high blood pressure almost always occurs. Levels of creatinine and urea-nitrogen in the blood rise further.

**Stage V.** The final stage is ESRD. The glomerular filtration rate drops to less than 10 milliliters per minute. Symptoms of kidney failure occur.

These stages describe the progression of kidney disease for most people with IDDM who develop ESRD. For people with IDDM, the average length of time required to progress from onset of kidney disease to stage IV is 17 years. The average length of time to progress to ESRD is 23 years. Progression to ESRD may occur more rapidly (5-10 years) in people with untreated high blood pressure. If proteinuria does not develop within 25 years, the risk of developing advanced kidney disease begins to decrease. Advancement to stages IV and V occurs less frequently in people with NIDDM than in people with IDDM. Nevertheless, about 60 percent of people with diabetes who develop ESRD have NIDDM.

### *Effects of High Blood Pressure*

High blood pressure, or hypertension, is a major factor in the development of kidney problems in people with diabetes. Both a family history of hypertension and the presence of hypertension appear to increase chances of developing kidney disease. Hypertension also accelerates the progress of kidney disease where it already exists.

Hypertension usually is defined as blood pressure exceeding 140 millimeters of mercury-systolic and 90 millimeters of mercury-diastolic. Professionals shorten the name of this limit to "140 over 90." The terms systolic and diastolic refer to pressure in the arteries during contraction of the heart (systolic) and between heartbeats (diastolic).

Hypertension can be seen not only as a cause of kidney disease, but also as a result of damage created by the disease. As kidney disease proceeds, physical changes in the kidneys lead to increased blood pressure. Therefore, a dangerous spiral, involving rising blood pressure and factors that raise blood pressure, occurs. Early detection and treatment of even mild hypertension are essential for people with diabetes.

## Preventing and Slowing Kidney Disease

### Blood Pressure Medicines

Scientists have made great progress in developing methods that slow the onset and progression of kidney disease in people with diabetes. Drugs used to lower blood pressure (antihypertensive drugs) can slow the progression of kidney disease significantly. One drug, an angiotensin-converting enzyme (ACE) inhibitor, has proven effective in preventing progression to stages IV and V.[1] Calcium channel blockers, another class of antihypertensive drugs, also show promise.

An example of an effective ACE inhibitor is captopril, which the Food and Drug Administration approved for treating kidney disease of Type I diabetes. The benefits of captopril extend beyond its ability to lower blood pressure; it may directly protect the kidney's glomeruli. ACE inhibitors have lowered proteinuria and slowed deterioration even in diabetic patients who did not have high blood pressure.

Some, but not all, calcium channel blockers may be able to decrease proteinuria and damage to kidney tissue. Researchers are investigating whether combinations of calcium channel blockers and ACE inhibitors might be more effective than either treatment used alone. Patients with even mild hypertension or persistent microalbuminuria should consult a physician about the use of antihypertensive medicines.

### Low-Protein Diets

A diet containing reduced amounts of protein may benefit people with kidney disease of diabetes. In people with diabetes, excessive consumption of protein may be harmful. Experts recommend that most patients with stage III or stage IV nephropathy consume moderate amounts of protein.

### *Intensive Management*

Antihypertensive drugs and low-protein diets can slow kidney disease when significant nephropathy is present, as in stages III and IV. A third treatment, known as intensive management or glycemic control, has shown great promise for people with IDDM, especially for those with early stages of nephropathy.

Intensive management is a treatment regimen that aims to keep blood glucose levels close to normal. The regimen includes frequently testing blood sugar, administering insulin on the basis of food intake and exercise, following a diet and exercise plan, and frequently consulting a health care team.

A number of studies have pointed to the beneficial effects of intensive management. Two such studies, funded by the National Institute of Diabetes and Digestive and Kidney Diseases (NIDDK) of the National Institutes of Health, are the Diabetes Control and Complications Trial (DCCT)[2] and a trial led by researchers at the University of Minnesota Medical School.[3]

The DCCT, conducted from 1983 to 1993, involved 1,441 participants who had IDDM. Researchers found a 50-percent decrease in both development and progression of early diabetic kidney disease (stages I and II) in participants who followed an intensive regimen for controlling blood sugar levels. The intensively managed patients had average blood sugar levels of 150 milligrams per deciliter—about 80 milligrams per deciliter lower than the levels observed in the conventionally managed patients.

In the Minnesota Medical School trial, researchers examined kidney tissues of long-term diabetics who received healthy kidney transplants. After 5 years, patients who followed an intensive regimen developed significantly fewer lesions in their glomeruli than did patients not following an intensive regimen. This result, along with findings of the DCCT and studies performed in Scandinavia, suggests that any program resulting in sustained lowering of blood glucose levels will be beneficial to patients in the early stages of diabetic nephropathy.

## *Dialysis and Transplantation*

When people with diabetes reach ESRD, they must undergo either dialysis or a kidney transplant. As recently as the 1970's, medical experts commonly excluded people with diabetes from dialysis and transplantation, in part because the experts felt damage caused by diabetes would offset benefits of the treatments. Today, because of better control of diabetes and improved rates of survival following treatment, doctors do not hesitate to offer dialysis and kidney transplantation to people with diabetes.

Currently, the survival of kidneys transplanted into diabetes patients is about the same as survival of transplants in people without diabetes. Dialysis for people with diabetes also works well in the short run. Even so, people with diabetes who receive transplants or dialysis experience higher morbidity and mortality because of coexisting complications of the diabetes—such as damage to the heart, eyes, and nerves.

## Looking to the Future

The incidences of both diabetes and ESRD caused by diabetes have been rising. Some experts predict that diabetes soon might account for half the cases of ESRD. In light of the increasing morbidity and mortality related to diabetes and ESRD, patients, researchers, and health care professionals will continue to benefit by addressing the relationship between the two diseases. The NIDDK is a leader in supporting research in this area.

Several areas of research supported by NIDDK hold great potential. Discovery of ways to predict who will develop kidney disease may lead to greater prevention, as people with diabetes who learn they are at risk institute strategies such as intensive management and blood pressure control. Discovery of better anti-rejection drugs will improve results of kidney transplantation in patients with diabetes who develop ESRD. For some people with IDDM, advances in transplantation—especially transplantation of insulin-producing cells of the pancreas—could lead to a cure for both diabetes and the kidney disease of diabetes.

## Good Care Makes a Difference

If you have diabetes:

- Ask your doctor about the DCCT and how its results might help you.
- Have your doctor measure your glycohemoglobin regularly. The $HbA_{1C}$ test averages your level of blood sugar for the previous 1-3 months.

- Follow your doctor's advice regarding insulin injections, medicines, diet, exercise, and monitoring your blood sugar.
- Have your blood pressure checked several times a year. If blood pressure is high, follow your doctor's plan for keeping it near normal levels.
- Ask your doctor whether you might benefit from receiving an ACE inhibitor.
- Have your urine checked yearly for microalbumin and protein. If there is protein in your urine, have your blood checked for elevated amounts of waste products such as creatinine.
- Ask your doctor whether you should reduce the amount of protein in your diet.

## References


1. Lewis, E.J., et al., The effect of angiotensin-converting-enzyme inhibition on diabetic nephropathy. *New England Journal of Medicine*, Vol. 329, No. 20, pp. 1456-1462, 1993.
2. *Diabetes Control and Complications Trial* [fact sheet], August 1994. National Diabetes Information Clearinghouse, 1 Information Way, Bethesda, MD 20892-3560.
3. Barbosa, J., et al., Effect of glycemic control on early diabetic renal lesions. *Journal of the American Medical Association*, Vol. 272, No. 8, pp. 600-606, 1994.

## Chapter 52

# *Microalbuminuria*

### *What is diabetic kidney disease?*

Kidney disease is one of the most serious complications of diabetes. After years of diabetes, the filtering units of the kidney (glomeruli) get scarred so that they cannot filter the blood efficiently. Eventually, the kidneys may fail completely so that the patient needs dialysis or a kidney transplant.

### *What causes diabetic kidney disease?*

We don't know for sure. Part of the problem is probably genetic (inherited). However, high blood glucose levels and high blood pressure also contribute.

### *If I have diabetes, how do I know if I am likely to get kidney disease?*

You cannot know for sure. However, certain things can make it more likely. These include: having a family member with diabetic kidney disease; high blood glucose levels: high blood pressure; and cigarette smoking.

---

### Are there tests that can tell if my kidneys have been hurt by diabetes?

Yes; blood and urine tests can show if your kidneys are affected.

### Are people who have Type I diabetes more likely to have kidney problems?

No; the risk of kidney problems is about equal in people with Type I and Type II diabetes. However, the risk of serious kidney failure (requiring dialysis or a kidney transplant) is higher in patients with Type I diabetes.

### Are people who have diabetes and high blood pressure more likely to have kidney problems?

Yes. High blood pressure can make diabetic kidney disease worse, and it can also cause kidney problems on its own.

### What does microalbuminuria mean?

Microalbuminuria means that the kidney has some damage, and is starting to spill some albumin (a kind of protein) in the urine. Microalbuminuria is the first sign of diabetic kidney disease.

### How is microalbuminuria measured?

It can be measured by a specific urine test, either on a single urine specimen, or on a 24-hour urine collection. Any doctor can test for microalbuminuria. Routine urine analysis does not detect microalbuminuria.

### Who should have this test? How often?

Everyone with diabetes who is between 12 and 70 years of age should have a urine test for microalbuminuria at least once a year. If positive, this should be reconfirmed on a second urine specimen.

### Is it possible to have microalbuminuria without having any symptoms?

Yes; microalbuminuria itself does not cause any symptoms.

### *Are there signs that show an increased risk of microalbuminuria?*

Not really, though certain risk factors (high blood glucose, high blood pressure) may be a clue that microalbuminuria is likely.

### *What would be considered a positive result?*

For a 24-hour urine collection, 30 to 300 mg of albumin means microalbuminuria. In a single urine specimen, a level of more than 30 mg of albumin per gram of creatinine is considered positive.

### *Can other things (besides kidney disease) cause this test to be positive?*

Yes. Some other conditions, such as essential hypertension, can also cause albuminuria. If the test is done during periods of illness, heavy exercise, urinary tract infections or poor blood glucose control, it may show a positive result.

### *Is there a home test that measure microalbuminuria?*

No, there are no accurate home tests.

### *Is the test expensive? Does health insurance cover it?*

The test is relatively inexpensive, and most health insurance plans will cover it. If you are not sure, check with your doctor or your insurance company.

### *Should people with both Type I and Type II diabetes be tested for microalbuminuria?*

Yes. All people with diabetes are at risk for developing microalbuminuria.

### *Will tight control of glucose help?*

Yes. Tight control lowers the risk of all diabetic complications, including the development of microalbuminuria and diabetic kidney disease.

### *Are there other things I can do to prevent kidney disease?*

Keeping your blood pressure under good control and quitting cigarette smoking will both help to prevent diabetic kidney disease.

### *What dietary changes should I make?*

You should stay on a diabetic diet, as prescribed by your doctor. If you have not seen a dietitian, ask to see one to help you learn all the possible ways you can control your diet.

### *Does a positive test for microalbuminuria suggest other problems besides kidney disease?*

Microalbuminuria suggests a higher risk for heart disease, as well as kidney disease.

### *How many people who test positive for microalbuminuria develop kidney failure? How long does this take to occur?*

Most patients with Type I diabetes who test positive for microalbuminuria will develop kidney failure after a number of years. For Type II diabetes, the number of people who will develop kidney failure is not known, but some of these patients will eventually get kidney failure.

### *If my kidneys fail eventually, what treatments are available?*

Either dialysis or kidney transplantation can be used to treat kidney failure. Your doctor can provide you with more information about these treatments.

### *What is the National Kidney Foundation and how does it help?*

More than 20 million Americans have some form of kidney or urologic disease. Millions more are at risk. The National Kidney Foundation, Inc., a major voluntary health organization, is working to find the answers through prevention, treatment and cure. Through its 52 Affiliates nationwide, the Foundation conducts programs in research, professional education, patient and community services, public education and organ donation. The work of the National Kidney Foundation is funded entirely by public donations.

Chapter 53

# *End-Stage Renal Disease: Choosing a Treatment That's Right for You*

## *Introduction*

This chapter is for people whose kidneys fail to work. This condition is called end-stage renal disease (ESRD).

Today, there are new and better treatments for ESRD that replace the work of healthy kidneys. By learning about your treatment choices, you can work with your doctor to pick the one that's best for you. No matter which type of treatment you choose, there will be some changes in your life. But with the help of your health care team, family, and friends, you may be able to lead a full, active life.

This chapter describes the choices for treatment: hemodialysis, peritoneal dialysis, and kidney transplantation. It gives the pros and cons of each. It also discusses diet and paying for treatment. It gives tips for working with your doctor, nurses, and others who make up your health care team. It provides a list of groups that offer information and services to kidney patients. It also lists magazines, books, and brochures that you can read for more information about treatment.

You and your doctor will work together to choose a treatment that's best for you. This chapter can help you make that choice.

## *When Your Kidneys Fail*

Healthy kidneys clean the blood by filtering out extra water and wastes. They also make hormones that keep your bones strong and

---

National Institute of Diabetes and Digestive and Kidney Diseases (NIDDK), NIH Pub. No. 96-2412, July 1995.

blood healthy. When both of your kidneys fail, your body holds fluid. Your blood pressure rises. Harmful wastes build up in your body. Your body doesn't make enough red blood cells. When this happens, you need treatment to replace the work of your failed kidneys.

## Hemodialysis

### Purpose

Hemodialysis is a procedure that cleans and filters your blood. It rids your body of harmful wastes and extra salt and fluids. It also controls blood pressure and helps your body keep the proper balance of chemicals such as potassium, sodium, and chloride.

### How It Works

Hemodialysis uses a dialyzer, or special filter, to clean your blood. The dialyzer connects to a machine. During treatment, your blood

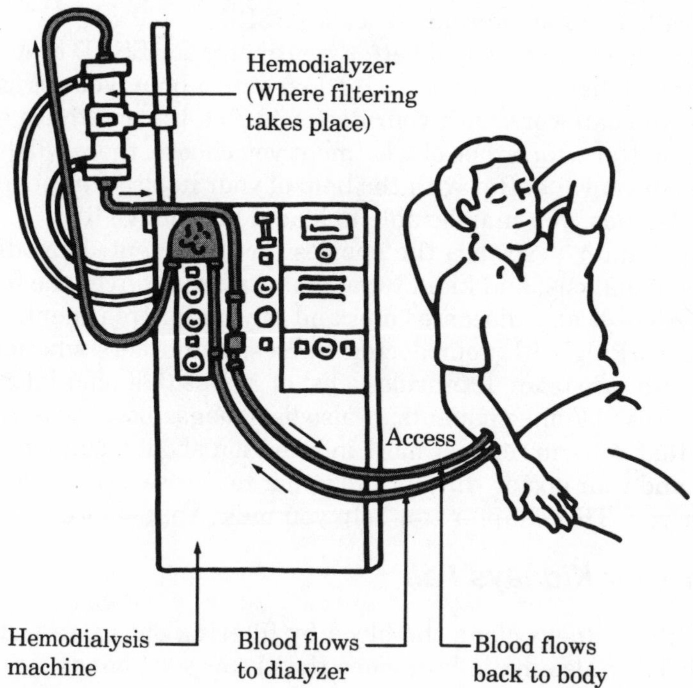


**Figure 53.1.** *Hemodialysis Treatment*

travels through tubes into the dialyzer. The dialyzer filters out wastes and extra fluids. Then the newly cleaned blood flows through another set of tubes and back into your body.

### *Getting Ready*

Before your first treatment, an access to your bloodstream must be made. The access provides a way for blood to be carried from your body to the dialysis machine and then back into your body. The access can be internal (inside the body—usually under your skin) or external (outside the body).

### *Who Performs It*

Hemodialysis can be done at home or at a center. At a center, nurses or trained technicians perform the treatment. At home, you perform hemodialysis with the help of a family member or friend. If you decide to do home dialysis, you and your partner will receive special training.

### *The Time It Takes*

Hemodialysis usually is done three times a week. Each treatment lasts from 2 to 4 hours. During treatment, you can read, write, sleep, talk, or watch TV.

### *Possible Complications*

Side effects can be caused by rapid changes in your body's fluid and chemical balance during treatment. Muscle cramps and hypotension are two common side effects. Hypotension, a sudden drop in blood pressure, can make you feel weak, dizzy, or sick to your stomach.

It usually takes a few months to adjust to hemodialysis. You can avoid many of the side effects if you follow the proper diet and take your medicines as directed. You should always report side effects to your doctor. They often can be treated quickly and easily.

### *Your Diet*

Hemodialysis and a proper diet help reduce the wastes that build up in your blood. A dietitian can help you plan meals according to your doctor's orders. When choosing foods, you should remember to:

- Eat balanced amounts of foods high in protein such as meat and chicken. Animal protein is better used by your body than the protein found in vegetables and grains.
- Watch the amount of potassium you eat. Potassium is a mineral found in salt substitutes, some fruits, vegetables, milk, chocolate, and nuts. Too much or too little potassium can be harmful to your heart.
- Limit how much you drink. Fluids build up quickly in your body when your kidneys aren't working. Too much fluid makes your tissues swell. It also can cause high blood pressure and heart trouble.
- Avoid salt. Salty foods make you thirsty and cause your body to hold water.
- Limit foods such as milk, cheese, nuts, dried beans, and soft drinks. These foods contain the mineral phosphorus. Too much phosphorus in your blood causes calcium to be pulled from your bones. Calcium helps keep bones strong and healthy. To prevent bone problems, your doctor may give you special medicines. You must take these medicines everyday as directed.

### Pros and Cons

Each person responds differently to similar situations. What may be a negative factor for one person may be positive for another. However, in general, the following are pros and cons for each type of hemodialysis.

*In-Center Hemodialysis Pros*

- You have trained professionals with you at all times.
- You can get to know other patients.

*In-Center Hemodialysis Cons*

- Treatments are scheduled by the center.
- You must travel to the center for treatment.

*Home Hemodialysis Pros*

- You can do it at the hours you choose. (But you still must do it as often as your doctor orders.)

- You don't have to travel to a center.
- You gain a sense of independence and control over your treatment.

*Home Hemodialysis Cons*

- Helping with treatments may be stressful to your family.
- You need training.
- You need space for storing the machine and supplies at home.

### *Working with Your Health Care Team*

Questions you may want to ask:

- Is hemodialysis the best treatment choice for me? Why or why not?
- If I am treated at a center, can I go to the center of my choice?
- What does hemodialysis feel like? Does it hurt?
- What is self-care dialysis?
- How long does it take to learn home hemodialysis? Who will train my partner and me?
- What kind of blood access is best for me?
- As a hemodialysis patient, will I be able to keep working? Can I have treatments at night if I plan to keep working?
- How much should I exercise?
- Who will be on my health care team? How can they help me?
- Who can I talk with about sexuality, family problems, or money concerns?
- How/where can I talk to other people who have faced this decision?
- Write down other questions you may have.

## Peritoneal Dialysis

### *Purpose*

Peritoneal dialysis is another procedure that replaces the work of your kidneys. It removes extra water, wastes, and chemicals from your body. This type of dialysis uses the lining of your abdomen to filter your blood. This lining is called the peritoneal membrane.

### *How It Works*

A cleansing solution, called dialysate, travels through a special tube into your abdomen. Fluid, wastes, and chemicals pass from tiny blood vessels in the peritoneal membrane into the dialysate. After several hours, the dialysate gets drained from your abdomen, taking the wastes from your blood with it. Then you fill your abdomen with fresh dialysate and the cleaning process begins again.

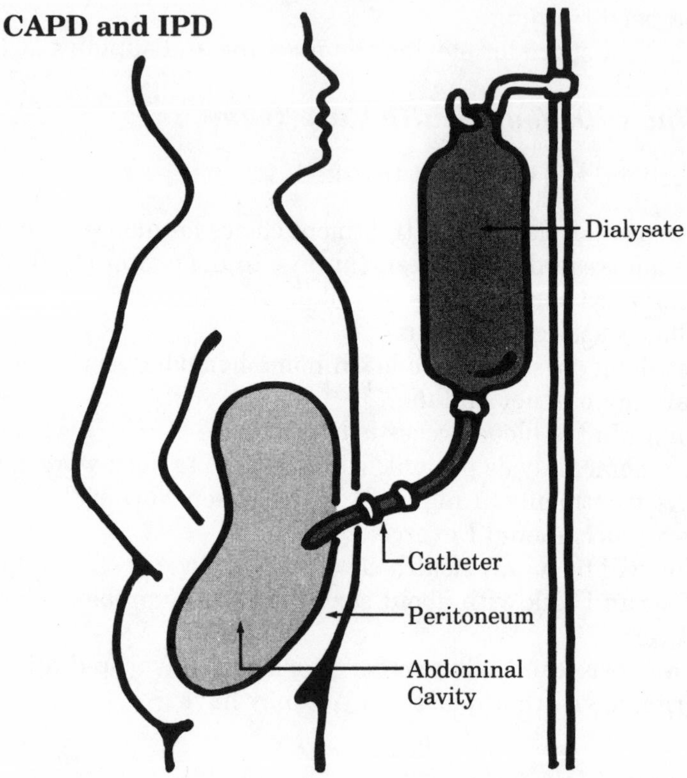


***Figure 53.2.*** *CAPD and IPD peritoneal dialysis.*

## *Getting Ready*

Before your first treatment, a surgeon places a small, soft tube called a catheter into your abdomen. This catheter always stays there. It helps transport the dialysate to and from your peritoneal membrane.

## *Types of Peritoneal Dialysis*

There are three types of peritoneal dialysis.

1. **Continuous Ambulatory Peritoneal Dialysis (CAPD).** CAPD is the most common type of peritoneal dialysis. It needs no machine. It can be done in any clean, well-lit place. With CAPD, your blood is always being cleaned. The dialysate passes from a plastic bag through the catheter and into your abdomen. The dialysate stays in your abdomen with the catheter sealed. After several hours, you drain the solution back into the bag. Then you refill your abdomen with fresh solution through the same catheter. Now the cleaning process begins again. While the solution is in your body, you may fold the empty plastic bag and hide it under your clothes, around your waist, or in a pocket.

   **Update to Section on Peritoneal Dialysis.** In recent years, peritoneal dialysis techniques have improved. A new system for continuous ambulatory peritoneal dialysis (CAPD) no longer requires the patient to carry the empty dialysate bag while the solution is in the patient's body, as described earlier in this chapter. In the new system, after the solution has drained into the patient's peritoneum, he or she can disconnect the tubing from the catheter in his or her abdomen. When it is time to change the solution, the patient reconnects the tubing to the catheter.

   For additional information about different types of dialysis, you may wish to contact your nephrologist or the clearinghouse at the following address:

   National Kidney and Urologic Diseases
   Information Clearinghouse
   3 Information Way
   Bethesda, MD 20892-3580

2. **Continuous Cyclic Peritoneal Dialysis (CCPD).** CCPD is like CAPD except that a machine, which connects to your catheter, automatically fills and drains the dialysate from your abdomen. The machine does this at night while you sleep.

3. **Intermittent Peritoneal Dialysis (IPD).** IPD uses the same type of machine as CCPD to add and drain the dialysate.

IPD can be done at home, but it's usually done in the hospital. IPD treatments take longer than CCPD.

### Who Performs It

CAPD is a form of self-treatment. It needs no machine and no partner. However, with IPD and CCPD, you need a machine and the help of a partner (family member, friend, or health professional).

### The Time It Takes

With CAPD, the dialysate stays in your abdomen for about 4 to 6 hours. The process of draining the dialysate and replacing fresh solution takes 30 to 40 minutes. Most people change the solution four times a day.

With CCPD, treatments last from 10 to 12 hours every night.

With IPD, treatments are done several times a week, for a total of 36 to 42 hours per week. Sessions may last up to 24 hours.

### Possible Complications

Peritonitis, or infection of the peritoneum, can occur if the opening where the catheter enters your body gets infected. You can also get it if there is a problem connecting or disconnecting the catheter from the bags. Peritonitis can make you feel sick. It can cause a fever and stomach pain.

To avoid peritonitis, you must be careful to follow the procedure exactly. You must know the early signs of peritonitis. Look for reddening or swelling around the catheter. You should also note if your dialysate looks cloudy. It is important to report these signs to your doctor so that the peritonitis can be treated quickly to avoid serious problems.

### Your Diet

Diet for peritoneal dialysis is slightly different than diet for hemodialysis.

- You may be able to have more salt and fluids.
- You may eat more protein.
- You may have different potassium restrictions.
- You may need to cut back on the number of calories you eat. This limitation is because the sugar in the dialysate may cause you to gain weight.

### Pros and Cons

There are pros and cons to each type of peritoneal dialysis.

*CAPD Pros*

- You can perform treatment alone.
- You can do it at times you choose.
- You can do it in many locations.
- You don't need a machine.

*CAPD Cons*

- It disrupts your daily schedule.

*CCPD Pros*

- You can do it at night, mainly while you sleep.

*CCPD Cons*

- You need a machine and help from a partner.

*IPD Pros*

- Health professionals usually perform treatments.

*IPD Cons*

- You may need to go to a hospital.
- It takes a lot of time.
- You need a machine.

### Working with Your Health Care Team

Questions you may want to ask:

- Is peritoneal dialysis the best treatment choice for me? Why or why not? Which type?
- How long will it take me to learn peritoneal dialysis?
- What does peritoneal dialysis feel like? Does it hurt?
- How will peritoneal dialysis affect my blood pressure?
- How do I know if I have peritonitis? How is peritonitis treated?
- As a peritoneal dialysis patient, will I be able to continue working?

- How much should I exercise?
- Who will be on my health care team? How can they help me?
- Who can I talk with about sexuality, finances, or family concerns?
- How/where can I talk to other people who have faced this decision?
- Write down other questions you may have.

## Dialysis Is Not a Cure

Hemodialysis and peritoneal dialysis are treatments that try to replace your failed kidneys. These treatments help you feel better and live longer, but they are not cures for ESRD. While patients with ESRD are now living longer than ever, ESRD can cause problems over the years. Some problems are bone disease, high blood pressure, nerve damage, and anemia (having too few red blood cells). Although these problems won't go away with dialysis, doctors now have new and better ways to treat or prevent them. You should discuss these treatments with your doctor.

## Kidney Transplantation

### Purpose

Kidney transplantation is a procedure that places a healthy kidney from another person into your body. This one new kidney does all the work that your two failed kidneys cannot do.

### How It Works

A surgeon places the new kidney inside your body between your upper thigh and abdomen. The surgeon connects the artery and vein of the new kidney to your artery and vein. Your blood flows through the new kidney and makes urine, just like your own kidneys did when they were healthy. The new kidney may start working right away or may take up to a few weeks to make urine. Your own kidneys are left where they are, unless they are causing infection or high blood pressure.

### Getting Ready

You may receive a kidney from a member of your family. This kind of donor is called a living-related donor. You may receive a kidney from a person who has recently died. This type of donor is called a cadaver donor. Sometimes a spouse or very close friend may donate a kidney. This kind of donor is called a living-unrelated donor.

It is very important for the donor's blood and tissues to closely match yours. This match will help prevent your body's immune system from fighting off, or rejecting, the new kidney. A lab will do special tests on blood cells to find out if your body will accept the new kidney.

### *The Time It Takes*

The time it takes to get a kidney varies. There are not enough cadaver donors for every person who needs a transplant. Because of this, you must be placed on a waiting list to receive a cadaver donor kidney. However, if a relative gives you a kidney, the transplant operation can be done sooner.

The surgery takes from 3 to 6 hours. The usual hospital stay may last from 10 to 14 days. After you leave the hospital, you will go to the clinic for regular followup visits.

If a relative or close friend gives you a kidney, he or she will probably stay in the hospital for one week or less.

### *Possible Complications*

Transplantation is not a cure. There is always a chance that your body will reject your new kidney, no matter how good the match. The chance of your body accepting the new kidney depends on your age, race, and medical condition.

Normally, 75 to 80 percent of transplants from cadaver donors are working one year after surgery. However, transplants from living relatives often work better than transplants from cadaver donors. This fact is because they are usually a closer match.

Your doctor will give you special drugs to help prevent rejection. These are called immunosuppressants. You will need to take these drugs every day for the rest of your life. Sometimes these drugs cannot stop your body from rejecting the new kidney. If this happens, you will go back to some form of dialysis and possibly wait for another transplant.

Treatment with these drugs may cause side effects. The most serious is that they weaken your immune system, making it easier for you to get infections. Some drugs also cause changes in how you look. Your face may get fuller. You may gain weight or develop acne or facial hair. Not all patients have these problems, and makeup and diet can help.

Some of these drugs may cause problems such as cataracts, extra stomach acid, and hip disease. In a smaller number of patients, these drugs also may cause liver or kidney damage when used for a long period of time.

### *Your Diet*

Diet for transplant patients is less limiting than it is for dialysis patients. You may still have to cut back on some foods, though. Your diet probably will change as your medicines, blood values, weight, and blood pressure change.

- You may need to count calories. Your medicine may give you a bigger appetite and cause you to gain weight.
- You may have to limit eating salty foods. Your medications may cause salt to be held in your body, leading to high blood pressure.
- You may need to eat less protein. Some medications cause a higher level of wastes to build up in your bloodstream.

### *Pros and Cons*

There are pros and cons to kidney transplantation.

*Pros*

- It works like a normal kidney.
- It helps you feel healthier.
- You have fewer diet restrictions.
- There's no need for dialysis.

*Cons*

- It requires major surgery.
- You may need to wait for a donor.
- One transplant may not last a lifetime. Your body may reject the new kidney.
- You will have to take drugs for the rest of your life.

### *Working with Your Health Care Team*

Questions you may want to ask:

- Is transplantation the best treatment choice for me? Why or why not?
- What are my chances of having a successful transplant?
- How do I find out if a family member or friend can donate?
- What are the risks to a family member or friend if he or she donates?
- If a family member or friend doesn't donate, how do I get placed on a waiting list for a kidney? How long will I have to wait?
- What are the symptoms of rejection?
- Who will be on my health care team? How can they help me?
- Who can I talk to about sexuality, finances, or family concerns?
- How/where can I talk to other people who have faced this decision?
- Write down other questions you may have.

## Conclusion

It's not always easy to decide which type of treatment is best for you. Your decision depends on your medical condition, lifestyle, and personal likes and dislikes. Discuss the pros and cons of each with your health care team. If you start one form of treatment and decide you'd like to try another, talk it over with your doctor. The key is to learn as much as you can about your choices. With that knowledge, you and your doctor will choose a treatment that suits you best.

## Paying for Treatment

Treatment for ESRD is expensive, but the Federal Government helps pay for much of the cost. Often, private insurance or state programs pay the rest.

### *Medicare*

Medicare pays for 80 percent of the cost of your dialysis treatments or transplant, no matter how old you are. To qualify,

- you must have worked long enough to be insured under Social Security (or be the child of someone who has) or
- you already must be receiving Social Security benefits.

You should apply for Medicare as soon as possible after beginning dialysis. Often, a social worker at your hospital or dialysis center will help you apply.

### *Private Insurance*

Private insurance often pays for the entire cost of treatment. Or it may pay for the 20 percent that Medicare does not cover. Private insurance also may pay for your prescription drugs.

### *Medicaid*

Medicaid is a state program. Your income must be below a certain level to receive Medicaid funds. Medicaid may pay for your treatments if you cannot receive Medicare. In some states, it also pays the 20 percent that Medicare does not cover. It also may pay for some of your medicines. To apply for Medicaid, talk with your social worker or contact your local health department.

### *Veterans Administration (VA) Benefits*

If you are a veteran, the VA can help pay for treatment. Contact your local VA office for more information.

### *Social Security Income (SSI) and Social Security Disability Income (SSDI)*

These benefits are available from the Social Security Administration. They assist you with the costs of daily living. To find out if you qualify, talk to your social worker or call your local Social Security office.

## *Organizations That Can Help*

There are several groups that offer information and services to kidney patients. You may wish to contact the following:

**American Kidney Fund**
Suite 1010
6110 Executive Boulevard
Rockville, MD 20852
(800) 638-8299

**American Association of Kidney Patients**
Suite LL1
1 Davis Boulevard
Tampa, FL 33606
(813) 251-0725

**National Kidney Foundation, Inc.**
30 East 33rd Street
New York, NY 10016
(800) 622-9010

**National Kidney and Urologic Diseases Information Clearinghouse**
Box NKUDIC
9000 Rockville Pike
Bethesda, MD 20892
(301) 654-4415

Additional diabetes organizations are listed in Chapter 67.

## Additional Reading

If you would like to learn more about ESRD and its treatment, you may be interested in reading:

*Your New Life With Dialysis—A Patient Guide for Physical and Psychological Adjustment*
Edith T. Oberley, M.A., and
Terry D. Oberley, M.D., Ph.D.
Fourth edition, 1991
Charles C. Thomas Publishers
2600 South First Street
Springfield, IL 62794-9265

*Understanding Kidney Transplantation*
Edith T. Oberley, M.A., and
Neal R. Glass, M.D., F.A.C.S.
Charles C. Thomas Publishers, 1987
2600 South First Street
Springfield, IL 62794-9265

*Kidney Disease: A Guide for Patients and Their Families*
American Kidney Fund
Suite 1010
6110 Executive Boulevard
Rockville, MD 20852
(800) 638-8299

*National Kidney Foundation Patient Education Brochures*
Includes information on treatment, diet, work, and exercise.
National Kidney Foundation, Inc.
30 East 33rd Street
New York, NY 10016
(800) 622-9010

*Medicare Coverage of Kidney Dialysis and Kidney Transplant Services: A Supplement to Your Medicare Handbook*. Publication Number HCFA-02183.
U.S. Department of Health and Human Services
Health Care Financing Administration
Suite 500
1331 H Street, NW
Washington, DC 20005
(301) 966-7843

*Renalife Magazine*
American Association of Kidney Patients (AAKP)
Suite LL1
1 Davis Boulevard
Tampa, FL 33606
(813) 251-0725
Published quarterly.

*Family Focus Newsletter*
National Kidney Foundation, Inc.
30 East 33rd Street
New York, NY 10016
(800) 622-9010

*For Patients Only Magazine*
Suite 400
20335 Ventura Boulevard
Woodland Hills, CA 91364
(818) 704-5555
Published six times per year.

# Part Seven

# Research Initiatives

Chapter 54

# *Diabetes Control and Complications Trial (DCCT)*

## *What Is the DCCT?*

The DCCT is a clinical study conducted from 1983 to 1993 by the National Institute of Diabetes and Digestive and Kidney Diseases (NIDDK). The study showed that keeping blood sugar levels as close to normal as possible slows the onset and progression of eye, kidney, and nerve diseases caused by diabetes. In fact, it demonstrated that *any* sustained lowering of blood sugar helps, even if the person has a history of poor control.

The largest, most comprehensive diabetes study ever conducted, the DCCT involved 1,441 volunteers with insulin-dependent diabetes mellitus (IDDM) and 29 medical centers in the United States and Canada. Volunteers had diabetes for at least 1 year but no longer than 15 years. They also were required to have no, or only early signs of, diabetic eye disease.

The study compared the effects of two treatment regimens—standard therapy and intensive control—on the complications of diabetes. Volunteers were randomly assigned to each treatment group.

### *DCCT Study Findings*

Lowering blood sugar reduces risk:

- Eye disease—76% reduced risk

---

National Diabetes Information Clearinghouse, NIH Publication No. 97-3874, September 1994.

- Kidney disease—50% reduced risk
- Nerve disease—60% reduced risk
- Cardiovascular disease—35% reduced risk

### *Elements of Intensive Management in the DCCT*

- Testing blood sugar levels 4 or more times a day
- Four daily insulin injections or use of an insulin pump
- Adjustment of insulin doses according to food intake and exercise
- A diet and exercise plan
- Monthly visits to a health care team composed of a physician, nurse educator, dietitian, and behavioral therapist.

## How Did Intensive Treatment Affect Diabetic Eye Disease?

All DCCT participants were monitored for diabetic retinopathy, an eye disease that affects the retina. Study results showed that intensive therapy reduced the risk for developing retinopathy by 76 percent. In participants with some eye damage at the beginning of the study, intensive management slowed the progression of the disease by 54 percent.

The retina is the light-sensing tissue at the back of the eye. According to the National Eye Institute, one of the National Institutes of Health, as many as 24,000 persons with diabetes lose their sight each year. In the United States, diabetic retinopathy is the leading cause of blindness in adults under age 65.

## How Did Intensive Treatment Affect Diabetic Kidney Disease?

Participants in the DCCT were tested to assess the development of diabetic kidney disease (nephropathy). Findings showed that intensive treatment prevented the development and slowed the progression of diabetic kidney disease by 50 percent.

Diabetic kidney disease is the most common cause of kidney failure in the United States and the greatest threat to life in adults with IDDM. After having diabetes for 15 years, one-third of people with IDDM develop kidney disease. Diabetes damages the small blood vessels in the kidneys, impairing their ability to filter impurities from blood for excretion in the urine. Persons with kidney damage must have a kidney transplant or rely on dialysis to cleanse their blood.

## *How Did Intensive Treatment Affect Diabetic Nerve Disease?*

Participants in the DCCT were examined to detect the development of nerve damage (diabetic neuropathy). Study results showed the risk of nerve damage was reduced by 60 percent in persons on intensive treatment.

Diabetic nerve disease can cause pain and loss of feeling in the feet, legs, and fingertips. It can also affect the parts of the nervous system that control blood pressure, heart rate, digestion, and sexual function. Neuropathy is a major contributing factor in foot and leg amputations among people with diabetes.

## *How Did Intensive Treatment Affect Diabetes-Related Cardiovascular Disease?*

DCCT participants were not expected to have many heart-related problems because their average age was only 27 when the study began. Nevertheless, they underwent cardiograms, blood pressure tests, and laboratory tests of blood fat levels to look for signs of cardiovascular disease. The study proved that volunteers on intensive treatment had significantly lower risks of developing high blood cholesterol, a cause of heart disease. The risk was 35 percent lower in these volunteers, suggesting that intensive treatment can help prevent heart disease.

## *What Are the Risks of Intensive Treatment?*

In the DCCT, the most significant side effect of intensive treatment was an increase in the risk for low blood sugar episodes severe enough to require assistance from another person. This is called severe hypoglycemia. Because of this risk, DCCT researchers do not recommend intensive therapy for children under age 13, people with heart disease or advanced complications, older adults, and people with a history of frequent severe hypoglycemia. Persons in the intensive management group also gained a modest amount of weight, suggesting that intensive treatment may not be appropriate for people with diabetes who are overweight.

DCCT researchers estimate that intensive management doubles the cost of managing diabetes because of increased visits to health care professionals and the need for more frequent blood testing at home. However, this cost is offset by the reduction in medical expenses related to long-term complications and by the improved quality of life of people with diabetes.

Results of the DCCT are reported in the *New England Journal of Medicine*, 329(14), September 30, 1993. Other articles related to the DCCT will be published in various journals during the next few years. For reprints of articles, please write to:

National Diabetes Information Clearinghouse
1 Information Way
Bethesda, Maryland 20892-3560

## Chapter 55

# *Diabetes Prevention Trial—Type 1*

### *What Is the DPT-1?*

The Diabetes Prevention Trial DPT-1 is a randomized, controlled, clinical trial designed to determine if it is possible to prevent or delay the onset of Type 1, or Insulin-Dependent Diabetes Mellitus (IDDM), in people predicted to be at risk for this disease. The DPT-1 is a multi-centered study sponsored by the National Institute of Diabetes and Digestive and Kidney Diseases (NIDDK), in cooperation with the National Institute of Child Health and Human Development, the National Institute of Allergy and Infectious Diseases, the National Center for Research Resources, the Juvenile Diabetes Foundation International and the American Diabetes Association. The DPT-1 started in early 1994 and will be carried out at medical centers around the nation for 6 years.

### *How Can We Predict Who Will Get Diabetes?*

IDDM is caused by a defect in an individual's immune system which triggers the body to destroy its own insulin producing cells. Insulin is a hormone that regulates how the body uses and stores food for energy and is necessary to sustain life. It is made in the pancreas

---

Information in this chapter is from the Barbara Davis Center for Childhood Diabetes, 4200 East 9th Avenue, Denver, CO 80262, (303) 315-8796, reprinted with permission granted in 1998; and the National Institute of Diabetes and Digestive and Kidney Diseases (NIDDK).

by a special cell called the islet, or beta cell. Lack of insulin causes high blood sugars which may result in symptoms such as weight loss, thirst, and increased urination. The onset of these symptoms is often abrupt. However, the initial trigger leading to beta cell loss occurs years earlier. Beta cell destruction is a gradual process of slow deterioration. Eventually diabetes develops, but only after most of the beta cells have been destroyed. Today there are blood tests which help us predict just who will develop IDDM and when:

**Islet Cell Autoantibodies (ICAs):** This is a blood test that measures the levels of antibodies against islet cells long before the onset of IDDM. Close relatives of a person with IDDM who test positive for ICAs are much more likely to develop IDDM than are relatives who test negative. The DPT-1 will use this as a screening test to determine if you are eligible for further testing.

**Insulin Autoantibodies (IAAs):** This blood test measures antibodies produced by the body against its own insulin. When associated with ICA, these signify an increased risk of developing IDDM.

**First-Phase Insulin Release (FPIR):** This is a more sophisticated blood test performed by an intravenous glucose tolerance test (IVGTT). This test measures the degree of beta cell damage that has already occurred.

Taken together, information from these three tests allow researchers to estimate a person's relative risk of developing IDDM within the next five years. (**Note:** All blood tests are free to you.)

## What Type of Treatments Will Be Tested in the DPT-1?

If you are found to be ICA-positive at screening, you may be invited to undergo additional testing to determine what your chances are for developing IDDM within the next five years. Volunteers will be selected on the basis of their likelihood of developing diabetes for enrollment into one of two randomized, controlled prevention trials testing two different forms of insulin therapy.

**Insulin Injection Trial:** This trial is for individuals who have more than a 50% chance of developing diabetes within five years. This trial will test the effectiveness of giving low-doses of long-acting insulin administered twice daily coupled with periodic intervals of intensified insulin treatment. This treatment has a minimal risk of causing low blood sugars. One half of those enrolled in this trial will be randomly assigned to the treatment being tested; the other half will not be given any form of treatment but will be under close clinical observation.

Both groups will benefit by having the opportunity for early diagnosis of diabetes well before any clinical symptoms appear enabling initiation of standard diabetes therapy much sooner than would usually occur. Participants in this trial will need to visit the Barbara Davis Center for Childhood Diabetes or other participating clinical research center twice a year for follow-up; one of these visits will require several days of hospitalization for administration of intensified insulin therapy for individuals receiving the insulin treatment.

**Oral Insulin Trial:** Started in 1996, another trial began for individuals who have between a 25% to 50% chance of developing diabetes within five years. This trial will test whether taking a capsule containing insulin crystals, will reduce the chances of developing IDDM. (The capsule can be swallowed whole, or its contents can be sprinkled on food.)

One half of the participating patients will randomly be assigned to receive this "active" drug and the other half will receive an inactive capsule containing a harmless substance (placebo). Neither the participant nor the researchers will know which treatment has been assigned. (Of course, this information can be immediately available if necessary.)

Both groups will benefit from the opportunity for early diagnosis of diabetes, should it develop during the course of the study, and initiation of early standard treatment. Participants in this study will need to visit the Barbara Davis Center for Childhood Diabetes or other participating clinical research center twice a year for follow-up; however, there is no hospitalization associated with this treatment.

**Please Note:** Volunteers cannot choose, but rather must qualify, for enrollment into either the Insulin Injection Trial or the Oral Insulin Trial on the basis of their likelihood of developing IDDM within the next five years. Also, while there is no cost to the participant for either of these treatments or for the required hospitalization, participants may have to pay their own expenses for travel to a clinical center.

## *Why Should I Volunteer for the Study?*

Clinical evidence exists which strongly suggests it may be possible to prevent IDDM. Researchers have already observed in preliminary studies that giving insulin injections to high risk individuals has the potential to halt, slow, or delay the progression of the disease. The DPT-1 trial is the first controlled clinical trial designed to determine if this treatment can be used to prove this encouraging possibility. Individuals with IDDM are dependent upon multiple daily injections to stay well. They also require multiple daily blood sugar tests and meal planning to maintain the good blood sugar levels needed to delay the complications of the disease. The severe long-term complications of IDDM include blindness, kidney failure, amputation, nerve damage, heart disease and stroke.

Since only 3-6% of all relatives of individuals with IDDM will be at risk for developing diabetes, it is estimated that at least 60,000 people will need to be screened to complete these two trials which will test two different treatments to prevent IDDM.

If you are screened for the DPT-1, you will learn if you are at risk for developing IDDM. If so, you will then have the opportunity to participate in a study that will determine whether or not it is possible to delay the onset of the disease.

Please recognize that your participation in this study will require a significant personal commitment in time and energy. Treatment for those who qualify for the trial may require that you take either daily insulin injections, or capsules, and that you travel to a clinical center for evaluation and testing on a regular basis. (Some treatments will also require hospitalization.) However, unlike people who already have diabetes, you will not have to make any other changes in your lifestyle or eating habits since you will not have diabetes, although the treatment may be similar.

If you are eligible and decide to volunteer for the study, your participation will help us answer critical questions about these preventive treatments and show whether it is possible to prevent IDDM. Not only may you be helping yourself, but you may be helping many other people who could benefit in the future by what we learn during these studies.

## Who Is Eligible?

For the ***Insulin Injection Trial***, a person must be:

- ***Between the ages of 4 and 45*** and be a ***first-degree relative*** (an immediate family member) of an individual with IDDM (Type 1 diabetes) such as a son, daughter, parent, brother or sister. ***Or***

- ***Between the ages of 4 and 20*** and be a ***second- or third-degree relative*** (a more distant family member) of an individual with IDDM such as a cousin, niece, nephew, aunt, uncle or grandchild.

For the ***Oral Insulin Trial***, a person must be:

- ***Between the ages of 3 and 45*** for first-degree relatives and ***3 and 20*** for second-degree relatives.

**For both trials, a person must:**

- Test positive for islet-cell autoantibodies (ICAs) based on blood screening conducted at the DPT-1 central laboratory.
- Not have diabetes already.
- Have no previous history of being treated with insulin or oral diabetes medications.
- Have not received any prior therapy for prevention of IDDM such as insulin, nicotinamide, or immunosuppressive drugs (i.e., have not been involved in any previous clinical studies of these agents).
- Have no known serious diseases.
- If you are a woman, you must not be planning to become pregnant during the course of the study. (You will not be excluded from participation, but are not encouraged to volunteer in the first place if you plan to have a baby during the trial period).
- Be willing to follow the DPT-1 protocol for the trial for which you qualify:

  For the **Insulin Injection Trial**, this means taking the treatment assigned to you for up to four to six years. For those assigned to the *Experimental Treatment* group, this means taking two daily injections coupled with periodic intensified treatment and agreeing to go to a clinical center twice a year for testing and treatment. For volunteers assigned to the *Standard Treatment* group, this means agreeing to come to a clinical center twice a year for follow up testing.

For those enrolled in the **Oral Insulin Trial**, this means taking the treatment assigned to you (one daily capsule) for up to three to five years. You must also be willing to travel periodically to the Barbara Davis Center for Childhood Diabetes or other participating clinical center for follow up.

## Who Can Be Screened?

Only first degree relatives of people with IDDM (Type 1 diabetes) who are less than age 45, and second-degree relatives less than age 20, are eligible for screening, children below age 3 may be screened, but they will not be enrolled in either trial until the minimum age is reached.

IDDM differs from the more common form of the disease, noninsulin-dependent diabetes (NIDDM), or Type 2 diabetes. We are **not** screening relatives of persons with NIDDM because the treatments being tested in the DPT-1 will not benefit anyone with a family history of NIDDM since it is not an autoimmune disease. People with IDDM mostly develop diabetes before age 40, have always been treated with insulin injections, and often may have had sudden onset of severe symptoms (weight loss, hunger, thirst, increased urination) at the time of diagnosis.

In contrast, people develop NIDDM generally after age 40, are often overweight, and frequently use oral medications, diet and exercise without insulin injections to manage their diabetes. People who currently take insulin but were previously controlled without insulin on any of the other therapies most likely do not have IDDM.

We encourage you to bring information about the study and screening procedures to your family doctor who may wish to screen several family members at one time or to provide this opportunity for screening to other patients. We also encourage your doctor to call any of the participating centers listed below to discuss the study in further detail.

## Where Can I Go to Be Screened?

The first step toward participating in this study is to have your blood tested for islet-cell antibodies (ICAs). There are several ways to do this:

- You can arrange to have a free screening by contacting The Barbara Davis Center for Childhood Diabetes or another of the DPT-1 clinical centers listed below. Each center has a list of cooperating clinical sites where you may also go for a free screening nearest your home. (There are more than 300 screening sites nationwide).

- Or, you may ask your local physician to assist you. Simply provide your family doctor with information about the DPT-1 and blood sample instructions. (Screening kits are available by calling the Operations Coordinating Center or any of the participating clinical centers listed below).

## How Can I Find Out More about the DPT-1 Study?

- To receive information and blood screening forms, you can write or call the national DPT-1 Operations Coordinating Center at:

Diabetes Prevention Trial DPT-1
P.0. Box 016960 (D-110)
Miami, FL 33101
1-800-HALT-DM1 (1-800-425-8361)

- If you need further information, you can write or call any of the DPT-1 clinical centers listed below. Members of the DPT-1 clinical staff can answer any questions you may have about the study.

## DPT-1 Clinical Centers

### California

Childrens Hospital of Los Angeles
Box 61/ 4650 Sunset Boulevard
Los Angeles, CA 90027
Tel: 1-888-835-3761
Fax: (213) 953-1349
E-mail: jvalenzuela%smtgate@chlais.usc.edu

University of Southern California
LA County Medical Center
Endocrine & Diabetes Service, Rm. 19629B
Los Angeles, CA 90033
Tel: (213) 226-7626
Fax: (213) 226-5709
E-mail: azeidler@hsc.usc.edu

Stanford University
S-302 Medical Center
Stanford, CA 94305-5119
Tel: (650) 725-0497
Fax: (650) 725-8375
E-mail:
darrell@forsythe.stanford.edu
MN.DEL@forsythe.stanford.edu

### *Colorado*

Barbara Davis Center for
Childhood Diabetes
Box B140/ 4200 East 9th Avenue
University of Colorado
Denver, CO 80262
Tel: 1-800-572-3992
Fax: (303) 315-4124
E-mail: sherrie.harris@uchsc.edu

### *Florida*

University of Florida
Box 100275
Gainesville, FL 32610-0275
Tel: 1-800-749-7424, ext. 2-7836
or 1-800-552-0219
Fax: (352) 392-3053
E-mail:
Dennis.pathology@mail.health.ufl.edu

University of Miami
P.O. Box 016960 (D-110)
Miami, FL 33101
Tel: (305) 243-DPT-1 (305-243-3781)
Fax: (305) 243-3313
E-mail:
dmatheson@mednet.med.miami.edu

### *Massachusetts*

Joslin Diabetes Center/Children's
Hospital /Beth Israel Hospital
1 Joslin Place
Boston, MA 02215
Tel: 1-800-2-HALT-DM (1-800-242-5836)
Fax: (617) 732-2432
E-mail:
dconboy@joslin.harvard.edu

### *Minnesota*

University of Minnesota
Box 101/ 516 Delaware Street, SE
Minneapolis, MN 55455
Tel: 1-800-688-5252, ext. 58944
Fax: (612) 626-3133
E-mail:
robertso@lenti.med.umn.edu

### *Washington*

University of Washington
1660 S. Columbian Way #358285
Seattle, WA 98108
Tel: (206) 543-4561
Fax: (206) 764-2615
E-mail:
diabetes@u.washington.edu

## Chapter 56

# *Diabetes Prevention Program—Type 2*

On June 10, 1996 the National Institutes of Health (NIH) announced the first nationwide research study to determine whether Type 2 diabetes can be prevented or delayed in people likely to develop the disease.

Called the Diabetes Prevention Program, the study will examine whether lowering blood sugar levels in people with a condition called "impaired glucose tolerance" (IGT) can help prevent or delay development of Type 2 diabetes. IGT is a precursor to diabetes. People with IGT have high blood sugar, but not high enough to be diagnosed as diabetes.

The study is seeking 4,000 participants who have IGT—including people with a family history of diabetes, overweight individuals, and women who had diabetes during pregnancy, (gestational diabetes).

"Approximately 21 million Americans have higher than normal blood sugar levels or IGT. Most of these people don't know they have IGT and that they may be at risk for developing Type 2 diabetes sometime during their lives," said Phillip Gorden, M.D., director of the National Institute of Diabetes and Digestive and Kidney Diseases (NIDDK). "The Diabetes Prevention Program will study two new classes of diabetes drugs and lifestyle changes, all of which have been proven in smaller studies to lower blood sugar and help prevent progression of IGT to Type 2 diabetes."

---

National Institutes of Health Press Release June 10, 1996 and Diabetes Prevention Program, National Institute of Diabetes and Digestive and Kidney Diseases.

The study seeks 2,000 minority volunteers, including African Americans, Hispanic Americans, American Indians, and Asian and Pacific Island Americans, all of whom have disproportionately high rates of Type 2 diabetes. Twenty percent of volunteers will be age 65 or older and 20 percent will be women who have had gestational diabetes.

"This country has seen a tripling of diabetes over the past 30 years, and as baby boomers continue to age, gain weight and remain inactive, Type 2 diabetes will only become more common, more costly and more destructive," said Frank Vinicor, M.D., M.P.H., president of the American Diabetes Association. "We are proud to support the Diabetes Prevention Program and are confident it will yield results that will benefit millions of Americans at risk for this serious disease.

Volunteers will be randomly assigned to one of four groups: intensive lifestyle changes to reduce weight by seven percent; intervention with the drug metformin, currently used to treat Type 2 diabetes; intervention with the drug troglitazone, currently being tested for treatment of Type 2 diabetes; and the control group, who will take placebo pills in place of the two drugs and will receive information on diet and exercise.

"The Diabetes Prevention Program investigators are confident that one or more of the interventions will be effective in decreasing the development of Type 2 diabetes," said David M. Nathan, M.D., the study chairman.

Approximately 15 million Americans have Type 2 diabetes, and half don't know it yet. Another 21 million Americans have IGT and half of them go on to develop Type 2 diabetes. Diabetes costs the U.S. $92.6 billion a year. With Type 2 diabetes, the body cannot effectively use insulin, the hormone that regulates how cells use sugar from food. As a result, blood sugar levels can build to dangerously high levels, causing damage to the eyes, kidneys, nerves and heart. Diabetes is a leading cause of blindness, amputation, kidney failure, heart attacks and strokes in adults in the United States.

Twenty-five medical centers nationwide are participating in the Diabetes Prevention Program. Volunteers can call 1-888-377-5646 (1-888-DPP JOIN) for a list of participating centers. The announcement was made by the National Institute of Diabetes and Digestive and Kidney Diseases of NIH at the American Diabetes Association annual meeting.

The Diabetes Prevention Program is sponsored by the National Institute of Diabetes and Digestive and Kidney Diseases, part of the NIH. It also is supported by the National Institute of Child Health and Human Development, National Institute on Aging, Office of Research on Minority Health, Indian Health Service, Centers for Disease Control and Prevention, and the American Diabetes Association. Corporate support is being provided by: Bristol-Myers Squibb Company, Health o meter, Inc., Lifescan, Inc., Lipha Pharmaceuticals, Inc., Parke- Davis, and Sankyo Pharmaceutical Co.

### *What is the Diabetes Prevention Program?*

The Diabetes Prevention Program (DPP) is a nationwide research study looking at ways people like you can avoid getting diabetes. The study is sponsored by the Federal government's National Institutes of Health.

Right now there is no cure for diabetes. But doctors believe that diabetes may be avoided by eating healthy food, exercising more, or taking pills. We are looking for volunteers to help find out if this is true.

### *Who can join?*

Men and women age 25 or older who are likely to get diabetes.

### *What will I be asked to do?*

If you join the study, you may be asked to:

- Exercise and eat healthy food.
- Take pills that lower blood sugar and may help prevent diabetes.
- Visit our medical center on a regular basis over three to six years to have your blood sugar level, weight and blood pressure checked.

### *How may I benefit?*

- You will receive free physical exams.
- A team of caring doctors and nurses will see you regularly to help you stay in good health throughout the study.
- You may be able to avoid getting diabetes.
- You may help your family in the future by contributing to medical research.

### *What is diabetes?*

Diabetes causes too much sugar in the blood. It can lead to blindness, amputations, kidney failure and heart attacks. Diabetes affects people of all backgrounds, but is more common in overweight and older people, and in certain ethnic groups, including:

- African Americans
- Hispanic Americans
- American Indians
- Asian Americans
- Pacific Islanders

### *How can I join?*

To join the DPP, please call the medical center in your area:

**Southwest American Indian Center for Diabetes Prevention**
Salt River and Gila River Indian Communities
Phoenix, Arizona
602-200-5338

**University of California, Los Angeles**
Culver City, CA
310-559-0774

**University of California, San Diego**
LaJolla, California
619-642-0225

**University of Southern California**
Los Angeles, California
213-226-7959

**University of Colorado**
**Health Sciences Center**
Denver, Colorado
303-315-7854

**University of Miami**
**School of Medicine**
Miami, Florida
305-243-3411

**University of Hawaii**
Honolulu, Hawaii
808-537-7155

**Northwestern University Medical School**
Chicago, Illinois
312-908-9500

**University of Chicago Hospitals**
Chicago, Illinois
773-702-9655

**Indiana University—Purdue University at Indianapolis**
Indianapolis, Indiana
317-278-0854

**Pennington Biomedical Research Center**
Baton Rouge, Louisiana
504-763-2596

**Johns Hopkins**
**School of Medicine**
Baltimore, Maryland
410-281-2990

**Joslin Diabetes Center**
Boston, Massachusetts
617-735-1907

**Massachusetts General Hospital**
Boston, Massachusetts
617-724-3197

**Washington University**
**School of Medicine**
St. Louis, Missouri
1-800-434-7465 or 314-454-4111

**University of New Mexico School of Medicine**
Albuquerque, New Mexico
505-272-8269

Northern Navajo
**Medical Center**
Shiprock, New Mexico
505-368-6345

**Pueblo of Zuni**
Zuni, New Mexico
505-782-4555

**St. Luke's—Roosevelt Hospital**
New York, New York
212-523-8989

**Diabetes Center—Albert Einstein College of Medicine**
Bronx, New York
718-405-8274 or 1-800-974-9669

**University of Pittsburgh Medical Center**
Pittsburgh, Pennsylvania
412-383-2194

**Thomas Jefferson University**
**Jefferson Medical College**
Philadelphia, Pennsylvania
1-800-JEFFNOW or 215-955-0444

**University of Tennessee, Memphis**
Memphis, Tennessee
901-448-8400 or 1-800-916-2606

**University of Texas Health Science Center**
San Antonio, Texas
210-567-4799

**University of Washington**
Seattle, Washington
206-764-2768

**Medlantic Clinical Research Center**
Washington, D.C.
202-675-2082

Don't let diabetes catch up with you. Join the DPP today. If you have a family member with **Type 1 diabetes**, you may be eligible to participate in another study called the *Diabetes Prevention Trial*. Call 1-800-HALT-DM1 (1-800-425-8361)

# Chapter 57

# *New Study Supports Need for Lower Blood Pressure*

Results of a new study suggest that lowering blood pressure may curb kidney disease, especially in African Americans.

Researchers funded by the National Institute of Diabetes and Digestive and Kidney Diseases (NIDDK) report that reducing blood pressure to a mean arterial pressure of less than 92, or about 125/75 millimeters of mercury (mmHg), slowed kidney disease in people who had more than 1 gram of protein in the urine. At higher blood pressures the disease advanced more quickly, especially in blacks, who lost kidney function 7 times faster than whites, according to researchers. The study appears in the September 9 issue of *Hypertension*.

"What we found is that it is important to control blood pressure, especially in blacks with protein in the urine," said Lee A. Hebert, lead author of the study and head of nephrology at Ohio State University Medical Center in Columbus.

Hebert and colleagues compared the effects of normal (below 140/90) and low (about 125/75) blood pressure in a group of 53 African Americans and 495 whites with moderate kidney disease. These men and women are a subset of the original 840 patients who took part in NIDDK's Modification of Diet in Renal Disease (MDRD) Study, which ended in 1993.

However, because the study data came from a subset of MDRD patients and because some other studies have shown contradictory

---

National Institute of Diabetes and Digestive and Kidney Diseases. This undated factsheet was downloaded from NIDDK's website in June 1998 (www.niddk.nih.gov).

results and cardiovascular problems in some patients when they reduced blood pressure, doctors aren't ready to recommend the lower blood pressure level for all patients. "These results are important, but it's not appropriate to base major health policy on a secondary analysis," said Lawrence Agodoa, a nephrologist and co-author of the report. "You really need a larger study to settle the question."

"We think everyone with hypertension can help protect the kidneys and the heart by controlling blood pressure, but we still don't know what level is best," said Hebert. "And we don't know what will happen in kidney disease due to hypertension," he added. Relatively few people in the study had this type of disease even though it is the major cause of kidney disease in African Americans and causes a high percentage of kidney disease in whites.

In contrast to other kidney diseases, which "come from problems within the kidney itself," Hebert explains, "kidney disease from high blood pressure comes from the outside. If we can remove the external cause—the hypertension—we might be able to stop the kidney disease in its tracks."

Researchers hope to finally settle the debate with another NIDDK trial, the African American Study of Kidney Disease and Hypertension (AASK), which is now enrolling patients. AASK is comparing low and normal blood pressure and specific classes of blood pressure drugs to control hypertension and protect the kidneys.

Patients can call 1-800-277-2275 for more information on AASK.

# Chapter 58

# *Clinical Islet Transplant Initiative*

The Diabetes Research Institute is currently testing a number of approaches involving islet cell transplantation. Today, there are multiple DRI protocols already approved that enable researchers to offer islet cells as an option to patients who are eligible for participation. Some of these trials include *Islets after Kidney* (IAK), *Simultaneous Kidney and Islets with Bone Marrow* (SKI*),* and the *Islets and Bone Marrow Alone* (IBMA) trial, scheduled to begin in early 1998. This last trial will herald a new phase of clinical trial testing at the DRI, the result of years of cumulative years of work. Because the DRI team has performed more islet cell transplants than any other investigative team to date, the Institute is the ideal location for this next important phase of testing to begin.

This new phase of clinical trials will test a variety of approaches that share one common goal: improved islet acceptance without the adverse side effects associated with chronic use of anti-rejection medications. The DRI's Islet Transplant Initiative will draw on its existing collaborations with the Navy and other academic partners, such as the University of Minnesota, to bring the most promising technologies and approaches to patient application as rapidly as possible. New developments that have arisen as a result of this initiative include the testing of exciting new molecules such as anti-CD154 ligand, the use of multiple high-dose bone marrow infusions, and the possibility of a testing center for new encapsulation devices.

---

Diabetes Research Institute, University of Miami School of Medicine, February 1998; reprinted with permission.

The progress made in islet isolation techniques—from the standardization of pancreas retrieval procedures to the current FDA-DRI efforts to establish benchmarks for islet isolations performed in this country—will ensure that future islet transplants will be the safest they have ever been.

## Background

When DRI researchers cured diabetic dogs through islet transplantation in the early 1980's, the hope was to quickly transfer that technology into human application. The first patients selected for the initial clinical trials were those who received kidney transplants and already required immunosuppressive drugs to prevent rejection of their new organs. In 1985, the first clinical islet transplant was conducted in a young woman. The transplanted islets greatly improved her blood sugar control, and her insulin requirement was reduced by almost 75 percent. However, the islet graft failed after one year. This failure was attributed to two factors: the insufficient number of islets isolated and transplanted, and the possible destruction of the "foreign" cells by the recipient's immune system. These two obstacles impeded the progress of human clinical trials until 1990, when Dr. Camillo Ricordi developed the automated method for islet isolation and purification that is now used by researchers worldwide. The Ricordi method, as it is called, enabled researchers to isolate a much larger number of islet cells from each donor pancreas.

With the ability to transplant greater numbers of purified islets, leading scientists launched numerous new clinical trials. Drs. Mintz and Alejandro from the Diabetes Research Institute and Drs. Ricordi and Tzakis, then at the University of Pittsburgh, combined their efforts in a unique clinical trial. Patients with extensive abdominal cancer underwent multiple organ transplants to replace their affected organs. In each case, the pancreas had to be removed and, since earlier efforts to transplant the entire pancreas had failed, the surgical team turned to islet transplantation to prevent diabetes from occurring in these pancreatectomized patients.

Using the new isolation techniques and modified protocols for immunosuppression, eight patients underwent these "cluster" organ transplants. Each received islet cells through the portal vein to the newly transplanted liver. In all eight cases, islet function was achieved. Sadly, most of these patients eventually succumbed to cancer, their primary disease. However, the first patient, a 15 year old girl, survived for five years, never once needing an insulin injection.

When she died, an autopsy revealed that the transplanted islets had been healthy and producing insulin. This case proved that islet cells could be isolated from a pancreas in sufficient numbers, transplanted into a liver successfully, and produce enough insulin to normalize blood sugars for at least five years.

While subsequent clinical trials have been limited to patients requiring organ transplants and therefore, immunosuppressive therapy, there is evidence that the drugs used to prevent rejection may themselves adversely affect the transplanted islets. The DRI is currently studying several factors which may help protect newly transplanted islets and enhance engraftment (the establishment of a blood supply to cells). In addition, the DRI's transplant immunology team is conducting research to identify which particular bone marrow cells are responsible for enhancing donor-specific tolerance and which cells may be acting as triggers for the rejection process.

The landmark Diabetes Control and Complication Trial (DCCT), funded by the National Institutes of Health, determined that normalizing blood glucose levels over time can greatly reduce the risk of long-term complications. However, the intensive management required to improve diabetes control also increased the likelihood of severe hypoglycemia. At the International Pancreas and Islet Transplantation Association (IPITA) meetings held in Miami in June of 1995, scientists from five centers presented data on the glucose control of their patients after islet transplantation. That data revealed that test groups with even partially successful islet transplants were able to achieve better hemoglobin A1c results without episodes of hypoglycemia than either conventional or intensive insulin therapy test groups.

## Tolerance Induction

The goal of islet transplantation research has always been to provide this therapy to patients early in the course of their disease and be able to do so without requiring long-term immunosuppressive therapy. In an effort to enhance transplant acceptance and allow the recipient's immune system to become tolerant of a "foreign" tissue, the DRI and the Division of Transplantation have been involved in an extensive clinical trial using donor bone marrow infusions in order to re-educate the recipient's immune system to accept specific donor tissue. This study, under the direction of Drs. Ricordi and Tzakis, each leaders in their field, determined the safety and effectiveness of single, double and multiple donor bone marrow infusions in organ transplant recipients, as compared to a control group receiving no donor bone marrow. When two or more donor bone marrow infusions were given, there was more than 85 percent graft acceptance, compared to the no bone marrow control group, in which the acceptance rate was only 72 percent. Transplant survival was also shown to improve significantly with the addition of donor bone marrow infusions.

To reduce the risk of adverse effects of high-dose bone marrow infusions, the DRI has been working with two corporate entities to develop procedures for removing certain cells from the bone marrow. The first phase of this program has already been successfully completed and FDA approval is pending for the start of the next phase of clinical trials. Another strategic goal of these new islet cell and multiple donor bone marrow infusion trials will be to test new agents that can potentially block the rejection of transplanted islets. Participants in the trials will be carefully scrutinized to see if a state of chimerism (co-existence of donor and recipient cells) has been achieved. In addition, immunosuppression will gradually be withdrawn in all patients within the first post-transplant year.

## Chapter 59

# *Pathfinders for Health—Studies among the Pima Indians*

History paints a colorful portrait of the American Indians who live today in the Gila River Indian Community. Their ancestors were among the first people to set foot in the Americas 30,000 years ago. They have lived in the Sonoron Desert near the Gila River in what is now southern Arizona for at least 2,000 years.

Called the Pima Indians by exploring Spaniards who first encountered them in the 1600s, these early Americans called themselves "O'Odham," the River people, and those with whom they intermarried, "Tohono O'Odham," the Desert people.

Archaeological finds suggest that the Pima Indians descended from the Hohokam, "those who have gone," a prehistoric people who originated in Mexico. Strong runners, the Pima Indians were also master weavers and farmers who could make the desert bloom. Once trusted scouts for the U.S. Cavalry, the Pima Indians are pathfinders for health, helping scientists from the National Institute of Diabetes and Digestive and Kidney Diseases (NIDDK), a part of the National Institutes of Health (NIH), learn the secrets of diabetes, obesity, and their complications.

Migrating from Mexico, the people settled the land up to where the Gila River and the Salt River meet, in what is now Arizona. They established a sophisticated system of irrigation that made the desert fruitful with wheat, beans, squash and cotton. The women of the

---

National Institute of Diabetes and Digestive and Kidney Diseases (NIDDK), NIH Pub. No. 95-3821.

community made exquisite baskets so intricately woven that they were watertight.

They were also a generous people. They sheltered the Pee Posh (or Maricopa Indians) who fled attack by hostile tribes, and who also became part of the Gila River community. Anyone who followed the Gila river, the main southern route to the Pacific, encountered these peaceful and productive traders who gave hospitality to travelers for hundreds of years. "Bread is to eat, not to sell. Take what you want," they told Kit Carson in 1846.

Today, the Pima Indians of the Gila River Indian Community are still an agricultural people, nurturing orchards of orange trees, pistachios and olives. They are still giving, too. Eleven thousand strong, the members of the Gila River Indian Reservation have participated in 30 years of research that will help people avoid diabetes, have healthier eyes, hearts, and kidneys, and to understand how and why people gain weight and what can be done to prevent it.

"The Pima Indians are giving a great gift to the world by continuing to volunteer for research studies. Their generosity contributes to better health for all people, and we are all in their debt." says Dr. Peter Bennett, Chief of the Phoenix Epidemiology and Clinical Research Branch of the NIDDK.

The Pima Indians' help is so important to the ability of doctors to understand and treat diabetes, obesity, and kidney disease because of the uniqueness of the community. There are few like it in the world.

Young Pima Indians often marry other Pimas. Many Pima families have lived in the Gila River Indian Community for generations. Because of this, scientists can search for root causes of disease through several generations of many families. The length of NIDDK's study and the number of families involved allows scientists an invaluable perspective on how the disease progresses. The more generations studied, the deeper and better the understanding of how diabetes affects people, and the greater the opportunity to develop drug or genetic therapy, or lifestyle changes that will slow or prevent the coming of disease.

The research takes so long, says NIH scientist Dr. Bill Knowler, because diseases like obesity and diabetes are so hard to understand. There seem to be several different causes, and the complex interaction between the genes a person inherits and the lifestyle a person chooses can make it hard to find treatments and cure. Scientists are trying to find a path through this maze.

Thirty years of research show that exercising and eating lower fat, fiber-rich foods can at least delay diabetes. "If you delay it long enough," adds Dr. Knowler, "it's almost as good as preventing it."

This cooperative search between the Pima Indians and the NIH began in 1963 when the NIDDK (then called the National Institute of Arthritis, Diabetes and Digestive and Kidney Diseases), made a survey of rheumatoid arthritis among the Pimas and the Blackfeet of Montana. They discovered an extremely high rate of diabetes among the Pima Indians. Two years later, the Institute, the Indian Health Service, and the Pima community set out to find some answers to this mystery. They hoped to shed light on an even broader question: Why do Native Americans, Hispanics and other non-white peoples have up to ten times the rate of diabetes as Caucasians?

Three decades' collective efforts by scientists and volunteers have laid the foundation for eventually curing or preventing diabetes and its complications. The work begun in 1965 has yielded a definition of diabetes that is now used worldwide, and set out diagnostic criteria used by doctors from Sacaton, Arizona to Sicily to identify and treat diabetes and to anticipate how it is likely to develop.

Doctors can best treat a disease when they understand what causes it and how it progresses. By studying Pima volunteers for many years, NIH doctors learned that unhealthy weight is a strong predictor of diabetes. Eighty percent of people with diabetes are overweight. They also discovered that high levels of insulin in the blood, or hyperinsulinemia, is another strong risk factor.

Studying this clue, researchers working with patients found that high levels of insulin were linked to insulin resistance. Normally, the pancreas releases insulin to regulate the amount of sugar or glucose in the blood. People who have noninsulin-dependent or Type II diabetes (hereafter referred to simply as "diabetes") produce insulin, but their bodies don't respond to it effectively. NIH researchers have made it clear that people with insulin resistance are those most likely to get diabetes.

By studying Pima Indian volunteers, Dr. Clifton Bogardus and his colleagues established that glucose not needed for immediate energy is converted to glycogen and stored in skeletal muscle. However, several enzymes that drive this natural process appear different in insulin resistant people, according to the researchers, and they continue to study the biochemistry of insulin resistance to understand this breakdown and how it might be repaired.

By studying Pima Indian volunteers, researchers have determined that diabetes runs in families, as does insulin resistance, and obesity. Scientists believe that some people also have a gene that makes them more likely to have the kidney disease that occurs in people who have had diabetes a long time. Looking for these genes is a key part of the search now being conducted by NIH and the Pima Indians.

Researchers are working on this complex genetic puzzle by studying blood drawn from every member of the Pima community who comes into the NIH clinic at Hu Hu Kam Memorial Hospital for an examination. Blood is checked for healthy levels of blood sugar, cholesterol and other nutrients. Then, each person's blood and serum are typed and some is reduced to a very small pellet of DNA, the genetic material that instructs a person's cells to function one way or another. When NIH researchers find a family with one parent who is diabetic and one who is not, they are able to study the genes of both parents and their children in an effort to find the gene or genes shared by those who have diabetes.

After finding these genes, scientists hope to break the codes that cause insulin resistance, obesity, diabetes and kidney disease of diabetes. "If we can locate the genes contributing to disease—some enzyme being made or not being made," explains Dr. Knowler, "we can identify which people are at high risk for the disease and figure out ways to intervene." Finding these genes will help doctors identify youngsters at risk and begin prevention before disease sets in.

Another important finding has already made a difference in how diabetes patients are treated. The complications that come with long-term diabetes—kidney disease, eye disease, and amputations caused by nerve damage—are the major reason for illness and death among the Pima Indians. When Dr. Knowler began his research in Phoenix, few understood what he and his colleagues would discover by working with Pima volunteers: that high blood pressure predicts complications of diabetes such as eye and kidney disease, and that lowering blood pressure may slow the onset of diabetes and the progress of already existing kidney disease. Because of this work, doctors today are not only aware of the need to treat high blood pressure in people with diabetes, but they begin treating it sooner than in the past.

"Our greatest pride," says Dr. Knowler, "is in conducting research that affects clinical practice."

Other research with important implications for future generations is Dr. David Pettitt's study of high blood sugar and diabetes in pregnant women. By working with Pima volunteers, Dr. Pettitt found that children born to diabetic women are more likely to be overweight and more likely to develop diabetes than children of women who have not developed diabetes.

Dr. Eric Ravussin conducts studies that measure food intake, metabolism, and energy expenditure to evaluate their interaction and contribution to a genetic predisposition to obesity.

Now NIH and the Pima Indians are building on these accomplishments. "The search goes forward on two fronts," says Dr. Knowler.

"We're working hard on the genetics of the disease. We're optimistic we will find one or more genes. It's still hard to predict how we might prevent diabetes, but we might, for example, be able eventually to correct the genetic difference that causes disease. More immediately, identifying the diabetes genes would allow us to identify the people most likely to get the disease."

The second strategy is to encourage those who are at high risk to change behaviors that can lead to diabetes, such as eating a high fat diet, being physically inactive, and being overweight.

The NIH has begun a major nationwide program to prevent diabetes in people who increase exercise and eat lower fat foods. Fifty percent of the volunteers will be American Indians and other minorities, and once again, the Pima Indians will be prominent among them. Health for this and future generations: that's the NIH-Pima goal.

*—section by Jane DeMouy*

## The Pima Indians and Genetic Research

Why do so many Pima Indians have diabetes? The question is simple, but the answers are not. They are part of a very complex puzzle that NIH researchers are trying to decode through genetic research.

There are approximately 100,000 genes packed into 23 pairs of chromosomes in each person. Within a gene, chemicals form individual codes, like words, which tell the cells of the body what to do. It is the code within a gene that directs the body to grow skin, and determines whether the skin is brown, yellow, black or white; to form hair and bone; to circulate blood and hormones such as adrenalin and insulin; and to perform every other biological process in the body.

Some diseases are caused by bacteria or viruses that infect the body and make it sick. Others, such as diabetes, occur because a gene's code causes it to function differently under some circumstances. For instance, if a person has a gene that makes that person likely to get diabetes, eating a lot of high fat food over time may increase that person's chance of getting sick. On the other hand, eating lower fat foods such as fruits and vegetables and exercising each day may help to prevent the disease. A person can't choose his or her genes, but can choose what to eat and whether or not to exercise.

Finding the gene or genes that may increase a person's risk for getting diabetes and obesity is the most effective way scientists have to learn what's wrong in a diabetic person.

With the help of the Pima Indians, NIH scientists have already learned that diabetes develops when a person's body doesn't use insulin effectively. They know that other genes probably influence some people's bodies to burn energy at a slow rate, and/or to want to eat more, making it more likely that they will become overweight. Being overweight, in turn, puts a person at even higher risk for diabetes. Because they have learned this over 30 years of working with the Pima Indians, NIH scientists now are able to test ways to prevent the disease with low-fat diets and regular exercise.

When scientists find the codes for the genes that contribute to diabetes and obesity, they will be able to study how the genes work, and how the changes that result might contribute to disease. Then they will have the best clues available to design treatments and cures.

DNA, each human being's personal collection of genes, is as individual as a thumbprint. Because the code for a particular gene can be slightly different in each person, tracking genes is difficult, time-consuming work. It is possible to do this work only when scientists have the cooperation of large families.

Mormon families in Salt Lake City helped researchers find a gene for colon cancer, and a large group of related families in Venezuela contributed their blood and skin samples so researchers could identify the gene for Huntington's disease. Now Pima families from the Gila River Indian Community are making it possible for NIDDK researchers to search for diabetes and obesity genes.

If it were not for families of Pima Indian volunteers and technology developed in the last 10 years, it would not be possible to search for the genetic causes of so complex a disease as diabetes, according to Dr. Clifton Bogardus of NIDDK.

"We got into this work because of Pima families," Dr. Bogardus says. "NIDDK scientists, including Drs. Bennett, Knowler, and Pettitt, have studied well over 90 percent of the people on the reservation at least once. We know the families, and DNA has been collected from them routinely since the mid 1980s."

Shortly after that, other scientists began to develop ways of creating maps that show where genes are located on chromosomes in cells. They learned how to cut a fragment of DNA, and find its code. Because fragments of DNA will naturally attach to complementary fragments like a zipper, scientists learned how to identify unfamiliar pieces of DNA by using familiar fragments that were electronically labeled. If the labeled DNA found a match, scientists were able to use x-ray film to make a "picture" of the unfamiliar DNA fragment.

When researchers have volunteers from large families of several generations whose medical and genetic history is well known to them, blood samples from those volunteers are extremely valuable in learning about a disease. Using laboratory techniques, they can separate the volunteers' DNA from their blood, and compare DNA from family members who have disease and those who do not.

The researchers look for a piece of DNA shared only by members of a family who have disease. When they find the same genetic variation in many people with disease, that variation is called a marker. Because a marker and a gene that helps cause disease are often inherited together, researchers can then use that marker like a signpost to search for the sought-after gene itself.

Beginning in 1983 and continuing for 10 years, NIDDK studied the genetic codes of almost 300 non-diabetic Pima Indians in great detail. "We looked at body composition, how well a person produced insulin, how well that person's cells responded to insulin, and other factors. After a number of years, some of the volunteers developed diabetes and we were able to determine that insulin resistance and obesity were major predictors of disease," Dr. Bogardus explains.

Because diabetes is such a complex disease, Dr. Bogardus and his staff are attempting to narrow their search by first looking for the genetic causes of physical conditions that can lead to diabetes, such as the genes that influence a person's cells to secrete less and respond less to insulin that is needed to regulate blood sugar.

In 1993, they identified a gene called FABP2 that may contribute to insulin resistance. This gene makes an intestinal fatty acid binding protein using one of two amino acids. When the gene makes the protein with threonine, one of those amino acids, the body seems to absorb more fatty acids from the fat in meals. NIH scientists think that could lead to a higher level of certain fats and fatty acids in the blood, which could contribute to insulin resistance.

Another group of NIH scientists, led by Dr. Michael Prochazka and Dr. Bruce Thompson, are developing a genetic map for the Pima Indians, a tool that could be very useful in defining what causes so much diabetes in the community. They have already identified a number of markers different from those in the white population.

Researchers sometimes get unexpected results leading to further work, even when they have carefully thought out a project. While studying how a person's cells respond to insulin, biochemist Dr. David Mott identified an enzyme called protein phosphatase 1 that seems to play a role in insulin resistance. "Now it turns out there are actually three of these protein phosphatase enzymes," Dr. Bogardus explains, "so we're trying to figure out which of the three is the most important. We're also trying to find out if there's a difference in one of those three genes in the Pima Indians," he adds.

The NIH gene-seekers hope to answer many questions that could make better health an expectation for diabetes-prone Pima Indians. How do these genes work? What switches these genes on and off? How does a person's life style contribute to disease when these genes are present? Is one gene missing some important chemical? If so, is there a substitute for that chemical's activity?

When they have these answers, doctors may be able to say why the Pima Indians and other non-whites get diabetes so often. They will be better able to identify those who are likely to become diabetic. Most importantly, they will have the pieces of the diabetic puzzle that could be the key to preventing diabetes in new generations of Pima Indians.

*—section by Jane DeMouy*

## Breaking the Vicious Cycle

Researchers working with Pima volunteers have discovered that the baby of a mother who has diabetes during pregnancy has a very high risk of becoming overweight and developing diabetes as a young adult. This added risk is separate from any genetic tendency for diabetes the child may have inherited.

Earlier research has given doctors important information about how a mother's diabetes affects her unborn child, and how to prevent complications in babies whose mothers have diabetes. Scientists know that babies exposed in the womb to high levels of blood sugar (glucose) often have problems at birth. The more uncontrolled a mother's blood sugar is, the bigger the problems:

- Babies of diabetic women are more than three times more likely to have birth defects.
- Overfed through the placenta by high levels of blood sugar, the babies of diabetic mothers may grow too large for safe delivery through the birth canal, and often require delivery by C-section.
- Babies of diabetic women are more often born prematurely, and as a result, have more brain and nerve problems than those born to mothers with normal blood sugar.
- Babies of diabetic women often have changes in the insulin-producing cells of the pancreas, which may place them at risk for problems with glucose metabolism later in life.

- Their mothers are more likely to suffer from toxemia, a life-threatening condition that endangers both mother and infant.

By taking insulin and paying attention to diet and exercise, a woman with diabetes can help keep blood sugar levels as normal as possible during pregnancy. By doing this, she can usually avoid the short-term complications for herself and her baby. For this reason, it is important for a woman to have a glucose tolerance test before and during pregnancy. This test is now routine for pregnant woman all over America because of what NIH doctors have learned from Pima Indian volunteers.

Because of the long-term studies being conducted among the Pima Indians, doctors also now know that a mother's diabetes can affect her child's health many years later. This long-term research has a special place in science. It can give insights and answer questions when other research approaches fall short. Because some of the children born to Pima mothers after the study began are now 28 to 30 years old, researchers are able to understand how a mother's diabetes can influence a child's health in adulthood.

By observing these children over the years, NIH scientists discovered that the children of women with diabetes during pregnancy have a higher risk of becoming obese and getting diabetes earlier in life than those born to mothers who had normal blood sugar during pregnancy but developed diabetes later. Apart from any genetic tendency the children may have inherited, those exposed to high blood sugar in the uterus had an added risk for unhealthy weight and diabetes at a younger age.

"We now know there is a non-genetic cause of diabetes, the diabetic intrauterine environment, which poses problems for the child that extend well beyond those apparent at birth," says Dr. David Pettitt of NIH.

Animal studies also show that exposure to a high level of blood sugar in the uterus has long-lasting effects on offspring. Abnormal changes in pancreatic tissue were seen in rats whose mothers had chemically induced diabetes but no genetic tendency to the disease. As adults, both second and third generation offspring of these rats had abnormal glucose tolerance and gestational diabetes.

"It's a vicious cycle," says Dr. Pettitt. "Children whose mothers had diabetes during pregnancy have a higher risk of becoming obese and getting diabetes at a young age. Many will already have diabetes or abnormal glucose tolerance by the time they reach their childbearing years, thus perpetuating the cycle."

Can the cycle be broken? Researchers hope that recent discoveries will pave the way to preventing obesity and diabetes later in the child's life. Tight control of blood sugar reduces complications for mother and baby at birth. Today, many more babies born to mothers with diabetes survive than did 30 years ago, and doctors know a lot more about how to control diabetes. Strict control of blood sugar can only benefit mother and child. Whether it can also reduce the child's long-term risk of diabetes is a question no one can answer yet.

"The challenge for the future is to see if it's possible to achieve diabetes control good enough to prevent the developing fetus from recognizing that its mother has diabetes," says Dr. Pettitt. "If we can do that, the rate of diabetes in the next generation is likely to decline, an achievement that would benefit not only the immediate children but future generations."

In a joint quest spanning three decades, Pima Indians and NIDDK researchers have begun to unravel some of the mysteries surrounding the causes of diabetes. Each new insight adds to a growing body of knowledge that promises to benefit generations of Pima Indians and millions of others around the world who share a high risk of developing diabetes and its devastating complications.

*– section by Joan Chamberlain*

## Obesity Associated with High Rates of Diabetes in the Pima Indians

NIDDK research conducted in the Pima Indians for the past 30 years has helped scientists prove that obesity is a major risk factor in the development of diabetes. One-half of adult Pima Indians have diabetes and 95% of those with diabetes are overweight.

These studies, carried out with the help of the Pima Indians, have shown that before gaining weight, overweight people have a slower metabolic rate compared to people of the same weight. This slower metabolic rate, combined with a high fat diet and a genetic tendency to retain fat may cause the epidemic overweight seen in the Pima Indians, scientists believe.

Scientists use the "thrifty gene" theory proposed in 1962 by geneticist James Neel to help explain why many Pima Indians are overweight. Neel's theory is based on the fact that for thousands of years populations who relied on farming, hunting and fishing for food, such as the Pima Indians, experienced alternating periods of feast and famine. Neel said that to adapt to these extreme changes in caloric needs, these people developed a thrifty gene that allowed them to store fat during times of plenty so that they would not starve during times of famine.

This gene was helpful as long as there were periods of famine. But once these populations adopted the typical Western lifestyle, with less physical activity, a high fat diet, and access to a constant supply of calories, this gene began to work against them, continuing to store calories in preparation for famine. Scientists think that the thrifty gene that once protected people from starvation might also contribute to their retaining unhealthy amounts of fat.

Dr. Eric Ravussin, a visiting scientist at the Phoenix Epidemiology and Clinical Research Branch at NIDDK, has studied obesity in the Pima Indians since 1984. He believes the thrifty gene theory applies to the Pimas.

The Pima Indians maintained much of their traditional way of life and economy until the late 19th century, when their water supply was diverted by American farmers settling upstream, according to Ravussin. At that time, their 2,000-year-old tradition of irrigation and agriculture was disrupted, causing poverty, malnutrition and even starvation. The Pima community had to fall back on the lard, sugar and white flour the U.S. government gave them to survive, says Ravussin.

However, World War II brought great social and economic change for American Indians. Those who entered military service joined Caucasian units. Many other American Indians migrated from reservations to cities for factory employment and their estimated cash income more than doubled from 1940 to 1944.

When the war and the economic boom ended, most Native Americans returned to the reservations, but contact with the larger society had profoundly affected the Pimas' way of life. Ravussin says it is no surprise that the increase in unhealthy weight among the Pima Indians occurred in those born post-World War II.

During this century people world-wide experienced more prosperity and leisure time, and less physical work. Since the 1920s, all Americans have consumed more fat and sugar and less starch and fiber. The greatest changes have occurred in consumption of fat. In the 1890s, the traditional Pima Indian diet consisted of only about 15 percent fat and was high in starch and fiber, but currently almost 40 percent of the calories in the Pima diet is derived from fat. As the typical American diet became more available on the reservation after the war, people became more overweight.

"The only way to correct obesity is to eat less fat and exercise regularly," Ravussin says.

Recently, Ravussin visited a Pima community living as their ancestors did in a remote area of the Sierra Madre mountains of Mexico. These Mexican Pimas are genetically the same as the Pima Indians of Arizona. Out of 35 Mexican Pimas studied, only three had diabetes and the population as a whole was not overweight, according to Ravussin.

"We've learned from this study of the Mexican Pimas that if the Pima Indians of Arizona could return to some of their traditions, including a high degree of physical activity and a diet with less fat and more starch, we might be able to reduce the rate, and surely the severity, of unhealthy weight in most of the population," Ravussin says.

"However, this is not as easy as it sounds because of factors such as genetic influences that are difficult to change. Our research focuses on determining the most effective way to bring about permanent weight loss in light of these factors," Ravussin adds.

*—section by Lorraine H. Marchand*

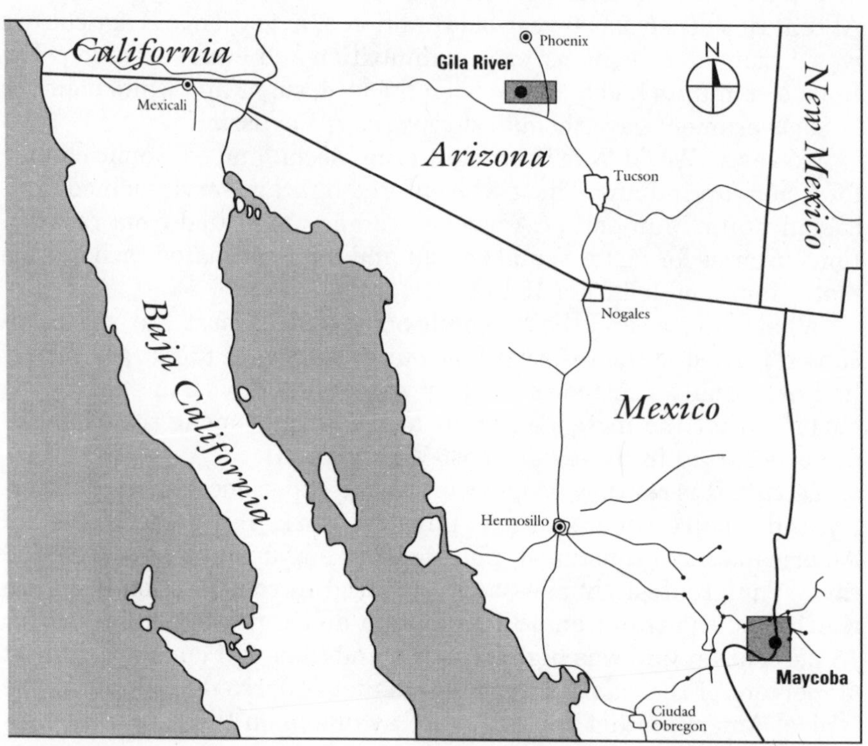


***Figure 59.1.*** *Shaded areas on the above map show where the Pima Indians live.*

## Advanced Technology Used to Measure Energy Expenditure

Since obesity clearly is an important risk factor for diabetes, researchers are working on developing effective methods for helping heavy people lose weight safely and permanently, and for preventing obesity in people with a genetic inclination to gain weight. To better understand why certain people have a tendency to be overweight and how their bodies react to various diets, NIH researchers are measuring many aspects of energy expenditure using precise and highly sophisticated technology.

### Metabolic Chamber

The most accurate methods of determining energy expenditure involve continuous measurements of heat output (direct calorimetry) or exhaled gas exchange (indirect calorimetry) in people confined to metabolic chambers. A metabolic chamber is a small room a person can live in for a 24 hour period, while metabolic rate is measured during meals, sleep, and light activities. Scientists measure the heat released from a person's body to determine how much energy each activity has burned for that person. In indirect calorimetry, researchers measure oxygen consumption, carbon dioxide production and nitrogen excretion to calculate a ratio that reflects energy expenditure.

Both measurements indicate whether a person has a "slow" or "fast" metabolic rate. A person with a lower metabolic rate burns calories slower and is at higher risk for gaining weight than people with higher metabolic rates.

### Indirect Methods Used in Free-Living Conditions

Since living in a chamber for a day or two restricts normal activity, researchers have developed methods to measure energy expenditure in free-living situations. They include monitoring heart rate and maintaining an activity diary. Using a person's activity diary, researchers can compute energy expenditure during various activities.

### Doubly Labeled Water Technique

A form of indirect calorimetry based on the elimination of deuterium and oxygen (18) from urine, the doubly labeled water technique measures the turnover of hydrogen and oxygen into water and carbon dioxide; energy expenditure is calculated from the difference. This method of determining energy expenditure is useful because it enables researchers to measure total carbon dioxide production over a long period of time—from five to 20 days—and yet only requires periodic sampling of urine. People being tested can continue their normal routines because the method does not require special arrangements or devices.

### *Resting Metabolic Rate*

Scientists have known for many years that there is a close correlation between the energy burned at rest (resting metabolic rate, or RMR) and body size. A low RMR is a risk factor for weight gain. In their search for the possible mechanisms underlying the variability in RMR among people, NIDDK researchers have explored the effects of gender, physical training, age, muscle metabolism) sympathetic nervous activity, and body temperature on RMR. In a large number of Caucasian volunteers, scientists found that females had a lower RMR than males because of the effect of sex hormones on metabolic rate. Other studies have demonstrated that diet, physical fitness and body temperature also influence RMR. Scientists also know that aging reduces RMR slightly.

### *Dexa Machine*

The Dexa Machine has replaced underwater weighing as the gold standard in measuring body composition because of its high degree of accuracy. It uses very low doses of radiation—about the amount a person would receive on a plane flight from Phoenix to Denver. A computer calculates the body's absorption of radiation and determines body density—the ratio of fat to muscle mass.

### *Measurement of Sympathetic Nervous Activity*

The sympathetic nervous system, which controls the blood flow and blood pressure in skeletal muscle, plays a role in human obesity through its effect on energy expenditure and food intake. One method used to assess this effect is to measure fasting muscle sympathetic nerve activity in the peroneal nerve and its relationship to energy expenditure and body composition. Researchers have found that sympathetic nervous activity is related to a person's metabolic rate and that reduced sympathetic nervous activity indicates a tendency to gain weight. Pima Indians have reduced sympathetic nervous activity compared to Caucasians of similar age, body weight and body composition.

### *Vending Machine*

Studies have shown that when overweight people are asked to record their daily food intake in a diary they tend to underestimate and record only two-thirds of what they actually ate. Researchers think this tendency to underestimate caloric intake may be part of the reason heavy people overeat. Therefore, NIDDK developed a special vending machine to accurately measure a person's food intake in a day. This computerized, automated food selection device calculates the person's caloric and fat intake and meal duration. Items in the vending machine include entrees such as chili, spaghetti and meat balls, chicken chimichangas, cheese pizza and macaroni and cheese, and snack items, including peanuts, sunflower seeds and french fries. Study volunteers may select foods of their choice but they are required to eat only from the vending machine for a set period of time.

### *Clamp*

The hyperinsulinemia euglycemic clamp is used to measure a person's insulin sensitivity. People with low insulin sensitivity are considered insulin resistant and are more likely to develop diabetes. People with a high degree of insulin sensitivity are less likely to develop diabetes.

## *Kidney Disease of Diabetes in the Pima Indians*

"The Gila River Indian Community may be the smallest town in the United States with its own dialysis center," says Dr. Bill Knowler about this community of 11,000 people. Dr. Knowler and his colleagues at the NIH suspect that the Pima Indians share a gene or genes that make them more likely to develop the kidney disease of diabetes (KDDM) that frequently leads to kidney failure.

The researchers have found that Pima Indians have over 20 times the rate of new cases of kidney failure as the general U.S. population, and diabetes is the culprit over 90 percent of the time. Furthermore, kidney disease is the leading cause of death from disease among Pima Indians who have diabetes.

American Indians have the highest rates of diabetes in the world. About half of adult Pima Indians have diabetes, which they get at a relatively young age. On average, Pima Indians are a mere 36 years old when they get diabetes, compared with Caucasians, who get it at about age 60. The longer a person has diabetes, the greater the risk for developing complications, such as kidney disease. However, recent research shows that keeping blood sugar as close to normal as possible can slow or even prevent complications.

Under normal conditions, the kidneys, nestled on each side of the body under the rib cage, maintain body fluid and salt balance and remove waste. They also help regulate blood pressure and release erythropoietin, a hormone that tells the bone marrow to make red blood cells.

The filtering units of the kidney, called glomeruli, are made up of clusters of tiny blood vessels. They act "like a screen that normally lets water and waste products filter through but holds back most of the protein," Dr. Knowler explains. "Early in the course of diabetes, we are seeing changes in the size of the holes of the screen, so that more protein escapes into the urine," he added. Called microalbuminuria, this excess protein may be one of the first clues that kidney damage has begun.

When the kidney's filters are damaged, the remaining ones have to work harder to make up for the loss. As more of the filters are damaged, the kidneys lose their ability to compensate. When the kidneys decline to only 5 or 10 percent of their original capacity, a person is diagnosed with end-stage kidney disease.

"The real tragedy of kidney disease is that it leads to kidney failure, which means that a person must go on dialysis or have a kidney transplant," Dr. Knowler says.

But recent studies bring hope that the years of collaboration between NIH, other scientists and the Pima community is beginning to bear fruit.

For example, the NIH researchers now know that Pima Indians are more likely to get kidney disease of diabetes if they have high blood pressure, even before onset of diabetes; if they have microalbuminuria, or a family history of protein in the urine or kidney disease; or if they have high blood sugar, or diabetes serious enough to require drug or insulin treatment. If the impact of these risk factors, such as high blood pressure, could be reduced, the onset of kidney disease might be prevented or slowed.

Even with this important information, investigators still needed to know what was happening inside the kidney before they could design treatment studies, according to Dr. Robert Nelson, a researcher from The Cleveland Clinic Foundation who works with Dr. Knowler.

Dr. Nelson explains that studies of patients with insulin-dependent, or Type I diabetes showed that the kidney filters blood faster and the blood moves faster within the kidney when diabetes sets in. It is the higher pressure that comes with those changes that may damage the sensitive filters and allow protein to leak into the urine.

Scientists thought that if the disease process worked the same in Pima Indians with Type II diabetes as in people with Type I diabetes, a special type of drug that reduces blood pressure within the kidney might help prevent or slow the kidney disease. Such a drug, an angiotensin-converting-enzyme (ACE) inhibitor, was recently approved by the Food and Drug Administration for the treatment of kidney disease of Type I diabetes.

Encouraged by this information, the Diabetic Renal Disease Study group, with Dr. Nelson directing patient care, set out to discover whether the kidney in Type II diabetes behaves as it does in Type I diabetes. After measuring kidney function in over 200 Pima Indians, with and without diabetes or kidney disease, the researchers found that the amount of blood filtered within the kidney *does* increase at the onset of Type II, as it does in Type I diabetes. A large European study of kidney function in people with Type II diabetes found the same thing.

After several years of studying how kidney disease of diabetes occurs, Dr. Nelson now believes there is enough evidence to conduct clinical studies to try to prevent its development or progression. A trial using an ACE inhibitor is now under way. Dr. Nelson says that although it seems slow in coming, the research is a "deliberate process" designed to get the best information possible in order to give the best care possible.

In the meantime, the best defense against kidney disease of diabetes—in any group of people—is to try to prevent diabetes from developing at all by maintaining healthy weight, exercising, and following a healthy diet. This is the goal of a new NIH Diabetes Prevention Program in which the Pimas and other American Indians are participating.

Once a person has diabetes, kidney disease might be prevented or slowed by controlling blood sugar levels and blood pressure, and by maintaining healthy weight.

Doctors and the Pima Indians continue to work together toward the day when the Gila River Indian Community will no longer need a dialysis center.

*—section by Mary Harris*

## Diabetic Eye Disease

Preventing diabetic eye disease, or retinopathy, is an important goal of the NIH Research Clinic at Sacaton. Long-term diabetes can cause blood vessels in the retina of the eye to break down, leading to loss of vision and even blindness. Doctors don't know the cause.

There are two things people with diabetes can do to slow, and perhaps prevent that complication, according to Dr. William Knowler: with the help of their doctors, he advises, they should try to keep their blood sugar and blood pressure as close to normal as possible. Secondly, they should have regular eye exams with eye drops to detect any early signs of eye disease, such as small problems in the blood vessels of the retina.

These early signs, called "background retinopathy," usually do not affect eyesight by themselves, but they can lead to a more dangerous stage, called proliferative retinopathy. In this second stage, new blood vessels build up in the retina and branch out into the vitreous humor in the middle of the eye. These blood vessels break and bleed easily, causing a blood clot that steals sight.

The detailed eye exams that can help prevent blindness are available to all residents of the Gila River Indian Community at the NIH Clinic in Sacaton every two years. A patient with background retinopathy should have eye exams more often. The sooner retinopathy is found, the better, says Dr. Knowler.

If retinopathy advances and the changes are spotted soon enough, eye doctors do have treatments to prevent blindness in some cases. They can use lasers to seal damaged blood vessels, preventing them from forming the blood clots that can cause blindness. However, these treatments must be given at just the right time, before serious damage is done to the eye. Until researchers discover the causes of diabetic disease, Dr. Knowler says, "keeping appointments for eye exams can make the difference between keeping or losing eyesight."

## New Study Focuses on Prevention

While scientists are achieving important gains in the improved treatment of diabetes, preventing the disease is a top priority in the diabetes research community. By learning more about why certain people are at high risk for developing diabetes, scientists may be able to develop ways to stop the disease before it starts, or at least delay its development.

Researchers do not yet fully understand why American Indians, and especially the Pima Indians, are more likely to develop diabetes, but one thing is clear—those who are overweight are at high risk. Approximately 80 percent of people with diabetes are overweight.

Studies have shown that American Indians, Africans and Hispanics living in their native homelands—where the traditional diet is low in fat and daily activities involve walking, gardening, farming, and other forms of physical labor—have very low rates of unhealthy weight and diabetes.

When these groups adopt the high fat diet and inactive lifestyle typical of Western civilization, weight gain—and frequently, diabetes and its complications—become significant health problems. Researchers think that if these minority populations returned to their native diet and lifestyle, the risk of diabetes could be reduced and people who already have the disease might be healthier.

To test these and other theories on prevention, NIH has launched a nationwide, multi-center clinical study, the Diabetes Prevention Program, to see if diabetes can be prevented or delayed in people at high risk for developing the disease. The NIH is recruiting several hundred Native Americans at high risk for developing diabetes to participate in the six-year study. Volunteers will be selected from among several American tribes, including the Pima Indians. Dr. William Knowler, chief of the Diabetes and Epidemiology Section at NIDDK, and Dr. Venkat Narayan, an NIDDK visiting scientist, will direct the study in the Pima Indians.

To prepare for this multi-center study, NIH researchers conducted a pilot study with 95 Pima Indians who are diabetes-free and have normal glucose tolerance tests. Researchers wanted to determine if study participants would follow a diet and exercise program, and participate in a cultural education program about their native heritage to learn more about the healthy lifestyle of their ancestors.

"We wanted to find out how best to work with people to bring about lifestyle changes," says Dr. Narayan, co-director of the pilot study.

The two groups in the pilot study were called Pima Action and Pima Pride. Volunteers in the Pima Action group were encouraged to eat a lower-fat, higher-fiber diet. The staff encouraged study participants to increase their consumption of foods such as beans, fruits and vegetables, and suggested recipes that can be prepared at home. The educational program included discussing healthy traditional behaviors that involved nutrition and exercise.

Volunteers in the Pima Action group were also encouraged to exercise three hours a week. Individuals were expected to expend additional calories exercising in leisure and occupational activities they enjoyed, recording their activities in a journal. Program staff met with study volunteers at 3, 6 and twelve month intervals to measure their progress. To maintain motivation and morale, volunteers exercised or worked in groups when possible, and were followed by local trained staff.

While Pima Action focused on weight loss, Pima Pride was an educational program that encouraged study volunteers to discover how their ancestors' values and lifestyle are relevant to their lives. Participants in Pima Pride attended presentations by community members and others to learn more about their ancestors' healthy diets and lifestyles.

Results from the pilot study have been promising, says Dr. Narayan. "What we've seen so far indicates that study participants are eager to try to make healthy lifestyle changes. Individuals have been willing to participate in the study and follow the goals. We're encouraged that the larger study will be successful."

After completing analysis of the data from the pilot study, the researchers will make adjustments to the diet/exercise and cultural education programs. They are developing an intervention that may combine other treatments with the best aspects of the Pima Pride and Pima Action programs. Recruitment for the study should begin in 1996.

*—section by Lorraine H. Marchand*

# Chapter 60

# The Role of Magnesium Supplementation in the Treatment of Diabetes

Numerous research reports and clinical commentaries regarding magnesium deficiency have appeared in recent years. Linkages between magnesium deficiency and insulin resistance, carbohydrate intolerance, accelerated atherosclerosis, dyslipidemia, hypertension, and adverse outcomes in pregnancies complicating diabetes have been observed or postulated. Direct effects of insulin on magnesium metabolism and transport have also been described. Clinical trial results, though limited, have drawn attention to the potential benefits of magnesium replenishment.

To assess the relevancy of these observations to diabetes research and practice, the American Diabetes Association sponsored a consensus conference on magnesium supplementation in the treatment of diabetes on 15-16 May 1992 in Philadelphia, PA. Eight experts in diabetes and related disorders heard 13 presentations from U.S. and European investigators respected in the field of magnesium metabolism and its impact on health and disease. The consensus panel was asked to answer the following five questions focusing on diagnostic and therapeutic issues regarding magnesium and diabetes:

1. What is the relationship between magnesium levels and disease?

2. Is there a magnesium abnormality in diabetes? If so, what is its importance?

---

3. Is magnesium deficiency a risk factor in diabetes?
4. Should magnesium levels be measured in people with diabetes? If so, how and when?
5. Should people with diabetes receive magnesium supplementation? What is the safety and efficacy of such supplementation?

The following consensus responses were then developed by the panel.

### *Question 1: What is the Relationship Between Magnesium Levels and Disease?*

Magnesium, the second most abundant intracellular cation, plays a key role in cellular metabolism. It is important for cardiac contractility and conductivity, neurochemical transmission, skeletal muscle excitability, and the maintenance of normal intracellular calcium, potassium, and perhaps sodium levels.

Magnesium is found primarily in bone and muscle tissue, with ~1% in extracellular fluid. Normal serum concentrations are 1.5-2.0 mEq/L. Magnesium is found in various foods but particularly good sources include liver, nuts, leafy green vegetables, legumes, and whole grains. The RDA for magnesium is 350 mg for men and 280 mg for nongravid women. Although it is estimated that only 30% of dietary magnesium is absorbed from the gut, and that the overall intake of dietary magnesium has declined during this century, magnesium deficiency as a result of inadequate dietary intake is unusual in the U.S.

There are three main causes of magnesium deficiency: excessive urinary losses (e.g., diuretic therapy, diabetic ketoacidosis), decreased intestinal absorption (e.g., severe diarrhea, small bowel resection), and decreased dietary intake (e.g., prolonged parenteral nutrition). Hypermagnesemia may develop in people with renal insufficiency; the levels of toxicity are not clearly defined, but central nervous system depression appears at levels of ~8-10 mEq/L.

Available data suggest that magnesium concentrations (both serum and intracellular) are decreased in a number of disease states including hypertension, diabetes, perinatel morbidity in diabetic pregnancies, arrhythmias, and congestive heart failure. Additionally, there are data relating magnesium deficiency to insulin resistance. Some investigators believe that diminished magnesium concentrations may underlie the "insulin-resistance syndrome."

Data relating magnesium deficiency to human disease are limited. Much of the data has been generated either in nonprimate animal models or in cross-sectional studies in humans involving hospitalized or clinic-based control groups. Carefully designed case control studies involving population-based control subjects, cohort studies, or clinical trials have not been performed. However, a small number of limited clinical trials have been performed examining the effect of magnesium replacement in the periinfarction period on ventricular arrhythmias and mortality. A recent metaanalysis by Teo et al. (1) suggests a beneficial effect of magnesium replacement in reducing postmyocardial infarction mortality. The studies encompassed by the metaanalysis did not focus on diabetic subjects, although there is no reason to believe that the outcome should be different in diabetic compared with nondiabetic subjects.

In the absence of prospective studies, it is possible that decreased magnesium levels may represent a marker or epiphenomenon rather than a cause of disease. In a number of areas, such as hypertension and diabetes, cross-sectional studies are sufficiently promising that more rigorous intervention-based studies in human subjects should be undertaken.

## *Question 2: Is There Magnesium Abnormality in Diabetes? If So, What Is Its Importance?*

Hypomagnesemia has been demonstrated in both insulin-dependent and non-insulin-dependent diabetic patients. Magnesium deficiency in diabetes is most likely the result of increased urinary magnesium losses secondary to chronic glycosuria. However, short-term improvement in glycemic control has not been shown to restore the serum magnesium level. Long-term studies may be needed to resolve this discrepancy.

The impact of magnesium deficiency on insulin secretion and insulin action is speculative. Limited clinical studies have suggested a strong association between magnesium deficiency and insulin resistance. However, it is doubtful that magnesium deficiency plays a primary role in the pathophysiology of the abnormal carbohydrate metabolism of diabetes.

Acute hypomagnesemia may develop in diabetic ketoacidosis. Serum magnesium may parallel serum potassium. Elevated or normal levels of both potassium and magnesium may be seen in diabetic ketoacidosis at the time of presentation. After appropriate fluid and insulin treatment, magnesium levels may fall acutely, similar to serum potassium.

A role for magnesium deficiency in the development of the chronic complications of diabetes has not been established. However, the impact of hypomagnesemia in the pregnant diabetic patient deserves special consideration. Although the importance of magnesium depletion in malformations or stillbirths has not been firmly established, the neonates of hypomagnesemic mothers are especially susceptible to severe hypomagnesemia, hypocalcemia, and tetany.

### *Question 3: Is Magnesium Deficiency a Risk Factor for Diabetes?*

Currently, it would be premature to conclude that magnesium deficiency is a risk factor for the development of diabetes. However, strong associations have been shown between magnesium deficiency and insulin resistance. No study has demonstrated a causal relationship between the two. Also, there is no conclusive evidence in humans that magnesium deficiency chronically impairs insulin secretion. Therefore, the following areas of research should be pursued:

1. Prospective studies are needed to determine whether serum magnesium concentrations or other indices of magnesium nutrition predict the development of diabetes in population groups known to be at high risk.

2. Prospective studies are needed in diabetic patients to determine whether magnesium deficiency increases the risk of such complications as cardiovascular disease, retinopathy, or nephropathy.

3. Randomized controlled trials are necessary to demonstrate convincingly whether supplementation with magnesium will decrease the incidence of diabetes and its complications.

### *Question 4: Should Magnesium Levels Be Measured in People with Diabetes? If So How and When?*

Currently available technology severely limits our ability to detect magnesium deficiency. The only measurements available routinely are serum and urine magnesium. Serum magnesium measures only 0.3% of the total body magnesium, and may poorly reflect the magnesium content of various tissues. However, decreased serum magnesium levels do reflect a reduction in total-body magnesium content, except in circumstances of acute magnesium depletion, such as rapid diuresis or recent administration of aminoglycoside antibiotics. Thus, serum magnesium is a specific but insensitive measure of magnesium depletion. Techniques that may better reflect total-body magnesium, such as ion selective electrodes or phosphate NMR spectroscopy, are research based and are not generally available for clinical use.

Urine magnesium must be measured in a 24-h sample, because variable excretion rates throughout the day make shorter measurements unreliable. The usefulness of urine testing in the diabetic patient is further limited by the fact that glycosuria enhances magnesium excretion. A magnesium tolerance (retention) test may provide more useful information about total-body magnesium stores. This test requires the parenteral administration of a calculated dose of magnesium, followed by 24-h urine collection, with calculation of the percentage of the magnesium load retained.

Until accurate indices of magnesium deficiency are available, routine evaluation of the magnesium status of otherwise healthy individuals with diabetes is not recommended. Nevertheless, it is appropriate to measure the serum magnesium in certain patients especially at risk of magnesium deficiency. These include patients with congestive heart failure or acute myocardial infarction, ketoacidosis, ethanol abuse, long-term parenteral nutrition, potassium or calcium deficiency, chronic use of certain drugs (e.g., diuretics, aminoglycosides, or digoxin), or pregnancy.

### *Question 5: Should People with Diabetes Receive Magnesium Supplementation? What Is the Safety and Efficacy of Such Supplementation?*

Although considerable evidence has been published associating magnesium deficiency with insulin resistance, diabetes, and hypertension, well-designed prospective studies demonstrating safety and beneficial results of magnesium replacement therapy have not been performed. Adequate dietary magnesium intake can generally be achieved by a nutritionally balanced meal plan as recommended by the American Diabetes Association.

Immediate beneficial effects from intravenous magnesium administration in the acute periinfarction period owing to a reduction of cardiac arrhythmias and of short-term postinfarction mortality have been demonstrated. Because myocardial infarction is the cause of death in most diabetic patients, magnesium administration to reduce peri-infarction mortality should be considered. A more complete evaluation of magnesium therapy in acute myocardial infarction will be forthcoming from clinical trials in progress.

In the preceding section, patients at high risk of magnesium deficiency were identified. In such patients documented with hypomagnesemia, oral magnesium chloride of dependable potency and bioavailability should be administered until such time as the serum magnesium level is normalized or the condition producing the hypomagnesemia is reversed. In patients with renal insufficiency and diminished glomerular filtration, oral magnesium replacement therapy must be carefully monitored because of the risk of hypermagnesemia. The risk-benefit ratio of such therapy should be weighed before initiating treatment.

The panel recommends that patients with diabetes at increased risk of magnesium deficiency as described above, but in whom such deficiencies cannot be demonstrated by clinically available tests, not receive magnesium supplementation. Investigational efforts that use newer technologies (e.g., NMR spectroscopy, ion selective electrodes) for demonstrating magnesium deficiency, which are presently unavailable in routine clinical practice, have suggested a high prevalence of such deficiencies in non-insulin dependent diabetes. Whether the results of these studies can be extended to the entire population of non-insulin dependent diabetes patients or only to selected patients remains unknown and therefore the benefit of treatment is uncertain.

## Conclusion

In conclusion, the weight of experimental data presented to the consensus panel suggests that magnesium deficiency may play a role in insulin resistance, carbohydrate intolerance, and hypertension. Serum magnesium levels, although readily available, are relatively insensitive assessments of magnesium deficiency. The implementation of newer ion selective electrodes or phosphate NMR assays for ionized or free intracellular magnesium may extend our understanding of magnesium deficiency. However, based on available data, only diabetic patients at high risk of hypomagnesemia should have total serum magnesium assessed, and such levels should be repleted only if hypomagnesemia can be demonstrated.

## Reference

1. Teo KK, Yusuf S, Collins R, Held PH, Peto R: Effects of intravenous magnesium in suspected acute myocardial infarction: overview of randomized trials. *Br Med J* 303:1499-503, 1991

# Chapter 61

# *Gastric Bypass Improves Glucose Tolerance*

Roux-en-Y gastric bypass (GBP) and vertical banded gastroplasty (VBG), two stomach operations, significantly improve prediabetic conditions in morbidly obese patients, according to investigators at the Medical College of Virginia (MCV) of Virginia Commonwealth University in Richmond. Morbidly obese persons—individuals whose ideal body weight is exceeded by at least 100 pounds—are subject to non-insulin-dependent diabetes mellitus (NIDDM) in addition to heart disorders, sleep problems, degenerative osteoarthritis, and many other diseases.

"Gastric bypass surgery remarkably improves glucose intolerance and hyperinsulinemia," says Dr. John M. Kellum, professor of surgery at MCV. Prediabetic individuals, who later may develop NIDDM, show elevated blood glucose and insulin concentrations after glucose meals, he says.

The two operations in their present form have been used since the early 1980's to treat morbid obesity. In GBP surgery the stomach is compartmentalized by stapling. The resulting compartments are a very small (approximately 15 mL volume) upper pouch, into which the esophagus empties, and the rest of the stomach, which is sealed off. The gastric bypass is created by draining this small upper pouch into a loop of small intestine. Consequently, after a patient has undergone this operation the amount of food he or she can eat at any one time is restricted, and the food that is eaten bypasses most of the

"Research Highlights," *Research Resources Reporter*, July 1991.

stomach and goes into the small intestine via the surgically created bypass. "The operation changes the normal route of nutrients," says Dr. Kellum, and results in decreased absorption of nutrients.

In VBG the upper portion of the patient's stomach is constricted by means of surgical staples, so the amount of food the patient can eat at any time is restricted. VBG does not change the normal route of nutrients, nor does it curtail the normal 4-hour processing in the stomach.

"Both operations are associated with a feeling of early satiety," says Dr. Harvey J. Sugerman, David Hume Professor of Surgery at MCV and one of Dr. Kellum's collaborators.

In a study to better understand the hormonal effects of these two types of surgery, Dr. Kellum and his associates performed GBP or VBG on 16 morbidly obese patients (5 men and 11 women 20 to 58 years old). The patients were in good health except for their obesity; none was diabetic or received insulin.

Nine patients underwent GBP and seven underwent VBG. Patients were assigned to the procedures on the basis of dietary habits, as determined by a registered dietician. The patients receiving GBP were "sweets eaters," individuals whose intake of simple sugars was greater than 15 percent of their total caloric intake. The MCV researchers say that GBP is more effective than VBG for patients whose morbid obesity is at least in part caused by diets high in sweets.

Patients receiving either operation showed significant weight loss by 6 months after surgery. GBP patients, who averaged 278 pounds before surgery, lost approximately 66 percent of their weight. VBG patients, whose preoperative weight averaged 291 pounds, lost 41 percent of their weight.

The measurements of the effects of surgery on gastrointestinal hormones were based on physiologic responses to test meals. On consecutive days prior to the operations and for approximately 11 months following the procedures, patients ate standardized test meals. The carbohydrate meal consisted of a bottle of Glucola, a liquid containing 100 grams of glucose. The protein-fat meal was composed of pureed veal. Each meal contained 400 calories. Following an overnight fast, blood samples were taken 10 minutes prior to the meal and at several intervals during the 3 hours following it.

In GBP patients the increases in blood glucose and insulin in response to the carbohydrate meal were almost 50 percent lower after the operation than before. VBG patients showed a less pronounced improvement in glucose tolerance. "Preoperatively the GBP patients were relatively resistant to insulin even though they released high amounts of insulin. This is a prediabetic condition," says Dr. Kellum. Because the insulin was not able to help metabolize the sugar "the high levels of glucose in the blood were converted to fat," Dr. Kellum explains.

The blood glucose levels in response to the protein-fat meal appeared to be unaffected by the operation in both patient groups.

The cause of the improvements in GBP patients is unclear. "We are unsure whether the improved glucose tolerance is due more to weight loss than to a direct effect of the operation," says Dr. Sugerman. Loss of weight, whether resulting from surgery or eating less food, is known to improve glucose tolerance and hyperinsulinemia. But Dr. Sugerman also notes that the operation may decrease the levels of gastric inhibitory polypeptide (GIP), a hormone that helps trigger the release of insulin in response to glucose. GIP is highly concentrated in the duodenum, a portion of the small intestine connected directly to the stomach. When the duodenum is bypassed, as it is in GBP patients, the levels of GIP drop, resulting in a lower insulin release. Dr. Kellum notes that because fasting or dieting also can lead to a decrease in GIP levels, the drop in insulin release is most likely the result of the combined effects of weight loss and the operation itself.

In addition, bypassing part of the stomach and the duodenum may result in decreased absorption of carbohydrates simply because the food is rapidly emptied from the stomach into the small intestine, according to the investigators.

The rapid emptying of food into the small intestine may initiate the "dumping syndrome" in GBP patients, a disorder marked by bloating, nausea, sweating, diarrhea, flushing, and an aversion to sweets. The exact mechanism responsible for the syndrome is uncertain, according to Dr. Sugerman. Patients who underwent VBG did not report symptoms of the dumping syndrome.

Enteroglucagon, a peptide released in the small intestine, appears to be a marker for the dumping syndrome. The blood levels of this hormone increased markedly in GBP patients after the carbohydrate meal, and the increase correlated well with clinical symptoms of the dumping syndrome, according to the investigators. Enteroglucagon performs a function similar to glucagon, a pancreatic hormone that increases the level of blood glucose.

In future studies Dr. Kellum plans to evaluate a possible role of cholecystokinin (CCK), a hormone that has been called the satiety hormone because its infusion into the brain of sheep inhibited feeding behavior. In the present study, however, Dr. Kellum noted that the blood levels of CCK did not change in either group of patients, thus casting doubt on its role as a human satiety hormone.

—*by Harvey Black*

## Additional Reading


1. Kellum, J. M., Kuemmerle, J. F., O'Dorisio, T. M., et al., Gastrointestinal hormone responses to meals before and after gastric bypass and vertical banded gastroplasty. *Annals of Surgery* 211:763-771, 1990.
2. Meryn, S., Stein, D., and Strauss, E. W., Pancreatic polypeptide, pancreatic glucagon and enteroglucagon in morbid obesity and following gastric bypass operation. *International Journal of Obesity* 10:37-42, 1986.
3. Sirinek, K. R., O'Dorisio, T. M., Hill, D., and McFee, A. S., Hyperinsulinism, glucose-dependent insulinotropic polypeptide, and the enteroinsular axis in morbidly obese patients before and after gastric bypass. *Surgery* 100:781-787, 1986.


The studies described in this article were supported by the General Clinical Research Centers Program of the National Center for Research Resources.

Chapter 62

# *Alternative Therapies for Diabetes*

Alternative therapies are treatments that are neither widely taught in medical schools nor widely practiced in hospitals. Alternative treatments that have been studied to manage diabetes include acupuncture, biofeedback, guided imagery, and vitamin and mineral supplementation. The success of some alternative treatments can be hard to measure. Many alternative treatments remain either untested or unproven through traditional scientific studies.

## *Acupuncture*

*Acupuncture* is a procedure in which a practitioner inserts needles into designated points on the skin. Some Western scientists believe that acupuncture triggers the release of the body's natural painkillers. Acupuncture has been shown to offer relief from chronic pain. Acupuncture is sometimes used by people with neuropathy, the painful nerve damage of diabetes.

## *Biofeedback*

*Biofeedback* is a technique which helps a person become more aware of and learn to deal with the body's response to pain. This alternative therapy emphasizes relaxation and stress-reduction techniques.

---

National Diabetes Information Clearinghouse, undated.

*Guided imagery* is a relaxation technique that some professionals who use biofeedback do. With guided imagery, a person thinks of peaceful mental images, such as ocean waves. A person may also include the images of controlling or curing a chronic disease, such as diabetes. People using this technique believe their condition can be eased with these positive images.

## Chromium

The benefit of added *chromium* for diabetes has been studied and debated for several years. Several studies report that chromium supplementation may improve diabetes control. Chromium is needed to make glucose tolerance factor, which helps insulin improve its action. Because of insufficient information on the use of chromium to treat diabetes, no recommendations for supplementation yet exist.

## Magnesium

Although the relationship between *magnesium* and diabetes has been studied for decades, it is not yet fully understood. Studies suggest that a deficiency in magnesium may worsen the blood sugar control in Type 2 diabetes. Scientists believe that a deficiency of magnesium interrupts insulin secretion in the pancreas and increases insulin resistance in the body's tissues. Evidence suggests that a deficiency of magnesium may contribute to certain diabetes complications.

## Vanadium

*Vanadium* is a compound found in tiny amounts in plants and animals. Early studies showed that vanadium normalized blood glucose levels in animals with Type 1 and Type 2 diabetes. A recent study found that when people with diabetes were given vanadium, they developed a modest increase in insulin sensitivity and were able to decrease their insulin requirements. Currently researchers want to understand how vanadium works in the body, discover potential side effects, and establish safe dosages.

To learn more about alternative therapies for diabetes treatment, contact the National Institutes of Health's Office of Alternative Medicines Clearinghouse at (888) 644-6226.

## *Additional Information on Alternative Therapies for Diabetes*

The National Diabetes Information Clearinghouse collects resource information on diabetes for Combined Health Information Database (CHID). CHID is a database produced by health-related agencies of the Federal Government. This database provides titles, abstracts, and availability information for health information and health education resources.

To provide you with the most up-to-date resources, information specialists at the clearinghouse created an automatic search of CHID. To obtain this information you may view the results of the automatic search on Alternative Therapies for Diabetes at http://www.aerie.com.

Or, if you wish to perform your own search of the database, you may access the CHID Online web site and search CHID yourself at http://chid.nih.gov.

This information is provided by the National Diabetes Information Clearinghouse, a service of the National Institute of Diabetes and Digestive and Kidney Diseases.

# *Part Eight*

# *Additional Help and Information*

## Chapter 63

# *The Diabetes Dictionary*

This dictionary of diabetes terms defines words that are often used when talking or writing about diabetes. It is designed for people who have diabetes and their families and friends. It provides basic information about the disease, its long-term effects, and its care.

The words are listed in alphabetical order. Some words have many meanings; only those meanings that relate to diabetes are included. A term will refer the reader to another definition only when the second definition gives additional information about a topic that is directly related to the first term.

### A

**ACE Inhibitor:** A type of drug used to lower blood pressure. Studies indicate that it may also help prevent or slow the progression of kidney disease in people with diabetes.

**Acetohexamide:** A pill taken to lower the level of glucose (sugar) in the blood. Only some people with noninsulin-dependent diabetes take these pills. *See also*: Oral hypoglycemic agents.

**Acetone:** A chemical formed in the blood when the body uses fat instead of glucose (sugar) for energy. If acetone forms, it usually means

---

NIH Pub. No. 94-3016, August 1994. Prepared by: National Diabetes Information Clearinghouse, National Institute of Diabetes and Digestive and Kidney Diseases, National Institutes of Health, 1 Information Way, Bethesda, Maryland, 20892-3560.

that the cells do not have enough insulin, or cannot use the insulin that is in the blood, to use glucose for energy. Acetone passes through the body into the urine. Someone with a lot of acetone in the body can have breath that smells fruity and is called "acetone breath." *See also*: Ketone bodies.

**Acidosis:** Too much acid in the body. For a person with diabetes, this can lead to diabetic ketoacidosis. *See also*: Diabetic ketoacidosis.

**Acute:** Happens for a limited period of time; abrupt onset; sharp, severe.

**Adrenal Glands:** Two organs that sit on top of the kidneys and make and release hormones such as adrenalin (epinephrine). This and other hormones, including insulin, control the body's use of glucose (sugar).

**Adult-Onset Diabetes:** Former term for noninsulin-dependent or type II diabetes. *See also*: Noninsulin-dependent diabetes mellitus.

**Adverse Effect:** A harmful result.

**Albuminuria:** More than normal amounts of a protein called albumin in the urine. Albuminuria may be a sign of kidney disease, a problem that can occur in people who have had diabetes for a long time.

**Aldose Reductase Inhibitor:** A class of drugs being studied as a way to prevent eye and nerve damage in people with diabetes. Aldose reductase is an enzyme that is normally present in the eye and in many other parts of the body. It helps change glucose (sugar) into a sugar alcohol called sorbitol. Too much sorbitol trapped in eye and nerve cells can damage these cells, leading to retinopathy and neuropathy. Drugs that prevent or slow (inhibit) the action of aldose reductase are being studied as a way to prevent or delay these complications of diabetes.

**Alpha Cell:** A type of cell in the pancreas (in areas called the islets of Langerhans). Alpha cells make and release a hormone called glucagon, which raises the level of glucose (sugar) in the blood.

**Amino Acid:** The building blocks of proteins; the main material of the body's cells. Insulin is made of 51 amino acids joined together.

**Amyotrophy:** A type of diabetic neuropathy that causes muscle weakness and wasting.

**Angiopathy:** Disease of the blood vessels (arteries, veins, and capillaries) that occurs when someone has diabetes for a long time. There are two types of angiopathy: *macro*angiopathy and *micro*angiopathy. In *macro*angiopathy, fat and blood clots build up in the large blood vessels, stick to the vessel walls, and block the flow of blood. In *micro*angiopathy, the walls of the smaller blood vessels become so thick and weak that they bleed, leak protein, and slow the flow of blood through the body. Then the cells, for example, the ones in the center of the eye, do not get enough blood and may be damaged.

**Anomalies:** Birth defects; abnormalities.

**Antagonist:** One agent that opposes or fights the action of another. For example, insulin lowers the level of glucose (sugar) in the blood, whereas glucagon raises it; therefore, insulin and glucagon are antagonists.

**Antibodies:** Proteins that the body makes to protect itself from foreign substances. In diabetes, the body sometimes makes antibodies to work against pork or beef insulins because they are not exactly the same as human insulin or because they have impurities. The antibodies can keep the insulin from working well and may even cause the person with diabetes to have an allergic or bad reaction to the beef or pork insulins.

**Antidiabetic Agent:** A substance that helps a person with diabetes control the level of glucose (sugar) in the blood so that the body works as it should. *See also*: Insulin; oral hypoglycemic agents.

**Antigens:** Substances that cause an immune response in the body. The body "sees" the antigens as harmful or foreign. To fight them, the body produces antibodies, which attack and try to eliminate the antigens.

**Antiseptic:** An agent that kills bacteria. Alcohol is a common antiseptic. Before injecting insulin, many people use alcohol to clean their skin to avoid infection.

**Arteriosclerosis:** A group of diseases in which the walls of the arteries get thick and hard. In one type of arteriosclerosis, fat builds up inside the walls and slows the blood flow. These diseases often occur in people who have had diabetes for a long time. *See also*: Atherosclerosis.

**Artery:** A large blood vessel that carries blood from the heart to other parts of the body. Arteries are thicker and have walls that are stronger and more elastic than the walls of veins. *See also*: Blood vessels.

**Artificial Pancreas:** A large machine used in hospitals that constantly measures glucose (sugar) in the blood and, in response, releases the right amount of insulin. Scientists are also working to develop a small unit that could be implanted in the body, functioning like a real pancreas.

**Aspartame:** A man-made sweetener that people use in place of sugar because it has very few calories.

**Asymptomatic:** No symptoms; no clear sign of disease present.

**Atherosclerosis:** One of many diseases in which fat builds up in the large- and medium-sized arteries. This buildup of fat may slow down or stop blood flow. This disease can happen to people who have had diabetes for a long time.

**Autoimmune Disease:** Disorder of the body's immune system in which the immune system mistakenly attacks and destroys body tissue that it believes to be foreign. Insulin-dependent diabetes is an autoimmune disease because the immune system attacks and destroys the insulin-producing beta cells.

**Autonomic Neuropathy:** A disease of the nerves affecting mostly the internal organs such as the bladder muscles, the cardiovascular system, the digestive tract, and the genital organs. These nerves are not under a person's conscious control and function automatically. Also called visceral neuropathy. *See also*: Neuropathy.

## B

**Background Retinopathy:** Early stage of diabetic retinopathy; usually does not impair vision. Also called "nonproliferative retinopathy."

**Basal Rate:** Refers to a continuous supply of low levels of insulin, as in insulin pump therapy.

**Beta Cell:** A type of cell in the pancreas in areas called the islets of Langerhans. Beta cells make and release insulin, a hormone that controls the level of glucose (sugar) in the blood.

**Beta Cell Transplantation:** *See*: Islet cell transplantation.

**Biosynthetic Human Insulin:** A man-made insulin that is very much like human insulin. *See also*: Human insulin.

**Biphasic Insulin:** A type of insulin that is a mixture of intermediate- and fast-acting insulin.

**Blood Glucose:** The main sugar that the body makes from the three elements of food—proteins, fats, and carbohydrates—but mostly from carbohydrates. Glucose is the major source of energy for living cells and is carried to each cell through the bloodstream. However, the cells cannot use glucose without the help of insulin.

**Blood Glucose Meter:** A machine that helps test how much glucose (sugar) is in the blood. A specially coated strip containing a fresh sample of blood is inserted in a machine, which then calculates the correct level of glucose in the blood sample and shows the result in a digital display. Some meters have a memory that can store results from multiple tests.

**Blood Glucose Monitoring:** A way of testing how much glucose (sugar) is in the blood. A drop of blood, usually taken from the fingertip, is placed on the end of a specially coated strip, called a testing strip. The strip has a chemical on it that makes it change color according to how much glucose is in the blood. A person can tell if the level of glucose is low, high, or normal in one of two ways. The first is by comparing the color on the end of the strip to a color chart that is printed on the side of the test strip container. The second is by inserting the strip into a small machine, called a meter, which "reads" the strip and shows the level of blood glucose in a digital window display.

Blood testing is more accurate than urine testing in monitoring blood glucose levels because it shows what the current level of glucose is, rather than what the level was an hour or so previously.

**Blood Pressure:** The force of the blood on the walls of arteries. Two levels of blood pressure are measured—the higher, or *systolic*, pressure, which occurs each time the heart pushes blood into the vessels, and the lower, or *diastolic*, pressure, which occurs when the heart rests. In a blood pressure reading of 120/80, for example, 120 is the *systolic* pressure and 80 is the *diastolic* pressure. A reading of 120/80 is said to be the normal range. Blood pressure that is too high can cause health problems such as heart attacks and strokes.

**Blood-Sampling Devices:** A small instrument for pricking the skin with a fine needle to obtain a sample of blood to test for glucose (sugar). *See also*: Blood glucose monitoring.

**Blood Sugar:** *See*: Blood glucose

**Blood Urea Nitrogen (BUN):** A waste product of the kidneys. Increased levels of BUN in the blood may indicate early kidney damage.

**Blood Vessels:** Tubes that act like a system of roads or canals to carry blood to and from all parts of the body. The three main types of blood vessels are arteries, veins, and capillaries. The heart pumps blood through these vessels so that the blood can carry with it oxygen and nutrients that the cells need or take away waste that the cells do not need.

**Bolus:** An extra boost of insulin given to cover expected rise in blood glucose (sugar) such as the rise that occurs after eating.

**Borderline Diabetes:** A term no longer used. *See*: Impaired glucose tolerance.

**Brittle Diabetes:** A term used when a person's blood glucose (sugar) level often swings quickly from high to low and from low to high. Also called labile and unstable diabetes.

**Bronze Diabetes:** A genetic disease of the liver in which the body takes in too much iron from food. Also called "hemocromatosis."

**Bunion:** A bump or bulge on the first joint of the big toe caused by the swelling of a sac of fluid under the skin. Shoes that fit well can keep bunions from forming. Bunions can lead to other problems such as serious infections. *See also*: Foot care.

## C

**C.D.E. (Certified Diabetes Educator):** A health care professional who is qualified by the American Association of Diabetes Educators to teach people with diabetes how to manage their condition. The health care team for diabetes should include a diabetes educator, preferably a C.D.E.

**C-Peptide:** A substance that the pancreas releases into the bloodstream in equal amounts to insulin. A test of C-peptide levels will show how much insulin the body is making.

**Calcium Channel Blocker:** A drug used to lower blood pressure.

**Callus:** A small area of skin, usually on the foot, that has become thick and hard from rubbing or pressure. Calluses may lead to other problems such as serious infection. Shoes that fit well can keep calluses from forming. *See also*: Foot care.

**Calorie:** Energy that comes from food. Some foods have more calories than others. Fats have many calories. Most vegetables have few. People with diabetes are advised to follow meal plans with suggested amounts of calories for each meal and/or snack. *See also*: Meal plan; exchange fists.

**Capillary:** The smallest of the body's blood vessels. Capillaries have walls so thin that oxygen and glucose can pass through them and enter the cells, and waste products such as carbon dioxide can pass back into the blood to be carried away and taken out of the body. Sometimes people who have had diabetes for a long time find that their capillaries become weak, especially those in the kidney and the retina of the eye. *See also*: Blood vessels.

**Capsaicin:** A topical ointment made from chili peppers used to relieve the pain of peripheral neuropathy.

**Carbohydrate:** One of the three main classes of foods and a source of energy. Carbohydrates are mainly sugars and starches that the body breaks down into glucose (a simple sugar that the body can use to feed its cells). The body also uses carbohydrates to make a substance called glycogen that is stored in the liver and muscles for future use. If the body does not have enough insulin or cannot use the insulin it has, then the body will not be able to use carbohydrates for energy the way it should. This condition is called diabetes. *See also*: Fats; protein.

**Cardiologist:** A doctor who sees and takes care of people with heart disease; a heart specialist.

**Cardiovascular:** Relating to the heart and blood vessels (arteries, veins, and capillaries); the circulatory system.

**Carpal Tunnel Syndrome:** A nerve disorder affecting the hand that may occur in people with diabetes; caused by a pinched nerve.

**Cataract:** Clouding of the lens of the eye. In people with diabetes, this condition is sometimes referred to as "sugar cataract."

**Cerebrovascular Disease:** Damage to the blood vessels in the brain, resulting in a stroke. The blood vessels become blocked because of fat deposits or they become thick and hard, blocking the flow of blood to the brain. Sometimes, the blood vessels may burst, resulting in a hemorrhagic stroke. People with diabetes are at higher risk of cerebrovascular disease. *See also*: Macrovascular disease; stroke.

**Charcot Foot:** A foot complication associated with diabetic neuropathy that results in destruction of joints and soft tissue. Also called "Charcot's joint" and "neuropathic arthropathy."

**Chemical Diabetes:** A term no longer used. *See*: Impaired glucose tolerance.

**Chlorpropamide:** A pill taken to lower the level of glucose (sugar) in the blood. Only some people with noninsulin-dependent diabetes take these pills. *See also*: Oral hypoglycemic agents.

**Cholesterol:** A fat-like substance found in blood, muscle, liver, brain, and other tissues in people and animals. The body makes and needs some cholesterol. Too much cholesterol, however, may cause fat to build up in the artery walls and cause a disease that slows or stops the flow of blood. Butter and egg yolks are foods that have a lot of cholesterol.

**Chronic:** Present over a long period of time. Diabetes is an example of chronic disease.

**Circulation:** The flow of blood through the heart and blood vessels of the body.

**Clinical Trial:** A scientifically controlled study carried out in people, usually to test the effectiveness of a new treatment.

**Coma:** A sleep-like state; not conscious. May be due to a high or low level of glucose (sugar) in the blood. *See also*: Diabetic coma.

**Comatose:** In a coma; not conscious.

**Complications of Diabetes:** Harmful effects that may happen when a person has diabetes. Some effects, such as hypoglycemia, can happen any time. Others develop when a person has had diabetes for a long time. These include damage to the retina of the eye (retinopathy), the blood vessels (angiopathy), the nervous system (neuropathy), and the kidneys (nephropathy). Studies show that keeping blood glucose levels as close to the normal, nondiabetic range as possible may help prevent, slow, or delay harmful effects to the eyes, kidneys, and nerves.

**Congenital Defects:** Problems or conditions that are present at birth.

**Congestive Heart Failure:** Heart failure caused by loss of pumping power by the heart, resulting in fluids collecting in the body. Congestive heart failure often develops gradually over several years, although it also can happen suddenly. It can be treated by drugs and in some cases, by surgery.

**Contraindication:** A condition that makes a treatment not helpful or even harmful.

**Controlled Disease:** Taking care of oneself so that a disease has less of an effect on the body. People with diabetes can "control" the disease by staying on their diets, by exercising, by taking medicine if it is needed, and by monitoring their blood glucose. This care will help keep the glucose (sugar) level in the blood from becoming either too high or too low.

**Conventional Therapy:** A system of diabetes management practiced by most people with diabetes; the system consists of one or two insulin injections each day, daily self-monitoring of blood glucose, and a standard program of nutrition and exercise. The main objective in this form of treatment is to avoid very high and very low blood glucose (sugar). Also called. "Standard Therapy."

**Coronary Disease:** Damage to the heart. Not enough blood flows through the vessels because they are blocked with fat or have become thick and hard; this harms the muscles of the heart. People with diabetes are at a higher risk of coronary disease.

**Coxsackie B4 Virus:** An agent that has been shown to damage the beta cells of the pancreas in lab tests. This virus may be one cause of insulin-dependent diabetes.

**Creatinine:** A chemical found in the blood and passed in the urine. A test of the amount of creatinine in blood or in blood and urine shows if the kidney is working fight or if it is diseased. This is called the creatinine clearance test.

**CSII: Continuous Subcutaneous Insulin Infusion:** *See*: Insulin pump.

**Cyclamate:** A man-made chemical that people used instead of sugar. The Food and Drug Administration banned the sale of cyclamates in 1973 because lab tests showed that large amounts of cyclamates can cause bladder cancer in rats.

## D

**Dawn Phenomenon:** A sudden rise in blood glucose levels in the early morning hours. This condition sometimes occurs in people with insulin-dependent diabetes and (rarely) in people with noninsulin-dependent diabetes. Unlike the Somogyi effect, it is not a result of an insulin reaction. People who have high levels of blood glucose in the mornings before eating may need to monitor their blood glucose during the night. If blood glucose levels are rising, adjustments in evening snacks or insulin dosages may be recommended. *See also*: Somogyi effect.

**Debridement:** The removal of infected, hurt, or dead tissue.

**Dehydration:** Great loss of body water. A very high level of glucose (sugar) in the urine causes loss of a great deal of water, and the person becomes very thirsty.

**Delta Cell:** A type of cell in the pancreas in areas called the islets of Langerhans. Delta cells make somatostatin, a hormone that is believed to control how the beta cells make and release insulin and how the alpha cells make and release glucagon.

**Desensitization:** A method to reduce or stop a response such as an allergic reaction to something. For instance, if a person with diabetes has a bad reaction to taking a full dose of beef insulin, the doctor gives the person a very small amount of the insulin at first. Over a period of time, larger doses are given until the person is taking the full dose. This is one way to help the body get used to the full dose and to avoid having the allergic reaction.

**Dextrose:** A simple sugar found in the blood. It is the body's main source of energy. Also called glucose. *See also*: Blood glucose.

**Diabetes Control and Complications Trial (DCCT):** A 10-year study (1983-1993) funded by the National Institute of Diabetes and Digestive and Kidney Diseases to assess the effects of intensive therapy on the long-term complications of diabetes. The study proved that intensive management of insulin-dependent diabetes prevents or slows the development of eye, kidney, and nerve damage caused by diabetes.

**Diabetes Insipidus:** A disease of the pituitary gland or kidney, not diabetes mellitus. Diabetes insipidus is often called "water diabetes" to set it apart from "sugar diabetes." The cause and treatment are not the same as for diabetes mellitus. 'Water diabetes" has diabetes in its name because most people who have it show most of the same signs as someone with diabetes mellitus—they have to urinate often, get very thirsty and hungry, and feel weak. However, they do not have glucose (sugar) in their urine.

**Diabetes Mellitus:** A disease that occurs when the body is not able to use sugar as it should. The body needs sugar for growth and energy for daily activities. It gets sugar when it changes food into glucose (a form of sugar). A hormone called insulin is needed for the glucose to be taken up and used by the body. Diabetes occurs when the body cannot make use of the glucose in the blood for energy because either the pancreas is not able to make enough insulin or the insulin that is available is not effective. The beta cells in areas of the pancreas called the islets of Langerhans usually make insulin.

There are two main types of diabetes mellitus: insulin-dependent (Type I) and noninsulin-dependent (Type II). In insulin-dependent diabetes (IDDM), the pancreas makes little or no insulin because the insulin-producing beta cells have been destroyed. This type usually appears suddenly and most commonly in younger people under age 30. Treatment consists of daily insulin injections or use of an insulin pump, a planned diet and regular exercise, and daily self-monitoring of blood glucose.

In noninsulin-dependent diabetes (NIDDM), the pancreas makes some insulin, sometimes too much. The insulin, however, is not effective (see Insulin Resistance). NIDDM is controlled by diet and exercise and daily monitoring of glucose levels. Sometimes oral drugs that lower blood glucose levels or insulin injections are needed. This type of diabetes usually develops gradually, most often in people over 40 years of age. NIDDM accounts for 90 to 95 percent of diabetes.

The signs of diabetes include having to urinate often, losing weight, getting very thirsty, and being hungry all the time. Other signs are blurred vision, itching, and slow healing of sores. People with untreated or undiagnosed diabetes are thirsty and have to urinate often because glucose builds to a high level in the bloodstream and the kidneys are working hard to flush out the extra amount. People with untreated diabetes often get hungry and tired because the body is not able to use food the way it should.

*Prevalence of Diagnosed Diabetes*

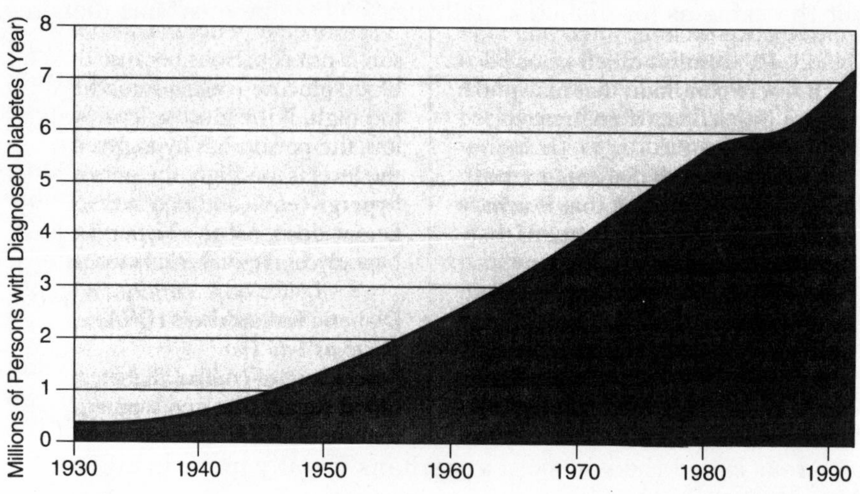


*Incidence of Diabetes*

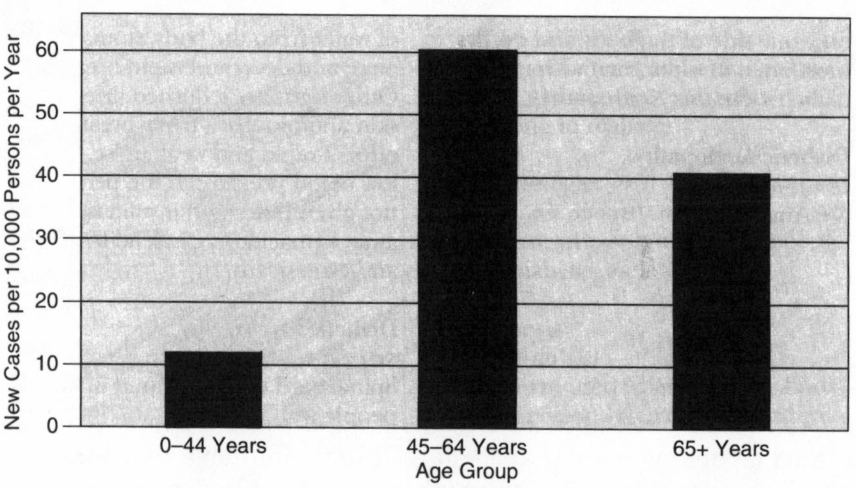


**Figure 63.1.**

In *insulin-dependent* diabetes, if the level of insulin is too low for a long period of time, the body begins to break down its stores of fat for energy. This causes the body to release acids (ketones) into the blood. The result is called ketoacidosis, a severe condition that may put a person into a coma if not treated right away.

The causes of diabetes are not known. Scientists think that *insulin-dependent* diabetes may be more than one disease and may have many causes. They are looking at hereditary (whether or not the person has parents or other family members with the disease) and at factors both inside and outside the body, including viruses.

*Noninsulin-dependent* diabetes appears to be closely associated with obesity and with the body resisting the action of insulin.

**Diabetic Amyotrophy:** A disease of the nerves leading to the muscles. This condition affects only one side of the body and occurs most often in older men with mild diabetes. *See also*: Neuropathy.

**Diabetic Angiopathy:** *See*: Angiopathy.

**Diabetic Coma:** A severe emergency in which a person is not conscious because the blood glucose (sugar) is too low or too high. If the glucose level is too low, the person has hypoglycemia; if the level is too high, the person has hyperglycemia and may develop ketoacidosis. *See also*: Hyperglycemia; hypoglycemia; diabetic ketoacidosis.

**Diabetic Ketoacidosis (DKA):** Severe, out-of-control diabetes (high blood sugar) that needs emergency treatment. DKA happens when blood sugar levels get too high. This may happen because of illness, taking too little insulin, or getting too little exercise. The body starts using stored fat for energy, and ketone bodies (acids) build up in the blood.

Ketoacidosis starts slowly and builds up. The signs include nausea and vomiting, which can lead to loss of water from the body, stomach pain, and deep and rapid breathing. Other signs are a flushed face, dry skin and mouth, a fruity breath odor, a rapid and weak pulse, and low blood pressure. If the person is not given fluids and insulin right away, ketoacidosis can lead to coma and even death.

**Diabetic Myelopathy:** Spinal cord damage found in some people with diabetes.

**Diabetic Nephropathy:** *See*: Nephropathy

**Diabetic Neuropathy:** *See*: Neuropathy

**Diabetic Osteopathy:** Loss of foot bone as viewed by x-ray; usually temporary. Also called "disappearing bone disease."

**Diabetic Retinopathy:** A disease of the small blood vessels of the retina of the eye. When retinopathy first starts, the tiny blood vessels in the retina become swollen, and they leak a little fluid into the center of the retina. The person's sight may be blurred. This condition is called background retinopathy. About 80 percent of people with background retinopathy never have serious vision problems, and the disease never goes beyond this first stage.

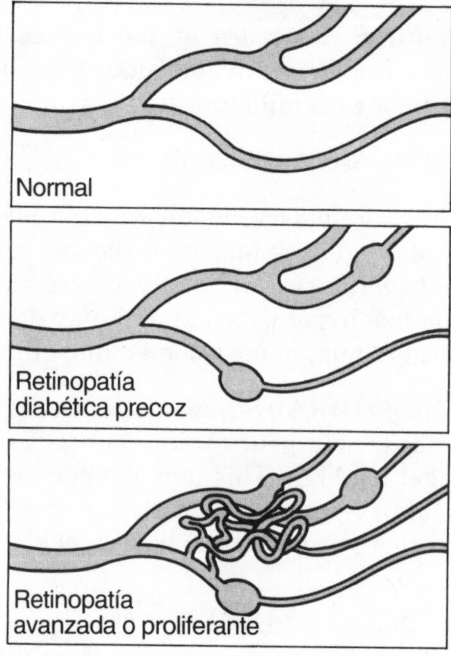


***Figure 63.2.*** *Diabetic Retinopathy*

However, if retinopathy progresses, the harm to sight can be more serious. Many new, tiny blood vessels grow out and across the eye. This is called *neovascularization*. The vessels may break and bleed into the clear gel that fills the center of the eye, blocking vision. Scar tissue may also form near the retina, pulling it away from the back of the eye. This stage is called *proliferative retinopathy*, and it can lead to impaired vision and even blindness. *See also*: Photocoagulation or vitrectomy for treatments.

**Diabetogenic:** Causing diabetes; some drugs cause blood glucose (sugar) to rise, resulting in diabetes.

**Diabetologist:** A doctor who sees and treats people with diabetes mellitus.

**Diagnosis:** The term used when a doctor finds that a person has a certain medical problem or disease.

**Dialysis:** A method for removing waste such as urea from the blood when the kidneys can no longer do the job. The two types of dialysis are: *hemodialysis* and *peritoneal dialysis*. In *hemodialysis*, the patient's blood is passed through a tube into a machine that filters out waste products. The cleansed blood is then returned to the body.

In *peritoneal dialysis* a special solution is run through a tube into the peritoneum, a thin tissue that lines the cavity of the abdomen. The body's waste products are removed through the tube. There are three types of peritoneal dialysis. Continuous ambulatory peritoneal dialysis (CAPD), the most common type, needs no machine and can be done at home. Continuous cyclic peritoneal dialysis (CCPD) uses a machine and is usually performed at night when the person is sleeping. Intermittent peritoneal dialysis (IPD) uses the same type of machine as CCPD, but is usually done in the hospital because treatment takes longer. Hemodialysis and peritoneal dialysis may be used to treat people with diabetes who have kidney failure.

**Diastolic Blood Pressure:** *See*: Blood pressure.

**Diet Plan:** *See*: Meal plan.

**Dietitian:** An expert in nutrition who helps people with special health needs plan the kinds and amounts of foods to eat. A registered dietitian (R.D.) has special qualifications. The health care team for diabetes should include a dietitian, preferably an R.D.

**Dilated Pupil Examination:** A necessary part of an examination for diabetic eye disease. Special drops are used to enlarge the pupils, enabling the doctor to view the back of the eye for damage.

**Distal Sensory Neuropathy:** *See*: Peripheral neuropathy.

**Diuretic:** A drug that increases the flow of urine to rid the body of extra fluid.

**DKA:** *See*: Diabetic ketoacidosis.

**DNA (Deoxyribonucleic Acid):** A chemical substance in plant and animal cells that tells the cells what to do and when to do it. DNA is the information about what each person inherits from his or her parents.

**Dupuytren's Contracture:** A condition that causes the fingers to curve inward and may also affect the palm. The condition is more common in people with diabetes and may precede diabetes.

## E

**Edema:** A swelling or puffiness of some part of the body such as the ankles. Water or other body fluids collect in the cells and cause the swelling.

**Electromyography (EMG):** Test used to diagnose neuropathy and check for nerve damage.

**Emergency Medical Identification:** Cards, bracelets, or necklaces with a written message used by people with diabetes or other medical problems to alert others in case of a medical emergency such as coma.

**Endocrine Glands:** Glands that release hormones into the bloodstream. They affect how the body uses food (metabolism). They also influence other body functions. One endocrine gland is the pancreas. It releases insulin so the body can use sugar for energy. *See also*: Gland.

**Endocrinologist:** A doctor who treats people who have problems with their endocrine glands. Diabetes is an endocrine disorder. *See also*: Endocrine glands.

**Endogenous:** Grown or made inside the body. Insulin made by a person's own pancreas is endogenous insulin. Insulin that is made from beef or pork pancreas or derived from bacteria is exogenous because it comes from outside the body and must be injected.

**End-Stage Renal Disease (ESRD):** The final phase of kidney disease; treated by dialysis or kidney transplantation. *See also*: Dialysis; nephropathy.

**Enzymes:** A special type of protein. Enzymes help the body's chemistry work better and more quickly. Each enzyme usually has its own chemical job to do such as helping to change starch into glucose (sugar).

**Epidemiology:** The study of a disease that deals with how many people have it, where they are, how many new cases develop, and how to control the disease.

**Epinephrine:** One of the secretions of the adrenal glands. It helps the liver release glucose (sugar) and limit the release of insulin. It also makes the heart beat faster and can raise blood pressure; also called adrenalin.

**Etiology:** The study of what causes a disease; also the cause or causes of a certain disease.

**Euglycemia:** A normal level of glucose (sugar) in the blood.

**Exchange Lists:** A grouping of foods by type to help people on special diets stay on the diet. Each group lists food in serving sizes. A person can exchange, trade, or substitute a food serving in one group for another food serving in the same group. The lists put foods in six groups: (1) starch/bread, (2) meat, (3) vegetables, (4) fruit, (5) milk, and (6) fats. Within a food group, each serving has about the same amount of carbohydrate, protein, fat, and calories.

**Exogenous:** Grown or made outside the body; for instance, insulin made from pork or beef pancreas is exogenous insulin for people.

## F

**Fasting Blood Glucose Test:** A method for finding out how much glucose (sugar) is in the blood. The test can show if a person has diabetes. A blood sample is taken in a lab or doctor's office. The test is usually done in the morning before the person has eaten. The normal, nondiabetic range for blood glucose is from 70 to 110 mg/dl, depending on the type of blood being tested. If the level is over 140 mg/dl, it usually means the person has diabetes (except for newborns and some pregnant women).

**Fats:** One of the three main classes of foods and a source of energy in the body. Fats help the body use some vitamins and keep the skin healthy. They also serve as energy stores for the body. In food, there are two types of fats: *saturated* and *unsaturated*.

*Saturated fats* are solid at room temperature and come chiefly from animal food products. Some examples are butter, lard, meat fat, solid shortening, palm oil, and coconut oil. These fats tend to raise the level of cholesterol, a fat-like substance in the blood.

*Unsaturated fats*, which include monounsaturated fats and polyunsaturated fats, are liquid at room temperature and come from plant oils such as olive, peanut, corn, cottonseed, sunflower, safflower, and soybean. These fats tend to lower the level of cholesterol in the blood. *See also*: Carbohydrate; protein.

**Fatty Acids:** A basic unit of fats. When insulin levels are too low or there is not enough glucose (sugar) to use for energy, the body burns fatty acids for energy. The body then makes ketone bodies, waste products that cause the acid level in the blood to become too high. This in turn may lead to ketoacidosis, a serious problem. *See also*: Diabetic ketoacidosis.

**Fiber:** A substance found in foods that come from plants. Fiber helps in the digestive process and is thought to lower cholesterol and help control blood glucose (sugar). The two types of fiber in food are soluble and insoluble. Soluble fiber, found in beans, fruits, and oat products, dissolves in water and is thought to help lower blood fats and blood glucose (sugar). Insoluble fiber, found in whole-grain products and vegetables, passes directly through the digestive system, helping to rid the body of waste products.

**Fluorescein Angiography:** A method of taking a picture of the flow of blood in the vessels of the eye by tracing the progress of an injected dye.

**Food Exchange:** *See*: Exchange lists.

**Foot Care:** Taking special steps to avoid foot problems such as sores, cuts, bunions, and calluses. Good care includes daily examination of the feet, toes, and toenails and choosing shoes and socks or stockings that fit well. People with diabetes have to take special care of their feet because nerve damage and reduced blood flow sometimes mean they will have less feeling in their feet than normal. They may not notice cuts and other problems as soon as they should.

**Fractional Urine:** Urine that a person collects for a certain period of time during 24 hours; usually from breakfast to lunch, from lunch to supper, from supper to bedtime, and from bedtime to rising. Also called "block urine."

**Fructose:** A type of sugar found in many fruits and vegetables and in honey. Fructose is used to sweeten some diet foods. It is considered a nutritive sweetener because it has calories.

**Fundus of the Eye:** The back or deep part of the eye, including the retina.

**Funduscopy:** A test to look at the back area of the eye to see if there is any damage to the vessels that bring blood to the retina. The doctor uses a device called an ophthalmoscope to check the eye.

## G

**Galactose:** A type of sugar found in milk products and sugar beets. It is also made by the body. It is considered a nutritive sweetener because it has calories.

**Gangrene:** The death of body tissue. It is most often caused by a loss of blood flow, especially in the legs and feet.

**Gastroparesis:** A form of nerve damage that affects the stomach. Food is not digested properly and does not move through the stomach in a normal way, resulting in vomiting, nausea, or bloating and interfering with diabetes management. *See also*: Autonomic neuropathy.

**Gene:** A basic unit of heredity. Genes are made of DNA, a substance that tells cells what to do and when to do it. The information in the genes is passed from parent to child—for example, a gene might tell some cells to make the hair red or the eyes brown.

**Genetic:** Relating to genes. *See also*: Gene; heredity.

**Gestation:** The length of pregnancy.

**Gestational Diabetes Mellitus (GDM):** A type of diabetes mellitus that can occur when a woman is pregnant. In the second half of the pregnancy, the woman may have glucose (sugar) in the blood at a higher than normal level. However, when the pregnancy ends, the blood glucose levels return to normal in about 95 percent of all cases.

**Gingivitis:** An inflammation of the gums that if left untreated may lead to periodontal disease, a serious gum disorder. Signs of gingivitis are inflamed and bleeding gums. *See also*: Periodontal disease.

**Gland:** A group of special cells that make substances so that other parts of the body can work. For example, the pancreas is a gland that releases insulin so that other body cells can use glucose (sugar) for energy. *See also*: Endocrine glands.

**Glaucoma:** An eye disease associated with increased pressure within the eye. Glaucoma can damage the optic nerve and cause impaired vision and blindness.

**Glomerular Filtration Rate:** Measure of the kidneys' ability to filter and remove waste products.

**Glomeruli:** Network of tiny blood vessels in the kidneys where the blood is filtered and waste products are removed.

**Glucagon:** A hormone that raises the level of glucose (sugar) in the blood. The alpha cells of the pancreas (in areas called the islets of Langerhans) make glucagon when the body needs to put more sugar into the blood.

An injectable form of glucagon, which can be bought in a drug store, is sometimes used to treat insulin shock. The glucagon is injected and quickly raises blood glucose levels. *See also*: Alpha cell.

**Glucose:** A simple sugar found in the blood. It is the body's main source of energy; also known as dextrose. *See also*: Blood glucose.

**Glucose Tolerance Test:** A test to see if a person has diabetes. The test is given in a lab or doctor's office in the morning before the person has eaten. A first sample of blood is taken from the person. Then the person drinks a liquid that has glucose (sugar) in it. After one hour, a second blood sample is drawn, and, after another hour, a third sample is taken. The object is to see how well the body deals with the glucose in the blood over time.

**Glycemic Response:** The effect of different foods on blood glucose (sugar) levels over a period of time. Researchers have discovered that some kinds of foods may raise blood glucose levels more quickly than other foods containing the same amount of carbohydrates.

**Glycogen:** A substance made up of sugars. It is stored in the liver and muscles and releases glucose (sugar) into the blood when needed by cells. Glycogen is the chief source of stored fuel in the body.

**Glycogenesis (or glucogenesis):** The process by which glycogen is formed from glucose. *See also*: Glycogen.

**Glycosuria:** Having glucose (sugar) in the urine.

**Glycosylated Hemoglobin Test:** A blood test that measures a person's average blood glucose (sugar) level for the 2- to 3-month period before the test. *See*: Hemoglobin A1C.

**Gram:** A unit of weight in the metric system. There are 28 grams in 1 ounce. In some diet plans for people with diabetes, the suggested amounts of food are given in grams.

## H

**HCF Diet:** A high-carbohydrate, high-fiber diet.

**Hemocromatosis:** *See*: Bronze diabetes.

**Hemodialysis:** A mechanical method of cleaning the blood for people who have kidney disease. *See also*: Dialysis.

**Hemoglobin A1C (HbA1C):** The substance of red blood cells that carries oxygen to the cells and sometimes joins with glucose (sugar). Because the glucose stays attached for the life of the cell (about 4 months), a test to measure hemoglobin A1C shows what the person's average blood glucose level was for that period of time.

**Heredity:** The passing of a trait such as color of the eyes from parent to child. A person "inherits" these traits through the genes.

**High Blood Pressure:** When the blood flows through the vessels at a greater than normal force. High blood pressure strains the heart; harms the arteries; and increases the risk of heart attack, stroke, and kidney problems. Also called hypertension.

**Hives (Urticaria):** A skin reaction that results in slightly elevated patches that are redder or paler than the surrounding skin and often are accompanied by itching.

**HLA Antigens:** Proteins on the outer part of the cell that help the body fight illness. These proteins vary from person to person. Scientists think that people with certain types of HLA antigens are more likely to develop insulin-dependent diabetes.

**Home Blood Glucose Monitoring:** A way a person can test how much glucose (sugar) is in the blood. Also called self-monitoring of blood glucose. *See also*: Blood glucose monitoring.

**Homeostatis:** When the body is working as it should because all of its systems are in balance.

**Hormone:** A chemical released by special cells to tell other cells what to do. For instance, insulin is a hormone made by the beta cells in the pancreas. When released, insulin tells other cells to use glucose (sugar) for energy.

**Human Insulin:** Man-made insulins that are similar to insulin produced by your own body. Human insulin has been available since October 1982.

**Hyperglycemia:** Too high a level of glucose (sugar) in the blood; a sign that diabetes is out of control. Many things can cause hyperglycemia. It occurs when the body does not have enough insulin or cannot use the insulin it does have to turn glucose into energy. Signs of hyperglycemia are a great thirst, a dry mouth, and a need to urinate often. For people with insulin-dependent diabetes, hyperglycemia may lead to diabetic ketoacidosis.

**Hyperinsulinism:** Too high a level of insulin in the blood. This term most often refers to a condition in which the body produces too much insulin. Researchers believe that this condition may play a role in the development of noninsulin-dependent diabetes and in hypertension. *See also*: Syndrome X.

**Hyperlipemia:** See: Hyperlipidemia.

**Hyperlipidemia:** Too high a level of fats (lipids) in the blood. *See also*: Syndrome X.

**Hyperosmolar Coma:** A coma (loss of consciousness) related to high levels of glucose (sugar) in the blood and requiring emergency treatment. A person with this condition is usually older and weak from loss of body fluids and weight. The person may or may not have a previous history of diabetes. Ketones (acids) are not present in the urine.

**Hypertension:** Blood pressure that is above the normal range. *See also*: High blood pressure.

**Hypoglycemia:** Too low a level of glucose (sugar) in the blood. This occurs when a person with diabetes has injected too much insulin, eaten too little food, or has exercised without extra food. A person with hypoglycemia may feel nervous, shaky, weak, or sweaty, and have a headache, blurred vision, and hunger. Taking small amounts of sugar, sweet juice, or food with sugar will usually help the person feel better within 10-15 minutes. *See also*: Insulin shock.

**Hypotension:** Low blood pressure or a sudden drop in blood pressure. A person rising quickly from a sitting or reclining position may have a sudden fall in blood pressure, causing dizziness or fainting.

## I

**IDDM:** *See*: Insulin-dependent diabetes mellitus.

**IGT:** *See*: Impaired glucose tolerance.

**Immunosuppressive Drugs:** Drugs that block the body's ability to fight infection or foreign substances that enter the body. A person receiving a kidney or pancreas transplant is given these drugs to stop the body from rejecting the new organ or tissue. Cyclosporin is a commonly used immunosuppressive drug.

**Impaired Glucose Tolerance (IGT):** Blood glucose (sugar) levels higher than normal but not high enough to be called diabetes. People with IGT may or may not develop diabetes. Other names (no longer used) for IGT are "borderline," "subclinical," "chemical," or "latent" diabetes.

**Implantable Insulin Pump:** A small pump placed inside of the body that delivers insulin in response to commands from a handheld device called a programmer.

**Impotence:** The loss of a man's ability to have an erect penis and to emit semen. Some men may become impotent after having diabetes for a long time because the nerves or blood vessels have become damaged. Sometimes the problem has nothing to do with diabetes and may be treated with counseling.

**Incidence:** How often a disease occurs; the number of new cases of a disease among a certain group of people for a certain period of time.

**Ingestion:** Taking food, water, or medicine into the body by mouth.

**Injection:** Putting liquid into the body with a needle and syringe. A person with diabetes injects insulin by putting the needle into the tissue under the skin (called subcutaneous). Other ways of giving medicine or nourishment by injection are to put the needle into a vein (intravenous) or into a muscle (intramuscular).

**Injection Sites:** Places on the body where people can inject insulin most easily. These are:

- The outer area of the upper arm.
- Just above and below the waist, except the area right around the navel (a 2-inch circle).
- The upper area of the buttock, just behind the hip bone.
- The front of the thigh, midway to the outer side, 4 inches below the top of the thigh to 4 inches above the knee.

These areas can vary with the size of the person.

**Injection Site Rotation:** Changing the places on the body where a person injects insulin. Changing the injection site keeps lumps or small dents from forming in the skin. These lumps or dents are called lipodystrophies. However, people should try to use the same body area for injections that are given at the same time each day—for example, always using the stomach for the morning injection or an arm for the evening injection. Using the same body area for these routine injections lessens the possibility of changes in the timing and action of insulin.

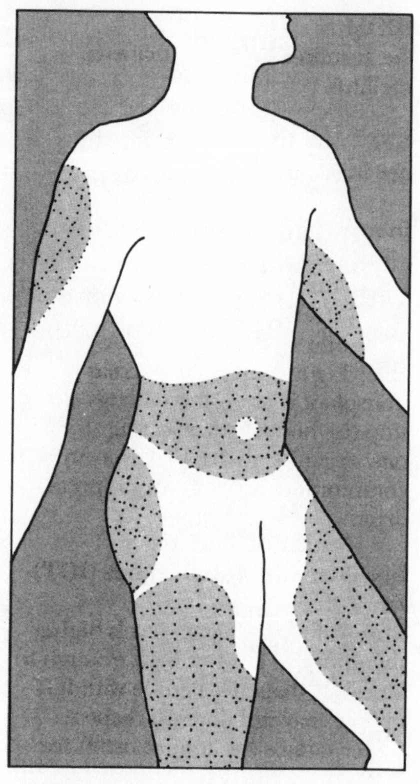

***Figure 63.3.*** *Injection Site Rotation*

**Insulin:** A hormone that helps the body use glucose (sugar) for energy. The beta cells of the pancreas (in areas called the islets of Langerhans) make the insulin. When the body cannot make enough insulin on its own, a person with diabetes must inject insulin made from other sources, i.e., beef, pork, human insulin (recombinant DNA origin), or human insulin (pork-derived, semisynthetic).

**Insulin Allergy:** When a person's body has an allergic or bad reaction to taking insulin made from pork or beef or from bacteria, or because the insulin is not exactly the same as human insulin or because it has impurities.

The allergy can be of two forms. Sometimes an area of skin becomes red and itchy around the place where the insulin is injected. This is called a local allergy.

In another form, a person's whole body can have a bad reaction This is called a systemic allergy. The person can have hives or red patches all over the body or may feel changes in the heart rate and in the rate of breathing. A doctor may treat this allergy by prescribing purified insulins or by desensitization. *See also*: Desensitization.

**Insulin Antagonist:** Something that opposes or fights the action of insulin. Insulin lowers the level of glucose (sugar) in the blood, whereas glucagon raises it; therefore, glucagon is an antagonist of insulin.

**Insulin Binding:** When insulin attaches itself to something else. This can occur in two ways. First, when a cell needs energy, insulin can bind with the outer part of the cell. The cell then can bring glucose (sugar) inside and use it for energy. With the help of insulin, the cell can do its work very well and very quickly. But sometimes the body acts against itself. In this second case, the insulin binds with the proteins that are supposed to protect the body from outside substances (antibodies). If the insulin is an injected form of insulin and not made by the body, the body sees the insulin as an outside or "foreign" substance. When the injected insulin binds with the antibodies, it does not work as well as when it binds directly to the cell.

**Insulin-Dependent Diabetes Mellitus (IDDM):** A chronic condition in which the pancreas makes little or no insulin because the beta cells have been destroyed. The body is then not able to use the glucose (blood sugar) for energy. IDDM usually comes on abruptly, although the damage to the beta cells may begin much earlier. The signs of IDDM are a great thirst, hunger, a need to urinate often, and loss of weight. To treat the disease, the person must inject insulin, follow a diet plan, exercise daily, and test blood glucose several times a day. IDDM usually occurs in children and adults who are under age 30. This type of diabetes used to be known as "juvenile diabetes," "juvenile-onset diabetes," and "ketosis-prone diabetes." It is also called type I diabetes mellitus.

**Insulin-Induced Atrophy:** Small dents that form on the skin when a person keeps injecting a needle in the same spot. They are harmless. *See also*: Lipoatrophy; injection site rotation.

**Insulin-Induced Hypertrophy:** Small lumps that form under the skin when a person keeps injecting a needle in the same spot. *See also*: Lipodystrophy; injection site rotation.

**Insulin Pen:** An insulin injection device the size of a pen that includes a needle and holds a vial of insulin. It can be used instead of syringes for giving insulin injections.

**Insulin Pump:** A device that delivers a continuous supply of insulin into the body. The insulin flows from the pump through a plastic tube that is connected to a needle inserted into the body and taped in place. Insulin is delivered at two rates: a low, steady rate (called the basal rate) for continuous day-long coverage, and extra boosts of insulin (called bolus doses) to cover meals or when extra insulin is needed. The pump runs on batteries and can be worn clipped to a belt or carried in a pocket. It is used by people with insulin-dependent diabetes.

**Insulin Reaction:** Too low a level of glucose (sugar) in the blood; also called hypoglycemia. This occurs when a person with diabetes has injected too much insulin, eaten too little food, or exercised without extra food. The person may feel hungry, nauseated, weak, nervous, shaky, confused, and sweaty. Taking small amounts of sugar, sweet juice, or food with sugar will usually help the person feel better within 10-15 minutes. *See also*: Hypoglycemia; insulin shock.

**Insulin Receptors:** Areas on the outer part of a cell that allow the cell to join or bind with insulin that is in the blood. When the cell and insulin bind together, the cell can take glucose (sugar) from the blood and use it for energy.

**Insulin Resistance:** Many people with noninsulin-dependent diabetes produce enough insulin, but their bodies do not respond to the action of insulin. This may happen because the person is overweight and has too many fat cells, which do not respond well to insulin. Also, as people age, their body cells lose some of the ability to respond to insulin. Insulin resistance is also linked to high blood pressure and high levels of fat in the blood.

Another kind of insulin resistance may happen in some people who take insulin injections. They may have to take very high doses of insulin every day (200 units or more) to bring their blood glucose (sugar) down to the normal range. This is also called "insulin insensitivity."

**Insulin Shock:** A severe condition that occurs when the level of blood glucose (sugar) drops quickly. The signs are shaking, sweating, dizziness, double vision, convulsions, and collapse. Insulin shock may occur when an insulin reaction is not treated quickly enough. *See also*: Hypoglycemia; insulin reaction.

**Insulinoma:** A tumor of the beta cells in areas of the pancreas called the islets of Langerhans. Although not usually cancerous, such tumors may cause the body to make extra insulin and may lead to a blood glucose (sugar) level that is too low.

**Intensive Intermittent Claudication:** Pain in the muscles of the leg that occurs off and on, usually while walking or exercising, and results in lameness (claudication). The pain results from a narrowing of the blood vessels feeding the muscle. Drugs are available to treat this condition.

**Intensive Management:** A form of treatment for insulin-dependent diabetes in which the main objective is to keep blood glucose (sugar) levels as close to the normal range as possible. The treatment consists of three or more insulin injections a day or use of an insulin pump; four or more blood glucose tests a day; adjustment of insulin, food intake, and activity levels based on blood glucose test results; dietary counseling; and management by a diabetes team. *See also*: Diabetes Control and Complications Trial; team management.

**Intramuscular Injection:** Putting a fluid into a muscle with a needle and syringe.

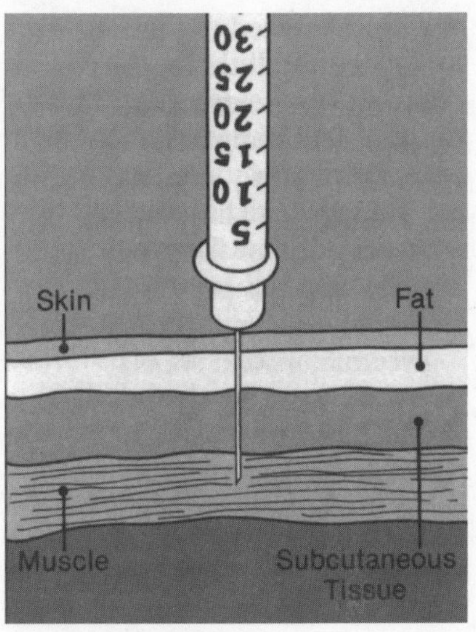


***Figure 63.4.*** *Intramuscular Injection*

**Intravenous Injection:** Putting a fluid into a vein with a needle and syringe.

**Islet Cell Transplantation:** Moving the beta (islet) cells from a donor pancreas and putting them into a person whose pancreas has stopped producing insulin. The beta cells make the insulin that the body needs to use glucose (sugar) for energy. Although transplanting islet cells may one day help people with diabetes, the procedure is still in the research stage.

**Islets of Langerhans:** Special groups of cells in the pancreas. They make and secrete hormones that help the body break down and use food. Named after Paul Langerhans, the German scientist who discovered them in 1869, these cells sit in clusters in the pancreas. There are five types of cells in an islet: beta cells, which make insulin; alpha cells, which make glucagon; delta cells, which make somatostaton; and PP cells and D, cells, about which little is known.

## J

**Jet Injector:** A device that uses high pressure to propel insulin through the skin and into the body.

**Juvenile Onset Diabetes:** Former term for insulin-dependent or type I diabetes. *See*: Insulin-dependent diabetes mellitus.

## K

**Ketoacidosis:** *See*: Diabetic ketoacidosis.

**Ketone Bodies:** Chemicals that the body makes when there is not enough insulin in the blood and it must break down fat for its energy. Ketone bodies can poison and even kill body cells. When the body does not have the help of insulin, the ketones build up in the blood and then "spill" over into the urine so that the body can get rid of them. The body can also rid itself of one type of ketone, called acetone, through the lungs. This gives the breath a fruity odor. Ketones that build up in the body for a long time lead to serious illness and coma. *See also*: Diabetic ketoacidosis.

**Ketonuria:** Having ketone bodies in the urine; a warning sign of diabetic ketoacidosis (DKA).

**Ketosis:** A condition of having ketone bodies build up in body tissues and fluids. The signs of ketosis are nausea, vomiting, and stomach pain. Ketosis can lead to ketoacidosis.

**Kidney Disease:** Any one of several chronic conditions that are caused by damage to the cells of the kidney. People who have had diabetes for a long time may have kidney damage. Also called nephropathy.

**Kidneys:** Two organs in the lower back that clean waste and poisons from the blood. The kidneys are shaped like two large beans, and they act as the body's filter. They also control the level of some chemicals in the blood such as hydrogen, sodium, potassium, and phosphate.

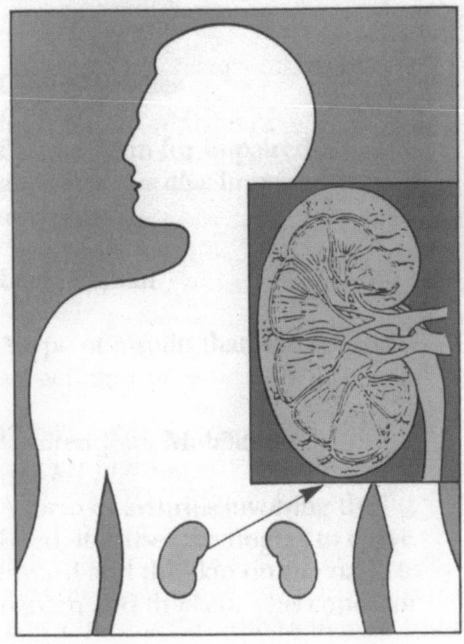

***Figure 63.5.*** *Kidneys*

**Kidney Threshold:** The point at which the blood is holding too much of a substance such as glucose (sugar) and the kidneys "spill" the excess sugar into the urine. *See also*: Renal threshold.

**Kussmaul Breathing:** The rapid, deep, and labored breathing of people who have ketoacidosis or who are in a diabetic coma. Kussmaul breathing is named for Adolph Kussmaul, the 19th century German doctor who first noted it. Also called "air hunger."

## L

**Labile Diabetes:** A term used to indicate when a person's blood glucose (sugar) level often swings quickly from high to low and from low to high. Also called brittle diabetes.

**Lactic Acidosis:** The buildup of lactic acid in the body. The cells make lactic acid when they use glucose (sugar) for energy. If too much lactic acid stays in the body, the balance tips and the person begins to feel ill. The signs of lactic acidosis are deep and rapid breathing, vomiting, and abdominal pain. Lactic acidosis may be caused by diabetic ketoacidosis or liver or kidney disease.

**Lactose:** A type of sugar found in milk and milk products (cheese, butter, etc.). It is considered a nutritive sweetener because it has calories.

**Lancet:** A fine, sharp-pointed blade or needle for pricking the skin.

**Laser Treatment:** Using a special strong beam of light of one color (laser) to heal a damaged area. A person with diabetes might be treated with a laser beam to heal blood vessels in the eye. *See also*: Photocoagulation.

**Latent Diabetes:** Former term for impaired glucose tolerance. *See also*: Impaired glucose tolerance.

**Lente Insulin:** A type of insulin that is intermediate-acting.

**Limited Joint Mobility:** A form of arthritis involving the hand; it causes the fingers to curve inward and the skin on the palm to tighten and thicken. This condition mainly affects people with IDDM.

**Lipid:** A term for fat. The body stores fat as energy for future use just like a car that has a reserve fuel tank. When the body needs energy, it can break down the lipids into fatty acids and burn them like glucose (sugar).

**Lipoatrophy:** Small dents in the skin that form when a person keeps injecting the needle in the same spot. *See also*: Lipodystrophy.

**Lipodystrophy:** Lumps or small dents in the skin that form when a person keeps injecting the needle in the same spot. Lipodystrophies are harmless. People who want to avoid them can do so by changing (rotating) the places where they inject their insulin. Using purified insulins may also help. *See also*: Injection site rotation.

## M

**Macroangiopathy:** *See*: Angiopathy.

**Macrosomia:** Abnormally large; in diabetes, refers to abnormally large babies that may be born to women with diabetes.

**Macrovascular Disease:** A disease of the large blood vessels that sometimes occurs when a person has had diabetes for a long time. Fat and blood clots build up in the large blood vessels and stick to the vessel walls. Three kinds of macrovascular disease are coronary disease, cerebrovascular disease, and peripheral vascular disease.

**Macular Edema:** A swelling (edema) in the macula, an area near the center of the retina of the eye that is responsible for fine or reading vision. Macular edema is a common complication associated with diabetic retinopathy. *See also*: Diabetic retinopathy; retina.

**Maturity-Onset Diabetes:** Former term for noninsulin-dependent or type II diabetes. *See*: Noninsulin-dependent diabetes mellitus.

**Meal Plan:** A guide for controlling the amount of calories, carbohydrates, proteins, and fats a person eats. People with diabetes can use such plans as the Exchange Lists or the Point System to help them plan their meals so that they can keep their diabetes under control. *See also*: Exchange lists; point system.

**Metabolism:** The term for the way cells chemically change food so that it can be used to keep the body alive. It is a two-part process. One part is called *catabolism*—when the body uses food for energy. The other is called *anabolism*—when the body uses food to build or mend cells. Insulin is necessary for the metabolism of food.

**Metformin:** A drug currently being tested as a treatment for noninsulin-dependent diabetes; belongs to a class of drugs called biguanides.

**Mg/dL:** Milligrams per deciliter. Term used to describe how much glucose (sugar) is in a specific amount of blood. In self-monitoring of blood glucose, test results are given as the amount of glucose in milligrams per deciliter of blood. A fasting reading of 70 to 110 mg/dL is considered in the normal (nondiabetic) range.

**Microaneurysm:** A small swelling that forms on the side of tiny blood vessels. These small swellings may break and bleed into nearby tissue. People with diabetes sometimes get microaneurysms in the retina of the eye.

**Microangiopathy:** *See*: Angiopathy.

**Microvascular Disease:** Disease of the smallest blood vessels that sometimes occurs when a person has had diabetes for a long time. The walls of the vessels become abnormally thick but weak, and therefore they bleed, leak protein, and slow the flow of blood through the body. Then some cells, for example, the ones in the center of the eye, may not get enough blood and may be damaged.

**Mixed Dose:** Combining two kinds of insulin in one injection. A mixed dose commonly combines regular insulin, which is fast acting, with a longer acting insulin such as NPH. A mixed dose insulin schedule may be prescribed to provide both short-term and long-term coverage.

**Mononeuropathy:** A form of diabetic neuropathy affecting a single nerve. The eye is a common site for this form of nerve damage. *See also*: Neuropathy.

**Morbidity Rate:** The sickness rate; the number of people who are sick or have a disease compared with the number who are well.

**Mortality Rate:** The death rate; the number of people who die of a certain disease compared with the total number of people. Mortality is most often stated as deaths per 1,000, per 10,000, or per 100,000 persons.

**Myocardial Infarction:** Also called a heart attack; results from permanent damage to an area of the heart muscle. This happens when the blood supply to the area is interrupted because of narrowed or blocked blood vessels.

**Myo-inositol:** A substance in the cell that is thought to play a role in helping the nerves to work. Low levels of myo-inositol may be involved in diabetic neuropathy.

## N

**National Institute of Diabetes and Digestive and Kidney Diseases (NIDDK):** One of the 17 institutes that make up the National Institutes of Health, an agency of the Public Health Service.

**Necrobiosis Lipoidica Diabeticorum:** A skin condition usually on the lower part of the legs. The lesions can be small or extend over a large area. They are usually raised, yellow, and waxy in appearance and often have a purple border. Young women are most often affected. This condition occurs in people with diabetes, or it may be a sign of diabetes. It also occurs in people who do not have diabetes.

**Neovascularization:** The term used when new, tiny blood vessels grow in a new place, for example, out from the retina. *See also*: Diabetic retinopathy.

**Nephrologist:** A doctor who sees and treats people with kidney diseases.

**Nephropathy:** Disease of the kidneys caused by damage to the small blood vessels or to the units in the kidneys that clean the blood. People who have had diabetes for a long time may have kidney damage.

**Nerve Conduction Studies:** Tests to determine nerve function; can detect early neuropathy.

**Neurologist:** A doctor who sees and treats people with problems of the nervous system.

**Neuropathy:** Disease of the nervous system. Many people who have had diabetes for a while have nerve damage. The three major forms of nerve damage are: peripheral neuropathy, autonomic neuropathy, and mononeuropathy. The most common form is peripheral neuropathy, which mainly affects the feet and legs. *See also*: Peripheral neuropathy; autonomic neuropathy; mononeuropathy.

**NIDDM:** *See*: Noninsulin-dependent diabetes mellitus.

**Noninsulin-Dependent Diabetes Mellitus (NIDDM):** The most common form of diabetes mellitus; about 90 to 95 percent of people who have diabetes have NIDDM. Unlike the insulin-dependent type of diabetes, in which the pancreas makes no insulin, people with noninsulin-dependent diabetes produce some insulin, sometimes even large amounts. However, either their bodies do not produce enough insulin or their body cells are resistant to the action of insulin (see Insulin Resistance). People with NIDDM can often control their condition by losing weight through diet and exercise. If not, they may need to combine insulin or a pill with diet and exercise. Generally, NIDDM occurs in people who are over age 40. Most of the people who have this type of diabetes are overweight. Noninsulin-dependent diabetes mellitus used to be called "adult-onset diabetes," "maturity-onset diabetes," "ketosis-resistant diabetes," and "stable diabetes." It is also called type II diabetes mellitus.

**Noninvasive Blood Glucose Monitoring:** A way to measure blood glucose without having to prick the finger to obtain a blood sample. Several noninvasive devices are currently being developed.

**Nonketotic Coma:** A type of coma caused by a lack of insulin. A nonketotic crisis means: (1) very high levels of glucose (sugar) in the blood; (2) absence of ketoacidosis; (3) great loss of body fluid; and (4) a sleepy, confused, or comatose state. Nonketotic coma often results from some other problem such as a severe infection or kidney failure.

**NPH Insulin:** A type of insulin that is intermediate-acting.

**Nutrition:** The process by which the body draws nutrients from food and uses them to make or mend its cells.

**Nutritionist:** *See*: Dietitian.

## O

**Obesity:** When people have 20 percent (or more) extra body fat for their age, height, sex, and bone structure. Fat works against the action of insulin. Extra body fat is thought to be a risk factor for diabetes.

**Obstetrician:** A doctor who sees and gives care to pregnant women and delivers babies.

**OGTT:** *See*: Oral glucose tolerance test.

**Ophthalmologist:** A doctor who sees and treats people with eye problems or diseases.

**Optometrist:** A person professionally trained to test the eyes and to detect and treat eye problems and some diseases by prescribing and adapting corrective lenses and other optical aids and by suggesting eye exercise programs.

**Oral Glucose Tolerance Test (OGTT):** A test to see if a person has diabetes. *See*: Glucose tolerance test.

**Oral Hypoglycemic Agents:** Pills or capsules that people take to lower the level of glucose (sugar) in the blood. The pills work for some people whose pancreas still makes some insulin. They can help the body in several ways such as causing the cells in the pancreas to release more insulin.

Six types of these pills are for sale in the United States. Four, known as "first-generation" drugs, have been in use for some time. Two types, called "second-generation" drugs, have been developed recently. They are stronger than first-generation drugs and have fewer side effects.

All oral hypoglycemic agents belong to a class of drugs known as sulfonylureas. Each type of pill is sold under two names: one is the generic name as listed by the Food and Drug Administration; the other is the trade name given by the manufacturer. They are:

First-Generation Agents:

*Generic Name*: Tolbutamide
*Trade Name*: Orinase

*Generic Name*: Acetohexamide
*Trade Name*: Dymelor

*Generic Name*: Tolazamide
*Trade Name*: Tolinase

*Generic Name*: Chlorpropamide
*Trade Name*: Diabinese

Second-Generation Agents:

*Generic Name*: Glipizide
*Trade Name*: Glucotrol

*Generic Name*: Glyburide
*Trade Name*: Diabeta, Micronase

**Overt Diabetes:** Diabetes in the person who shows clear signs of the disease such as a great thirst and the need to urinate often.

## P

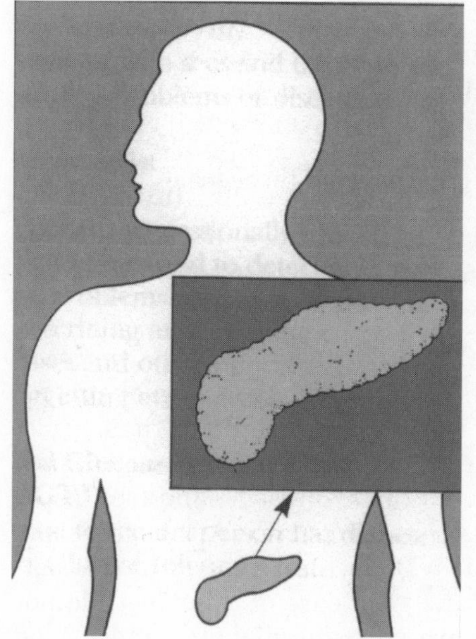

**Pancreas:** An organ behind the lower part of the stomach that is about the size of a hand. It makes insulin so that the body can use glucose (sugar) for energy. It also makes enzymes that help the body digest food. Spread all over the pancreas are areas called the islets of Langerhans. The cells in these areas each have a special purpose. The alpha cells make glucagon, which raises the level of glucose in the blood; the beta cells make insulin; the delta cells make somatostatin. There are also the PP cells and the $D_1$ cells, about which little is known.

***Figure 63.6.** Pancreas*

**Pancreas Transplant:** A surgical procedure that involves replacing the pancreas of a person who has diabetes with a healthy pancreas that can make insulin. The healthy pancreas comes from a donor who has just died or from a living relative. A person can donate half a pancreas and still live normally.

At present, pancreas transplants are usually performed in persons with insulin-dependent diabetes who have severe complications. This is because after the transplant the patient must take immunosuppressive drugs that are highly toxic and may cause damage to the body.

**Pancreatectomy:** A procedure in which a surgeon takes out the pancreas.

**Pancreatitis:** Inflammation (pain, tenderness) of the pancreas; it can make the pancreas stop working. It is caused by drinking too much alcohol, by disease in the gallbladder, or by a virus.

**Peak Action:** The time period when the effect of something is as strong as it can be such as when insulin in having the most effect on lowering the glucose (sugar) in the blood.

**Pediatric Endocrinologist:** A doctor who sees and treats children with problems of the endocrine glands; diabetes is an endocrine disorder. *See also*: Endocrine glands.

**Periodontal Disease:** Damage to the gums. People who have diabetes are more likely to have gum disease than people who do not have diabetes.

**Periodontist:** A specialist in the treatment of diseases of the gums.

**Peripheral Neuropathy:** Nerve damage, usually affecting the feet and legs; causing pain, numbness, or a tingling feeling. Also called "somatic neuropathy" or "distal sensory polyneuropathy."

**Peripheral Vascular Disease (PVD):** Disease in the large blood vessels of the arms, legs, and feet. People who have had diabetes for a long time may get this because major blood vessels in their arms, legs, and feet are blocked and these limbs do not receive enough blood. The signs of PVD are aching pains in the arms, legs, and feet (especially when walking) and foot sores that heal slowly. Although people with diabetes cannot always avoid PVD, doctors say they have a better chance of avoiding it if they take good care of their feet, do not smoke, and keep both their blood pressure and diabetes under good control. *See also*: Macrovascular disease.

**Peritoneal Dialysis:** A way to clean the blood of people who have kidney disease. *See also*: Dialysis.

**Pharmacist:** A person trained to prepare and distribute medicines and to give information about them.

**Photocoagulation:** Using a special strong beam of light (laser) to seal off bleeding blood vessels such as in the eye. The laser can also burn away blood vessels that should not have grown in the eye. This is the main treatment for diabetic retinopathy.

**Pituitary Gland:** An endocrine gland in the small, bony cavity at the base of the brain. Often called "the master gland," the pituitary serves the body in many ways—in growth, in food use, and in reproduction.

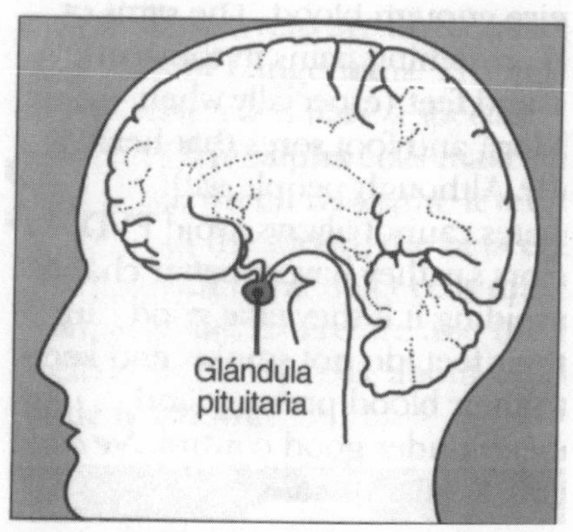


***Figure 63.7.*** *Pituitary Gland*

**Podiatrist:** A doctor who treats and takes care of people's feet.

**Podiatry:** The care and treatment of human feet in health and disease.

**Point System:** A way to plan meals that uses points to rate food. The foods are placed in four classes: calories, carbohydrates, proteins, and fats. Each food is given a point value within its class. A person with a planned diet for the day can choose foods in the same class that have the same point values for meals and snacks.

**Polydipsia:** A great thirst that lasts for long periods of time; a sign of diabetes.

**Polyphagia:** Great hunger; a sign of diabetes. People with this great hunger often lose weight.

**Polyunsaturated Fats:** A type of fat that comes from vegetables. *See also*: Fats.

**Polyuria:** Having to urinate often; a common sign of diabetes.

**Postprandial Blood Glucose:** Blood taken 1-2 hours after eating to see the amount of glucose (sugar) in the blood.

**Preeclampsia:** A condition that some women with diabetes have during the late stages of pregnancy. Two signs of this condition are high blood pressure and swelling because the body cells are holding extra water.

**Prevalence:** The number of people in a given group or population who are reported to have a disease.

**Previous Abnormality of Glucose Tolerance (PrevAGT):** A term for people who have had above-normal levels of blood glucose (sugar) when tested for diabetes in the past but who show as normal on a current test. PrevAGT used to be called either "latent diabetes" or "prediabetes."

**Prognosis:** Telling a person now what is likely to happen in the future because of having a disease.

**Proinsulin:** The substance made first in the pancreas that is then made into insulin. When insulin is purified from the pancreas of pork or beef, all the proinsulin is not fully removed. When some people use these insulins, the proinsulin can cause the body to react with a rash, to resist the insulin, or even to make dents or lumps in the skin at the place where the insulin is injected. The purified insulins have less proinsulin and other impurities than the other types of insulins.

**Proliferative Retinopathy:** A disease of the small blood vessels of the retina of the eye. *See also*: Diabetic retinopathy.

**Prosthesis:** A man-made substitute for a missing body part such as an arm or a leg; also an implant such as for the hip.

**Protein:** One of the three main classes of food. Proteins are made of amino acids, which are called the building blocks of the cells. The cells need proteins to grow and to mend themselves. Protein is found in many foods such as meat, fish, poultry, and eggs. *See also*: Carbohydrate; fats.

**Proteinuria:** Too much protein in the urine. This may be a sign of kidney damage.

**Pruritus:** Itching skin; may be a symptom of diabetes.

**Purified Insulins:** Insulins with much less of the impure proinsulin. It is thought that the use of purified insulins may help avoid or reduce some of the problems of people with diabetes such as allergic reactions.

## R

**Reagents:** Strips or tablets that people use to test the level of glucose (sugar) in their blood and urine or the level of acetone in their urine. These reagents are treated with chemicals that change color during the test. Each type of reagent has its own color code to show how much glucose or acetone there is at the time of the test.

**Rebound:** A swing to a high level of glucose (sugar) in the blood after having a low level. *See also*: Somogyi effect.

**Receptors:** Areas on the outer part of a cell that allow the cell to join or bind with insulin that is in the blood. *See also*: Insulin receptors.

**Regular Insulin:** A type of insulin that is fast acting.

**Renal:** A term that means having something to do with the kidneys.

**Renal Threshold:** When the blood is holding so much of a substance such as glucose (sugar) that the kidneys allow the excess to spill into the urine. This is also called "kidney threshold," "spilling point," and "leak point."

**Retina:** The center part of the back lining of the eye that senses light. It has many small blood vessels that are sometimes harmed when a person has had diabetes for a long time.

**Retinopathy:** A disease of the small blood vessels in the retina of the eye. *See also*: Diabetic retinopathy.

**Risk Factor:** Anything that raises the chance that a person will get a disease. With noninsulin-dependent diabetes, people have a greater risk of getting the disease if they weigh a lot more (20 percent or more) than they should.

## S

**Saccharin:** A man-made sweetener that people use in place of sugar because it has no calories.

**Saturated Fat:** A type of fat that comes from animals. *See also*: Fats.

**Secondary Diabetes:** When a person gets diabetes because of another disease or because of taking certain drugs or chemicals.

**Secrete:** To make and give off such as when the beta cells make insulin and then release it into the blood so that the other cells in the body can use it to turn glucose (sugar) into energy.

**Segmental Transplantation:** A surgical procedure in which a part of a pancreas that contains insulin-producing cells is placed in a person whose pancreas has stopped making insulin.

**Self-Monitoring of Blood Glucose:** A way as person can test how much glucose (sugar) is in the blood. Also called home blood glucose monitoring. *See also*: Blood glucose monitoring.

**Shock:** A severe condition that disturbs the body. A person with diabetes can go into shock when the level of blood glucose (sugar) drops suddenly. *See also*: Insulin shock.

**Sliding Scale:** Adjusting insulin on the basis of blood glucose tests, meals, and activity levels.

**Somatic Neuropathy:** *See*: Peripheral neuropathy.

**Somatostatin:** A hormone made by the delta cells of the pancreas (in areas called the islets of Langerhans). Scientists think it may control how the body secretes two other hormones, insulin and glucagon.

**Somogyi Effect:** A swing to a high level of glucose (sugar) in the blood from an extremely low level, usually occurring after an untreated insulin reaction during the night. The swing is caused by the release of stress hormones to counter low glucose levels. People who experience high levels of blood glucose in the morning may need to test their blood glucose levels in the middle of the night. If blood glucose levels are falling or low, adjustments in evening snacks or insulin doses may be recommended. This condition is named after Dr. Michael Somogyi, the man who first wrote about it. Also called "rebound."

**Sorbitol:** A sugar alcohol the body uses slowly. It is a sweetener used in diet foods. It is called a nutritive sweetener because it has four calories in every gram, just like table sugar and starch.

Sorbitol is also produced by the body. Too much sorbitol in cells can cause damage. Diabetic retinopathy and neuropathy may be related to too much sorbitol in the cells of the eyes and nerves.

**Spilling Point:** When the blood is holding so much of a substance such as glucose (sugar) that the kidneys allow the excess to spill into the urine. *See also*: Renal threshold.

**Split Dose:** Division of a prescribed daily dose of insulin into two or more injections given over the course of a day. Also may be referred to as multiple injections. Many people who use insulin feel that split doses offer more consistent control over blood glucose (sugar) levels.

**Stiff Hand Syndrome:** Thickening of the skin of the palm that results in loss of ability to hold hand straight. This condition occurs only in people with diabetes.

**Stroke:** Disease caused by damage to blood vessels in the brain. Depending on the part of the brain affected, a stroke can cause a person to lose the ability to speak or move a part of the body such as an arm or a leg. Usually only one side of the body is affected. *See also*: Cerebrovascular disease.

**Subclinical Diabetes:** A term no longer used. *See*: Impaired glucose tolerance.

**Subcutaneous Injection:** Putting a fluid into the tissue under the skin with a needle and syringe. *See also*: Injection.

**Sucrose:** Table sugar; a form of sugar that the body must break down into a more simple form before the blood can absorb it and take it to the cells.

**Sugar:** A class of carbohydrates that taste sweet. Sugar is a quick and easy fuel for the body to use. Types of sugar are lactose, glucose, fructose, and sucrose.

**Sulfonylureas:** Pills or capsules that people take to lower the level of glucose (sugar) in the blood. *See also*: Oral hypoglycemic agents.

**Symptom:** A sign of disease. Having to urinate often is a symptom of diabetes.

**Syndrome:** A set of signs or a series of events occurring together that make up a disease or health problem.

**Syndrome X:** Term describing a combination of health conditions that place a person at high risk for heart disease. These conditions are noninsulin-dependent diabetes, high blood pressure, high insulin levels, and high levels of fat in the blood.

**Syringe:** A device used to inject medications or other liquids into body tissues. The syringe for insulin has a hollow plastic or glass tube (barrel) with a plunger inside. The plunger forces the insulin through the needle into the body. Most insulin syringes now come with a needle attached. The side of the syringe has markings to show how much insulin is being injected.

**Systemic:** A word used to describe conditions that affect the entire body. Diabetes is a systemic disease because it involves many parts of the body such as the pancreas, eyes, kidneys, heart, and nerves.

**Systolic Blood Pressure:** *See*: Blood pressure.

## T

**Team Management:** Describes a diabetes treatment approach in which medical care is provided by a physician, diabetes nurse educator, dietitian, and behavioral scientist working together with the patient.

**Thrush:** An infection of the mouth. In people with diabetes, this infection may be caused by high levels of glucose (sugar) in mouth fluids, which helps the growth of fungus that causes the infection. Patches of whitish-colored skin in the mouth are signs of this disease.

**Tolazamide:** A pill taken to lower the level of glucose (sugar) in the blood. Only some people with noninsulin-dependent diabetes take these pills. *See also*: Oral hypoglycemic agents.

**Tolbutamide:** A pill taken to lower the level of glucose (sugar) in the blood. Only some people with noninsulin-dependent diabetes take these pills. *See also*: Oral hypoglycemic agents.

**Toxemia of Pregnancy:** A condition in pregnant women in which poisons such as the body's own waste products build up and may cause harm to both the mother and baby. The first signs of toxemia are swelling near the eyes and ankles (edema), headache, high blood pressure, and weight gain that the mother might confuse with the normal weight gain of being pregnant. The mother may have both glucose (sugar) and acetone in her urine. The mother should tell the doctor about these signs at once.

**Toxic:** Harmful; having to do with poison.

**Transcutaneous Electronic Nerve Stimulation (TENS):** A treatment for painful neuropathy.

**Trauma:** A wound, hurt, or injury to the body. Trauma can also be mental such as when a person feels great stress.

**Triglyceride:** A type of blood fat. The body needs insulin to remove this type of fat from the blood. When diabetes is under control and a person's weight is what it should be, the level of triglycerides in the blood is usually about what it should be.

**Twenty-Four Hour Urine:** The total amount of a person's urine for a 24-hour period.

**Type I Diabetes Mellitus:** *See*: Insulin-dependent diabetes mellitus.

**Type II Diabetes Mellitus:** *See*: Noninsulin-dependent diabetes mellitus.

## U

**U-100:** *See*: Unit of insulin.

**Ulcer:** A break in the skin; a deep sore. People with diabetes may get ulcers from minor scrapes on the feet or legs, from cuts that heal slowly, or from the rubbing of shoes that do not fit well. Ulcers can become infected.

**Ultralente Insulin:** A type of insulin that is long acting.

**Ultrasound:** Test used to monitor pregnancy and to diagnose neuropathy.

**Unit of Insulin:** The basic measure of insulin. U-100 insulin means 100 units of insulin per milliliter (ml) or cubic centimeter (cc) of solution. Most insulin made today in the United States is U-100.

**Unsaturated Fats:** A type of fat. *See also*: Fats.

**Unstable Diabetes:** A type of diabetes when a person's blood glucose (sugar) level often swings quickly from high to low and from low to high. Also called "brittle diabetes" or "labile diabetes."

**Urea:** One of the chief waste products of the body. When the body breaks down food, it uses what it needs and throws the rest away as waste. The kidneys flush the waste from the body in the form of urea, which is in the urine.

**Urine Testing:** Checking urine to see if it contains glucose (sugar) and ketones. Special strips of paper or tablets (called reagents) are put into a small amount of urine or urine plus water. Changes in the color of the strip show the amount of glucose or ketones in the urine. Urine testing is the only way to check for the presence of ketones, a sign of serious illness. However, urine testing is less desirable then blood testing for monitoring the level of glucose in the body. *See also*: Blood glucose monitoring; reagents.

**Urologist:** A doctor who sees men and women for treatment of the urinary tract and men for treatment of the genital organs.

## V

**Vaginitis:** An infection of the vagina usually caused by a fungus. A woman with this condition may have itching or burning and may notice a discharge. Women who have diabetes may develop vaginitis more often than women who do not have diabetes.

**Vascular:** Relating to the body's blood vessels (arteries, veins, and capillaries).

**Vein:** A blood vessel that carries blood to the heart. *See also*: Blood vessels.

**Visceral Neuropathy:** *See*: Autonomic neuropathy.

**Vitrectomy:** Removing the gel from the center of the eyeball because it has blood and scar tissue in it that blocks sight. An eye surgeon replaces the clouded gel with a clear fluid. *See also*: Diabetic retinopathy.

**Vitreous Humor:** The clear jelly (gel) that fills the center of the eye.

**Void:** To empty the bladder in order to obtain a urine sample for testing.

## X

**Xylitol:** A sweetener found in plants and used as a substitute for sugar; it is called a nutritive sweetener because it provides calories, just like sugar.

Chapter 64

# Looking for Diabetes Recipes and Cookbooks

Will I still be able to enjoy my favorite ethnic recipes? Do I have to avoid sugar all the time? What will I make for Thanksgiving? Can I still make foods taste good with herbs and spices?

Many questions arise about what recipes you can make after you find out you have diabetes. To answer these questions, the National Diabetes Information Clearinghouse (NDIC) put together this brief list of diabetes cookbooks and magazines. These cookbooks and magazines have a wide variety of recipes, and they are easy to find. The recipes give diabetes exchanges and nutrition information. All the cookbooks are up to date with today's tastes and trends in foods.

You can buy many other diabetes cookbooks. Other cookbooks focus on just one type of food such as desserts or beans, or one cuisine, such as Italian or Chinese. Also, there are many meal-planning tools.

## Where to Find These Cookbooks

You can buy many of these cookbooks in bookstores. If you cannot find a book on the shelf, ask the store manager to order it for you. Or you can order it from the publisher by calling the number under each listing. Also, you can look for these books in your local library.

---

National Institute of Diabetes and Digestive and Kidney Diseases (NIDDK), NIH Pub. No. 97-4253, October 1997. The list of items described on these pages is not all inclusive. Items are listed as a public service *only* and are not to be construed as having the favor or endorsement of the U.S. Department of Health and Human Services.

## Cookbooks

***The Art of Cooking for the Diabetic* (3rd edition).** Mary Abbott Hess, R.D. (1996). Contemporary Books: Chicago, IL, or New York, NY. 528 pp.

The beginning of the book describes the American Diabetes Association's 1994 nutrition recommendations. It also offers advice on exercise, alcohol, dining out, and traveling. The book includes 375 recipes, from appetizers to soups and salads, to breads, entrees, vegetables, grains, and desserts. All recipes contain nutrition information for carbohydrate, protein, fat, calories, fiber, sodium, and cholesterol.

For more information, call (312) 540-4500.

***The Complete Step-by-Step Diabetic Cookbook* (3rd edition).** Registered Dietitians from the University of Alabama at Birmingham. (1995). Oxmoor House: Birmingham, AL. 368 pp.

The book begins with information on food labeling, sugars, sugar substitutes, and foods for "sick days." The book gives you more than 300 recipes for beverages, eggs, entrees, starches, vegetables, sauces, and desserts. The nutrition information includes carbohydrate, protein, fat, calories, fiber, sodium, and cholesterol.

For more information, call (800) 633-4910.

***The Diabetic's Innovative Cookbook: A Positive Approach to Living with Diabetes.*** Joseph Juliano, M.D., and Dianne Young. (1994). Henry Holt and Company: New York, NY. 416 pp.

The first of two sections of this book are written by Joseph Juliano, M.D., a physician who has 30 years of experience with his own diabetes. He writes about how critical it is to follow a diabetes meal plan, how to eat at parties and restaurants, and what to do when you travel. He also discusses sweeteners, desserts, and the importance of eating fresh vegetables. The second part of the book is written by Dianne Young, a professional chef. She gives 145 recipes from breakfasts to soups, salsas, vegetables, and side dishes, rice and pasta, entrees and desserts. All recipes have nutrition information for calories, protein, carbohydrate, fat, and sodium.

For more information, call (800) 488-5233.

***Family Cookbook: Volume IV.*** (Three other volumes [I, II, III] of the family cookbooks are available. They were last revised in 1987.) American Diabetes Association and The American Dietetic Association. (1991). Prentice Hall Press: New York, NY. 403 pp.

The book offers a tour of regional cooking styles and a discussion of eating trends in America. The 1986 Exchange Lists for Meal Planning are given. The book includes more than 200 recipes from every region of America. Recipes for appetizers, soups, salads, breads, meats, fish, vegetables, desserts, and more are presented. All recipes contain nutrition information for calories, protein, fat, carbohydrate, sodium, potassium, fiber, and cholesterol.

For more information, call (800) 877-1600 ext. 5000.

***Healthy & Hearty Diabetic Cooking.*** The Canadian Diabetes Association Publisher. (1993). Diabetes Self-Management Books, R.A. Rappaport Publishing, Inc.: New York, NY. 337 pp.

The book explores the basic principles of how to microwave and how to make your favorite recipes healthier. It includes more than 200 recipes from appetizers to salad dressings, one-dish meals, meat, poultry, meatless main dishes, cookies, sauces, basics, and more. All the recipes have nutrition information for calories, carbohydrate, protein, fat, saturated fat, cholesterol, fiber, and sodium.

For more information, call (800) 366-3303.

***The Joy of Snacks* (2nd edition).** Nancy Cooper, R.D. (1991). Chronimed Publishing Company: Minneapolis, MN. 295 pp.

This book begins with a few cooking tips and hints about ingredients. It includes recipes for more than 200 snacks in 14 categories such as appetizers, dips and spreads, recipes especially for kids, rise 'n shine breakfasts, cookies and bars, frozen snacks, and convenient snack foods. All recipes have nutrition information for calories, carbohydrate, protein, fat, and sodium.

For more information, call (800) 848-2793.

***MicroWave Diabetes Cookbook.*** Betty Marks. (1991). Surrey Books: Chicago, IL. 200 pp.

This book begins with helpful hints for microwave cooking. It includes more than 130 recipes from appetizers to soups, fish, meat, poultry, grains, starches, vegetables, baked goods, and more. All recipes have nutrition information for cholesterol, carbohydrate, protein, sodium, fiber, total fat, saturated fat, polyunsaturated fat, monounsaturated fat, and calories.

For more information, call (800) 326-4430.

***Month of Meals*** (five books are available). American Diabetes Association. (1990-1994). American Diabetes Association: Alexandria, VA. 70 pp.

Each of the five books helps you add variety and interest to your meal plan with a month of suggested meals and snacks. You can mix and match meals and snacks based on the number of calories you need and what you like to eat. Some of the meals show you how to prepare and fit a recipe into a meal.

For more information, call (800) 232-6733.

***The UCSD Healthy Diet for Diabetes: A Comprehensive Nutritional Guide and Cookbook*** (University of California at San Diego). Susan Algert, R.D., Barbara Grasse, R.D., and Annie Durning, R.D. (1990). Houghton Mifflin Company: Boston, MA. 373 pp.

The first part of this book gives you the basics about diabetes and meal planning including tips on dining out, drinking alcohol, exercising, and monitoring blood sugar. The rest of the book contains 225 recipes from beverages, dips and chips to salads and dressings, vegetables and side dishes, grains, beans and pasta, meatless main dishes, desserts, and more. All recipes have nutrition information for calories, protein, fat, carbohydrate, fiber, cholesterol, sodium, and potassium.

For more information, call (212) 420-5842.

***Diabetic Meals In 30 Minutes—or Less!*** Robyn Webb, M.S. (1996). American Diabetes Association: Alexandria, VA. 180 pp.

This book helps you learn to make great-tasting meals in 30 minutes or less. It includes 140 recipes from appetizers to soups and salads, entrees, and desserts. All recipes have nutrition information for calories, carbohydrate, protein, fat, saturated fat, cholesterol, fiber, and sodium.

For more information, call (800) 232-6733.

## Magazines

Two popular magazines are written for people with diabetes. Recipes are in each issue. The recipes often have a seasonal or holiday theme. If you get the magazine or read it in a library, you will always have access to new recipes.

***Diabetes Forecast.*** American Diabetes Association. (Monthly periodical). American Diabetes Association: Alexandria, VA.

All recipes have nutrition information for calories, calories from fat, total fat, saturated fat, cholesterol, sodium, carbohydrate, fiber, sugars, protein, and diabetes exchanges.

For more information, call (800) DIABETES or (800) 342-2383.

***Diabetes Self-Management.*** (Bimonthly). R.A. Rappaport Publishing, Inc.: New York, NY.

All recipes have nutrition information for calories, carbohydrate, protein, fat, saturated fat, fiber, sodium, and diabetes exchanges.

For more information, call (800) 234-0923.

## Using the Combined Health Information Database

More diabetes cookbooks and meal-planning tools can be found by doing a literature search from the Diabetes subfile of the Combined Health Information Database (CHID). CHID is available online through the National Institute of Diabetes and Digestive and Kidney Diseases' home page at <http://www.niddk.nih.gov/>.

If you would like references to materials on other topics, you may request a special literature search of CHID from the National Diabetes Information Clearinghouse, 1 Information Way, Bethesda, MD 20892-3560; telephone: (301) 654-3327; fax: (301) 907-8906; e-mail: ndic@aerie.com

Chapter 65

# Additional Resources for Diabetes Information

## Materials Available

The following materials are available from the organizations listed. Contact the issuing agency for up-to-date ordering and price information. Complete contact information can be found in Chapter 67—Directory of Diabetes Organizations.

*Ace Inhibitors, Kidney Disease, and Diabetes*, DM-138 (information packet with documents of varying dates) National Diabetes Information Clearinghouse.

*Alcohol and Diabetes*, DM-158 (information packet with documents of varying dates) National Diabetes Information Clearinghouse.

*Alternative Methods of Insulin Delivery*, DM-143 (information packet with documents of varying dates) National Diabetes Information Clearinghouse.

"Buyers Guide to Diabetes Supplies," published every October in *Diabetes Forecast*. American Diabetes Association.

*Children with Diabetes*, DM-161 (information packet with documents of varying dates) National Diabetes Information Clearinghouse.

---

The listings in this chapter were selected and compiled from many sources deemed reliable. Inclusion does not constitute an endorsement; omission does not indicate judgement.

*Complementary and Alternative Therapies for Diabetes Treatment*, DM-172 (information packet with documents of varying dates) National Diabetes Information Clearinghouse.

*Consejos de cuidado dental para diabéticos*, 1990, National Diabetes Information Clearinghouse.

*Diabetes & Pedorthics: Conservative Foot Care*, Pedorthic Footwear Association

*Diabetes and Gastroparesis*, DM-151 (information packet with documents of varying dates) National Diabetes Information Clearinghouse.

*Diabetes and Heart Disease, High Blood Pressure, and Stroke*, DM-142 (information packet with documents of varying dates) National Diabetes Information Clearinghouse.

*Diabetes and Nutrition: Eating for Health*, (videocassette), 1994, American Association of Diabetes Educators.

*Diabetes and Skin Conditions*, DM-152 (information packet with documents of varying dates) National Diabetes Information Clearinghouse.

*Diabetes and the Glycemic Index*, DM-154 (information packet with documents of varying dates) National Diabetes Information Clearinghouse.

*Diabetes Care*, a professional journal, American Diabetes Association.

*Diabetes Care*: Special Issue "Diabetes and Exercise '90," by M. Berger, ed. November 1992, pp. 1676-1813, American Diabetes Association.

*Diabetes Dateline*, published four time per year, National Diabetes Information Clearinghouse.

*Diabetes Forecast*, a consumer magazine, American Diabetes Association.

*Diabetes in America*, Second Edition, (NIH Pub. No. 95-1468) 1995, National Institute of Diabetes and Digestive and Kidney Diseases.

*Diabetes Insipidus*, DM-139 (information packet with documents of varying dates) National Diabetes Information Clearinghouse.

*Diabetes Research and Training Centers*, 1995, National Diabetes Information Clearinghouse.

*Diabetes Spectrum*, a professional journal, American Diabetes Association.

*Diabetes*, a professional journal, American Diabetes Association.

*Diabetic Neuropathy: The Nerve Damage of Diabetes*, 1995, National Diabetes Information Clearinghouse.

*Diccionario de diabetes*, 1991, National Diabetes Information Clearinghouse.

*Diet and Diabetes*, DM-132 (information packet with documents of varying dates) National Diabetes Information Clearinghouse.

*Diet and Nutrition: Guides, Manuals, Fact Sheets, and Cookbooks for People with Diabetes,* a literature search, 1995. National Diabetes Information Clearinghouse.

*Diet, Exercise, and Diabetes*, 1990. Juvenile Diabetes Foundation International.

*Direct and Indirect Costs of Diabetes in the United States in 1992*, 1993, American Diabetes Association, 1993.

*Employment, Discrimination, and Diabetes*, DM-140 (information packet with documents of varying dates) National Diabetes Information Clearinghouse.

*Enfermedad periodontal en los diabéticos – Guía para los pacientes*, 1987, National Diabetes Information Clearinghouse

*Exchange Lists for Meal Planning*, 1995. American Diabetes Association.

*Financial Assistance and Insurance*, DM-144 (information packet with documents of varying dates) National Diabetes Information Clearinghouse.

*Healthy Food Guide: Diabetes and Hemodialysis*, 1993. American Dietetic Association.

*Healthy Food Guide: Diabetes and Peritoneal Dialysis*, 1993. American Dietetic Association.

"Hypoglycemia and Employment/Licensure" (Position Statement) 1995, American Diabetes Association.

*Hypoglycemia*, 1995, National Diabetes Information Clearinghouse.

*Impotence* (NIH Pub. No 95-3923) 1995, National Kidney and Urologic Diseases Information Clearinghouse.

*Impotence and Diabetes*, DM-147 (information packet with documents of varying dates) National Diabetes Information Clearinghouse.

*Information about Insulin*, undated, Juvenile Diabetes Foundation International.

*Insuficiencia renal crónica terminal: Elección del tratamiento que le conviene a usted*, 1992, National Diabetes Information Clearinghouse.

*Islet Cell Transplants*, DM-145 (information packet with documents of varying dates) National Diabetes Information Clearinghouse.

*Joint and Bone Conditions Related to Diabetes*, DM-150 (information packet with documents of varying dates) National Diabetes Information Clearinghouse.

*Kidney Disease of Diabetes*, 1995, National Diabetes Information Clearinghouse.

*Kids, Food, and Diabetes: Family Cookbook*, 1991. Juvenile Diabetes Foundation International.

*Monitoring Your Blood Sugar*, undated, Juvenile Diabetes Foundation International.

*Noninvasive Blood Glucose Monitoring*, DM-146 (information packet with documents of varying dates) National Diabetes Information Clearinghouse.

*¡Ojo con su Visiós!* 1995, National Diabetes Information Clearinghouse.

*Oral Hypoglycemic Agents and NIDDM*, DM-157 (information packet with documents of varying dates) National Diabetes Information Clearinghouse.

*Oral Medications and Type 2 Diabetes*, 1990, Juvenile Diabetes Foundation International.

*Peripheral Neuropathy*, DM-153 (information packet with documents of varying dates) National Diabetes Information Clearinghouse.

*Pregnancy and Diabetes*, undated, Juvenile Diabetes Foundation International.

*Prevention and Treatment of Complications of Diabetes Mellitus: A Guide for Primary Care Practitioners*, 1991, Centers for Disease control and Prevention, Division of Diabetes Translation.

*Self-Monitoring of Blood Glucose*, DM-160 (information packet with documents of varying dates) National Diabetes Information Clearinghouse.

*Success for a Lifetime with Diabetes*, (videocassette), 1993, American Association of Diabetes Educators.

*Travel and Diabetes*, DM-149 (information packet with documents of varying dates) National Diabetes Information Clearinghouse.

*What You Should Know about Diabetes*, undated, Juvenile Diabetes Foundation International.

*Your Podiatric Physician Talks about Diabetes,* American Podiatric Medical Association

## Articles Available

The following articles are available in periodic publications. To help identify subject material more readily, titles are listed first. Check your local library for availability.

"ADA Guidelines to Diabetes and Exercise," by E.S. Horton. *Diabetes Forecast*, June 1991, pp. 38-39.

"Alcohol, Alcohol, Everywhere: But Not a Drop to Drink?" by Marti Chitwood and Christine B. Welch. *Diabetes Forecast*, November 1992, pp. 39-42.

"All about Food Additives: What Goes in Your Food and Why," by M. Hudnall. *Diabetes Self-Management*, November-December 1993, pp. 22, 24-26.

"Assessment and Management of Foot Disease in Patients with Diabetes," by Gregory M. Caputo, Peter R. Cavanagh, Jan S. Ulbrecht, Gary W. Gibbons, and Adolf W. Karchmer. *The New England Journal of Medicine*, September 29, 1994, pp. 854-60.

"Association between Exercise and Other Preventive Health Behaviors among Diabetics," by J. H. Summerson, J.C. Konen, and

M.B. Dignan. *Public Health Reports*, September-October 1991, pp. 543-47.

"Brief Overview of Diabetes Mellitus and Exercise." *Diabetes Educator*, 17(3) 175-178, May-June 1991.

"Childhood Development: What's Normal and What's Not," by Linda M. Siminerio. *Diabetes Self-Management*, March/April 1992, pp. 43-45.

"Choosing a Pediatric Diabetes Program," by Paul Strumph. *Diabetes Self-Management*, January/February 1992, pp. 41-43.

"Comparison of Laboratory Test Frequency and Test Results Between African-Americans and Caucasians with Diabetes: Opportunity for Improvement," by Kimberlydawn Wisdom, Jon P. Fryzek, Suzanne L. Havstad, Robert M. Anderson, Michael C. Dreilling, and Barbara C. Tilley. *Diabetes Care*, June 1997, pp. 971-977.

"Dealing with Gastroparesis," by Robert S. Dinsmoor. *Diabetes Self-Management*, September/October 1990, pp. 24-27.

"Dermatologic Complications Associated with Diabetes," by Kenneth R. Reingold and Peter M. Elias. *Diabetes Spectrum*, Vol. 3, No. 5, 1990, pp. 282-87.

"Diabetes Foot Care: A Team Approach," by Lawrence B. Harkless and Lawrence A. Lavery. *Diabetes Spectrum*, Vol. 5, No. 3, 1992, pp. 136-137.

"Diabetes Self-Testing." *Diabetes Forecast*, May 1996, pp. 75-76.

"Diabetes: Nutrition Guidelines Emphasize Personal Touch," Mayo Foundation. *Mayo Clinic Health Letter*, August 1994, pp. 4-5.

"Diabetic Gastroparesis: A Review," by Per-Henrik Nilsson. *Journal of Diabetes and Its Complications*, Vol 10, 1996, pp. 113-22.

"Diets for Diabetes: More Choices Than Ever," by Judy Friesen, F. Xavier Pi-Sunyer, Susan L. Thom, and Kathleen Wishner. *Patient Care*, September 194, pp. 86-94.

"Digital Sclerosis," by Terry Meriden. *Diabetes Forecast*, April 1993, pp. 17-18.

"Disabilities Act Protects You against Job Discrimination," by Cheryl Hunt. *Diabetes in the News*, October 1993, pp. 22-24.

"Exercise and Decreased Risk of NIDDM," by E.S. Horton. *The New England Journal of Medicine*, July 18, 1991, pp. 196-97.

"Exercise as Prevention," by S.J. Ackerman. *Diabetes Forecast*, March 1992, pp. 35-36.

"Importance of Glycemic Index in Diabetes," by Janette C. Brand Miller. *American Journal of Clinical Nutrition*, 1994; 59(suppl) pp. 747S-52S.

"Improvement of Insulin Sensitivity by Short-Term Exercise Training in Hypertensive African American Women," by Michael D. Brown, Geoffrey E. Moore, Mary T. Korytkowski, Steve D. McCole, and James M. Hagberg. *Hypertension*, December 1997, pp. 1549-53.

"Insulin Administration." *Diabetes Care*, January 1995, pp. 29-32.

"Insulin Key to Diabetes but Not Full Cure," by Judith Randal. *FDA Consumer*, May 1992, pp. 15-19.

"Insulin Resistance—Mechanisms, Syndromes, and Implications," by David E. Moller and Jeffrey S. Flier. *The New England Journal of Medicine*, September 26, 1991, pp. 938-46.

"Insulin's Helping Hand," by Patricia Cane. *Diabetes Forecast*, May 1994, pp. 34-36.

"Issues in the Care of Infants and Toddlers with Insulin-Dependent Diabetes Mellitus," by Wendy Kushion, Patricia J. Salisbury, Kathleen W. Seitz, and Bruce E. Wilson. *Diabetes Educator*, Vol 17, No. 2, pp. 107-10.

"Loosing the Apron Strings: A Guide to Letting Go," by Melissa Strugger. *Diabetes Self-Management*, November/December, pp. 26-28.

"Meter Mysteries Solved," by Jennifer Bogosian. *Diabetes Forecast*, October 1994, pp. 26-28.

"New Diabetic Guidelines, Personal Health," by Jane E. Brody. *New York Times*, May 25, 1994.

"New Oral Therapies for Type 2 Diabetes," by Jonathan Q. Purnell and Irl B. Hirsch. *American Family Physician*, November 1, 1997, pp. 1835-42.

"New Sugar Guidelines," by Robert S. Dinsmoor. *Diabetes Self-Management*, July/August 1994, pp. 22-23.

"Parent + Teacher = Healthy Child," by Peggy Finston. *Diabetes Forecast*, September 1994, pp. 27-30.

"Real-World Management of Type 2 Diabetes," by Mayer B. Davidson, Veronica Piziak, Arthur H. Rubenstein, and Kathleen Wishner. *Patient Care*, September 30, 1994, pp. 68-85.

"Report of the Expert Committee on the Diagnosis and Classification of Diabetes Mellitus. *Diabetes Care*, July 1997, pp. 1183-97.

"Six Secrets of Successful Parenting," by Debbie Lloyd. *Diabetes Forecast*, May 1994, pp. 30-33.

"Skinful Secrets: Caring for Your Outermost Layer," by Darlene J. Paduano. *Diabetes Self-Management*, January/February 1992, pp.37-39.

"Starting Insulin Therapy in Patients with Type 2 Diabetes," by Rodney A. Hayward, Willard G. Manning, Sherrie H. Kaplan, Edward H. Wagner, and Sheldon Greenfield. *JAMA*, November 26, 1997, pp. 1663-69.

"Staying Fit During Pregnancy," by A. White. *Diabetes Forecast*, February 1992, pp. 44-46.

"Telling It Like It Is: A Look at the New Food Labels," by Lea Ann Holzmeister. *Diabetes Self-Management*, March/April 1994, pp. 40-45.

"Trends in the Prevalence and Incidence of Self-Reported Diabetes Mellitus—United States, 1980-1994," *Morbidity and Mortality Weekly Report*, October 31, 1997, pp.1014-1028.

"Update on Blood Glucose Monitoring," by Virginia Peragallo-Dittko. *Diabetes Self-Management*, May/June 1996, pp. 8-16.

"When Your Kid Doesn't Eat Right," by Linda Steranchak. *Diabetes Self-Management*, January/February 1995, pp. 28-32.

## Available on the Internet

The following documents and other websites of interest to people with diabetes are available on the internet.

American Association of Kidney Patients
www.aakp.org

American Kidney Fund Publications
www.arbon.com/kidney/brochure.htm

Children with Diabetes on-line community
www.castleweb.com/diabetes/

Diabetes and a Vegetarian Diet
http://envirolink.org/arrs/VRG/diabetes.html

Diabetes and Digestion, Canadian Diabetes Association
www.diabetes.ca:80/atoz/chol.htm

Diabetes in Skin Disease
http://telemedicine.org/diabetes.htm

Diabetes Mall
www.diabetesnet.com/index.html

Diabetes Monitor
www.mdcc.com/

Diabetes Omni-Link
www.diabetesomni-link.com/

Diabetes Well
www.diabeteswell.com:80/index.htm

Foot Care
www.diabeteslife.net:80/living/foot/index.html

Healing Handbook for Persons with Diabetes
www.ummed.edu/dept/diabetes/handbook

Human vs. Beef/Pork Insulin, Canadian Diabetes Association
http://www.diabetes.ca/atoz/bpi.htm

Impotence Resource Center
www.impotence.org

Insulin
http://207.82.194.117/living/medicate/insulin.html

Medilife's Diabetes Center
www.medilife.com/medilife/diabetes/index.htm

Staying Sexually Healthy, *The Monitor Newsletter*, Volume 7, No. 3
©1997 Lifescan: A Johnson & Johnson Company
http://www.lifescan.com/lsabout/mon97b.html

What to Do When You Have Gestational Diabetes
www.aafp.org/patientinfo/gest.html

## Chapter 66

# *Financial Help for Diabetes Care*

*Medicare* is usually for people over 65 years old. People who are disabled or have become disabled also can apply for Medicare, and there is limited coverage for people of all ages with kidney failure. To learn if you can get Medicare, and for details about what is covered, check with your local Social Security office or call the Medicare Hotline at (800) 638-6833. The Medicare Hotline will also tell you about special programs to help people with limited incomes.

*Medicaid* helps people who are under 65 with their medical needs. To qualify, you must meet the financial and other requirements of your State. What is covered also varies from State to State. Apply for help at your local or State health and public assistance office.

The *Department of Veterans Affairs* (VA) serves veterans who have service-related health problems or who need financial help. If you are a veteran and have questions about whether you can get VA health care, call (800) 827-1000. The operator will connect you with a regional VA information center.

Most county or city governments have *public health departments* that offer help to people who need medical care. Call your local government office to get more information.

In many communities, some *private, not-for-profit groups* with an interest in diabetes offer financial support to people who qualify based on their medical needs. If you have a medical need that a government agency is unable to fill, these agencies may be able to help. Your local library is a good source to learn about these groups.

---

National Diabetes Information Clearinghouse, March 1998.

Finally, be honest with your *health care providers*. Tell them if you are unable to pay for food, medicines, or diabetes supplies. Ask them if they know where you can get help. Your health care providers may be able to tell you about programs set up by diabetes supply companies or by your county or city.

## Additional Information on Financial Help for Diabetes Care

The National Diabetes Information Clearinghouse collects resource information on diabetes for Combined Health Information Database (CHID). CHID is a database produced by health-related agencies of the Federal Government. This database provides titles, abstracts, and availability information for health information and health education resources.

To provide you with the most up-to-date resources, information specialists at the clearinghouse created an automatic search of CHID. To obtain this information you may view the results of the automatic search on Financial Help for Diabetes Care at http://chid.aerie.com.

Or, if you wish to perform your own search of the database, you may access the CHID Online web site and search CHID yourself at http://chid.nih.gov.

This information is provided by the National Diabetes Information Clearinghouse, a service of the National Institute of Diabetes and Digestive and Kidney Diseases.

# Chapter 67

# *Directory of Diabetes Organizations*

This directory lists Government agencies, voluntary associations, and private organizations that provide diabetes information and resources. Some of these diabetes organizations offer educational materials and support to people with diabetes and the general public while others primarily serve health care professionals.

## *Department of Health and Human Services*

### *National Institutes of Health (NIH)*

**National Institute of Diabetes and Digestive and Kidney Diseases (NIDDK)**

The National Institute of Diabetes and Digestive and Kidney Diseases (NIDDK) is the Government's lead agency for diabetes research. NIDDK operates three information clearinghouses of potential interest to people seeking diabetes information and funds six Diabetes Research and Training Centers.

**National Diabetes Information Clearinghouse (NDIC)**
1 Information Way
Bethesda, MD 20892-3560
Tel: (301) 654-3327

---

National Diabetes Information Clearinghouse (NDIC), April 1997; supplemental additions made and contact information verified and updated in June 1998.

Fax: (301) 907-8906
E-mail: ndic@info.niddk.nih.gov
Website: http://www.niddk.nih.gov

**Mission:** To serve as a diabetes information, educational, and referral resource for health professionals and the public. NDIC is a service of NIDDK.

**Materials:** Diabetes education materials are available free or at little cost. Literature searches on myriad subjects related to diabetes are provided. NDIC publishes *Diabetes Dateline*, a quarterly newsletter.

**National Kidney and Urologic Diseases Information Clearinghouse (NKUDIC)**
3 Information Way
Bethesda, MD 20892-3580
Tel: (301) 654-4415
Fax: (301) 907-8906
E-mail: nkudic@aerie.com
Website: http://www.niddk.nih.gov

**Mission:** To provide information about kidney and urologic diseases to the public, patients and their families, and health care professionals. NKUDIC also works with related organizations to educate people about kidney and urologic diseases; answers inquiries; and develops, reviews, and distributes publications. NKUDIC is a service of NIDDK.

**Materials:** Education materials, including the fact sheet *Kidney Disease of Diabetes* and the booklet *End-Stage Renal Disease: Choosing a Treatment That's Right for You*; literature searches on a number of topics related to kidney and urologic diseases; and *KU Notes*, a semi-annual newsletter.

**Weight-Control Information Network (WIN)**
1 WIN Way
Bethesda, MD 20892-3665
Tel: (800) 946-8098
or (301) 984-7378
Fax: (301) 984-7196
E-mail: WINN@info.niddk.nih.gov
Website: http://www.niddk.nih.gov/health/nutrit/winn.htm

**Mission:** To address the health information needs of individuals through the production and dissemination of educational materials. In addition, WIN is developing communication strategies for a pilot program to encourage at-risk individuals to achieve and maintain a healthy weight by making changes in their lifestyle.

**Materials:** Fact sheets, pamphlets, reprints, consensus statements, reports, and literature searches on weight control, obesity, and weight-related nutritional disorders. WIN's newsletter, *WIN Notes*, is published semi-annually and provides health professionals with the latest research findings and progress about the WIN program.

**Diabetes Research and Training Centers (DRTCs)**

The National Institute of Diabetes and Digestive and Kidney Diseases (NIDDK) supports six DRTCs across the United States. [Editor's Note: Contact information could be verified for only the five DRTCs listed below.]

**Mission:** To offer educational seminars and workshops for health care professionals; develop and use an array of educational assessment and evaluation instruments; provide expert advice on developing and implementing diabetes programs; and provide referrals to people with diabetes.

**Materials:** Individual centers produce a variety of diabetes education materials. For information about publications and programs contact the individual center listed below:

*Einstein / Montefiore DRTC*
1300 Morris Park Avenue
Bronx, NY 10461
Tel: (718) 430-2908
or (718) 430-3345 (epidemiologist)
Fax: (718) 430-8634

*Michigan DRTC*
G1103 Towsley Center, Box 0201
University of Michigan Medical School
Ann Arbor, MI 48109-0201
Tel: (313) 763-1426

*University of Chicago DRTC*
Center for Research in Medical Education and Health Care
5841 S. Maryland Avenue, MC 6091
Chicago, IL 60637
Tel: (773) 753-1310
Fax: (773) 753-1316
E-mail: wmcnabb@medicine.bsd.uchicago.edu

*Vanderbilt University DRTC*
Vanderbilt Medical Center
305 Medical Arts Building
1211 21st Avenue South
Nashville, TN 37212
Tel: (615) 936-1149
Fax: (615) 936-1152

Washington University DRTC
(medical research only)
Division of Health Behavior Research
4444 Forest Park, Suite 6700
St. Louis, MO 63108
Tel: (314) 286-1900
Fax: (314) 286-1919

**National Eye Institute (NEI)**
National Eye Health Education Program
Box 20/20 Vision Place
Bethesda, MD 20892
Tel: (800) 869-2020 (for health professionals only) or (301) 496-5248
Fax: (301) 402-1065
E-mail: 2020@nei.nih.gov
Website: http://www.nei.nih.gov

**Mission:** NEI's National Eye Health Education Program (NEHEP) promotes public and professional awareness of the importance of early diagnosis and treatment of diabetes eye diseases. NEHEP is a partnership with various public and private organizations who plan and implement eye health education programs targeted to a variety of high-risk audiences.

**Materials:** NEI produces patient and professional education materials related to diabetic eye disease and its treatment, including literature for patients, guides for health professionals, and education kits for community health workers and pharmacists. The following are several titles that focus on diabetic eye disease: *Educating People with Diabetes* (kit), *Information Kit for Pharmacists*, and *Ojo con su Visión* (Watch Out for Your Vision) (in Spanish).

**National Heart, Lung, and Blood Institute (NHLBI) Information Center**
P.O. Box 30105
Bethesda, MD 20824-0105
Tel: (301) 251-1222
Fax: (301) 251-1223
E-mail: nhlbiic@dgsys.com
Website: http://www.nhlbi.nih.gov/ nhlbi/nhlbi.html

**Mission:** To respond to telephone and mail inquiries related to high blood pressure, cholesterol, asthma, heart attack, obesity, and sleep disorders as well as information requests associated with cardiovascular disease prevention and heart-health promotion.

**Materials:** Patient education materials are available on numerous topics including cholesterol, high blood pressure, asthma, heart disease, exercise, obesity, stroke, sarcoidosis, and Raynaud's phenomenon. Treatment guidelines for health professionals are available on high blood cholesterol, high blood pressure, and asthma. Professional materials are also available on heart and lung health in the workplace and schools. Serial publications include *Heart Memo*, which provides program updates about cholesterol, high blood pressure, and heart attack, and *Asthma Memo*, which describes the activities of the National Asthma Education and Prevention Program.

**National Oral Health Information Clearinghouse (NOHIC)**
1 NOHIC Way
Bethesda, MD 20892-3500
Tel: (301) 402-7364
Fax: (301) 907-8830
E-mail: nidr@aerie.com
Website: http://www.nidr.nih.gov

**Mission:** To serve as a resource for patients, health professionals, and the public who seek information on the oral health of special care patients: people with genetic or systemic disorders that compromise oral health; people whose medical treatment causes oral problems; and people with mental or physical disabilities that make dental hygiene difficult. A service of the National Institute of Dental Research, NOHIC gathers and disseminates information from many sources, including voluntary health organizations, educational institutions; Government agencies, and industry.

**Materials:** NOHIC provides a variety of services to help patients and professionals obtain information including patient education materials and literature searches. *OH Notes* is NOHIC's newsletter, which is published annually.

## Other Governmental Sources of Information

Agency for Health Care Policy and Research (AHCPR)
Parklawn Building, Room 18-12
5600 Fishers Lane
Rockville, MD 20857
Tel: (301) 443-4100
Tel: (301) 227-8364—Division of Information and Publications
Website: www.ahcpr.gov

**Materials:** Materials are available on medical treatment effectiveness, health care costs and utilizations, health care expenditures, health information systems, health technology assessment, and funding opportunities for grants and contracts. Single copies of publications are available free upon request from the AHCPR (send a self-addressed mailing list.) An annotated publications list is also available.

**Centers for Disease Control and Prevention (CDC)**
Division of Diabetes Translation
National Center for Chronic Disease Prevention and Health Promotion
K-10, 4770 Buford Highway NE.
Atlanta, GA 30341-3724
Tel: (770) 488-5000
Fax: (770) 488-5969
Website: http://www.cdc.gov/diabetes

(home page includes links to information about State diabetes-control programs).

**Mission:** To reduce the burden of diabetes in the United States by planning, conducting, coordinating, and evaluating Federal efforts to translate promising results of diabetes research into widespread clinical and public health practice.

**Materials:** CDC distributes several publications including the annual surveillance report and annotated bibliographies reviewing current literature on economic issues and knowledge regarding diabetes in the United States and territorial Latino populations. State-based diabetes control programs produce public and professional materials specific to their needs and strategies. Information about some of these materials are available on the home page.

**Indian Health Service (IHS)**
Diabetes Program, Headquarters West
5300 Homestead Road NE.
Albuquerque, NM 87110
Tel: (505) 764-0036
Website: www.ihs.gov/IHSmain.html

**Mission:** To develop, document, and sustain a health effort to prevent and control diabetes in American Indian and Alaska Native communities.

**Materials:** IHS makes many diabetes resources available including the *Diabetes Curriculum Packet*, nutrition education materials, general diabetes information, professional resources, training programs, posters, audiovisual materials, and other patient education materials. Education materials are directed toward populations served by IHS and are written at a lower reading level. Materials can be obtained upon request from the IHS Diabetes Headquarters Office.

**Office of Minority Health Resource Center (OMH-RC)**
P.O. Box 37337
Washington, DC 20013-7337
Tel: (800) 444-6472
Fax: (301) 589-0884
E-mail: info@omhrc.gov
Website: http://www.omhrc.gov

**Mission:** To improve the health of racial and ethnic populations through the development of health policies and programs. OMH-RC is the largest resource and referral service on minority health in the Nation.

**Materials:** OMH-RC offers information, publications, mailing lists, database searches, referrals, and more for African-American, Asian, Hispanic/Latino, Native American/ Alaska Native, and Pacific Islander populations. OMH-RC publishes the newsletter *Closing the Gap*.

**Veterans Health Administration (VHA)**
Diabetes Program, Headquarters
Dr. Leonard Pogach
VA Medical Center
East Orange, NJ 07019
Tel: (973) 676-1000, ext. 1282
Fax: (973) 677-4408

**Mission:** To decrease the prevalence of adverse health outcomes in veterans with diabetes by ensuring that each patient at each facility has access to preventive and treatment programs that meet national standards of care.

**Materials:** The VHA Diabetes Clinical Practice Guidelines are a comprehensive, evidence-based document that incorporates information from several existing, national consensus, evidence-based guidelines into a format that maximally facilitates clinical decision making. An algorithmic format was chosen because of evidence that such a format improves data collection and diagnostic and therapeutics decision making and changes patterns of resource use. Guidelines were developed in six major subject areas, including glycemic control, foot care, eye care, hypertension, lipids, and renal disease. A computer version of the algorithm is under discussion.

## Voluntary Associations

**American Association of Diabetes Educators (AADE)**
100 W. Monroe Street
Chicago, IL 60603
Tel: (312) 424-2426 or (800) 338-3633
Fax: (312) 424-2427
Diabetes Educator Access Line:
(800) TEAMUP4 (800-832-6874)
Website: http://www.aadenet.org

**Mission:** To advance the role of the diabetes educator and improve the quality of diabetes education and care.

**Materials:** AADE publishes *The Diabetes Educator*, a bimonthly journal for members. It also publishes *AADE News* nine times a year. Several other professional publications and videotapes are available for purchase.

**American Diabetes Association (ADA)**
National Service Center
1660 Duke Street
Alexandria, VA 22314
Tel: (703) 549-1500 (National Service Center)
or (800) 342-2383 (800 DIABETES)
(reaches affiliate office in the State in which call is placed)
E-mail: customerservice@diabetes.org
Website: http://www.diabetes.org

**Mission:** To prevent and cure diabetes and to improve the lives of all people affected by diabetes.

**Materials:** American Diabetes Association publishes many books and resources for health professionals and people with diabetes. In addition, they publish several magazines and journals. *Diabetes Forecast* is a monthly magazine for people with diabetes. *Diabetes*, *Diabetes Care*, and *Diabetes Spectrum* are professional journals. For further details and ordering information on American Diabetes Association's publications, contact the American Diabetes Association, Order Fulfillment Dept., P.O. Box 930850, Atlanta, GA 31193-0850; (800) 232-6733; or see <http://www.ada judd.com >.

**American Dietetic Association (ADA)**
216 W. Jackson Boulevard, Suite 800
Chicago, IL 60606-6995
Tel: (312) 899-0040
Fax: (312) 899-1979
Website: http://www.eatright.org

**Mission:** To serve the public through the promotion of optimal nutrition, health, and well-being.

**Materials:** The American Dietetic Association publishes a monthly professional journal, *The Journal of The American Dietetic Association* and a monthly newsletter, *ADA Courier*. In addition they publish many books and other resources for consumers and professionals. For additional information or to order materials, call (800) 877-1600 ext. 5000.

*Diabetes Care and Education Dietetic Practice Croup (DCE)*
(a subgroup of The American Dietetic Association). For information, contact The American Dietetic Association using the above information.

**Mission:** To promote quality nutrition care and education. As leaders in the diabetes community, DCE members make positive contributions to persons with diabetes and their families, the DCE membership, and other professional organizations and industry.

**Materials:** Professional and consumer publications have been created by DCE in conjunction with both The American Dietetic Association and American Diabetes Association. Materials can be ordered through either association. In addition, a bimonthly newsletter is published for members.

*National Center for Nutrition and Dietetics, Consumer Nutrition Hotline*
(part of The American Dietetic Association)
Tel: (800) 366-1655
Website: http://www.eatright.org

**Mission:** To promote optimal nutrition, health, and well-being for the consumer through the center's programs and services. A toll-free consumer nutrition hotline, which includes a referral service to registered dietitians, and a resource library is available.

**American Foundation for Urologic Disease Inc. (AFUD)**
1128 N. Charles Street
Baltimore, MD 21201
Tel: (800) 242-2383 or (410) 468-1800
E-mail: lesley@afud.org
Website: http://www.access.digex.net/~afud

**Mission:** To provide research grants, patient and public education, Government relations, and patient support group activities.

**Materials:** AFUD publishes an informational brochure about the organization; *Foundation Focus*, their quarterly newsletter; and several patient education brochures.

**American Heart Association**
7320 Greenville Avenue
Dallas, TX 75231
Tel: (800) 242-1793
Website: www.amhrt.org

**Description:** A private, voluntary organization that has literature on heart disease and how to prevent it. Contact the local affiliate of the American Heart Association listed in telephone directories.

**American Podiatric Medical Association (APMA)**
9312 Old Georgetown Road
Bethesda, MD 20814-1698
Tel: (301) 571-9200
Fax: (301) 530-2752
E-mail: askapma@apma.org
Website: http://www.apma.org
APMA Foot Care Information Center
Tel: (800) FOOT-CARE (800-366-8227)

**Mission:** To serve the professional needs and promote the standards and ethics of doctors of podiatric medicine and their services to the public.

**Materials:** APMA publishes a monthly magazine, *APMA News*; a monthly journal, *Journal of the American Podiatric Medical Association*; and a diabetes-specific booklet, *Your Podiatric Physician Talks About Diabetes*.

**The International Diabetes Federation (IDF)**
Rue Defacqz 1
B-1000 Brussels, Belgium
Tel: 32-2/538-5511
Fax: 32-2/538-5114
E-mail: idf@idf.org
Website: http://www.idf.org

**Mission:** To bring together people concerned with diabetes through their professional or personal lives, and use their combined strengths to further issues of importance to people with diabetes. To serve as a federation of diabetes associations in 114 countries around the world, in official relations with the World Health Organization (WHO) and the Pan American Health Organization (PAHO).

**Materials:** The IDF publishes *The IDF Newsletter*, *The IDF Bulletin*, and publications *Together We Are Stronger*, a guide to building successful diabetes associations, and *Lowering the Price of Ignorance*, a world view on diabetes education.

**International Diabetic Athletes Association (IDAA)**
1647 West Bethany Home Road #B
Phoenix, AZ 85015
Tel: (602) 433-2113 or (800) 898-4322
Fax: (602) 433-9331
E-mail: idaa@diabetes-exercise.org
Website: http://www.diabetes-exercise.org/

**Mission:** To enhance the quality of life for people with diabetes through exercise.

**Materials:** *The Challenge* is IDAA's quarterly newsletter. IDAA also provides pamphlets on diabetes and exercise.

**Juvenile Diabetes Foundation International (JDF)**
120 Wall Street
New York, NY 10005
Tel: (212) 785-9500 or (800) 533-2873
Fax: (212) 785-9595
E-mail: info@jdfcure.com
Website: http://www.jdfcure.com

**Mission:** To support and fund research to find a cure for diabetes and its complications. The Juvenile Diabetes Foundation is a nonprofit, voluntary health agency.

**Materials:** JDF publishes the quarterly journal *Countdown*, the quarterly newsletter *Research News*, and a series of patient education brochures about insulin-dependent and noninsulin-dependent diabetes.

**National Kidney Foundation Inc. (NKF)**
30 East 33rd Street
New York, NY 10016
Tel: (800) 622-9010 or (212) 889-2210
Fax: (212) 689-9261
Website: http://www.kidney.org

**Mission:** To eradicate all diseases of the kidney and urinary tract. To seek the means to prevent kidney disease, while ensuring that individuals with disease receive the finest care.

**Materials:** NKF has several publications including *The Kidney*, *American Journal of Kidney Diseases*, *CNSW Perspectives*, *CRN Quarterly*, *CNNT Action Update*, and *NKF Family Focus*. Additional patient and public education materials are available.

**Pedorthic Footwear Association (PFA)**
9861 Broken Land Parkway
Suite 255
Columbia, MD 21046-1151
Tel: (410) 381-7278 or (800) 673-8447
Fax: (410) 381-1167
Website: http://www.nsra.org
Website: http://www.pedorthics.org

**Mission:** To increase knowledge and understanding of pedorthics and its practice, to encourage development of new pedorthic tools and techniques, and to foster the professional development of pedorthic practitioners.

**Materials:** PFA publishes the bimonthly magazine *Pedoscope*; the brochures *Pedorthics: Foot Care through Proper Footwear* and *Diabetes & Pedorthics: Conservative Foot Care*; the videotape "Pedorthics"; reference guides; and manuals.

## Private Organizations

**International Diabetes Center (IDC) Institute for Research and Education Health System Minnesota**
3800 Park Nicollet Boulevard
Minneapolis, MN 55416-2699
Tel: (612) 993-3393
Fax: (612) 993-1302
E-mail: fruehs@found.hsmnet.com
Website: http://www.onhealth.com

**Mission:** To improve the quality of life of individuals with diabetes and those at risk of developing diabetes by undertaking clinical care, education, research, and outreach activities that stimulate and support health. IDC also seeks to improve the health care delivery system by continually developing, implementing, and evaluating outcomes of diabetes management.

**Materials:** IDC has a wide range of publications for people with diabetes and diabetes educators, including books, booklets and planners, and a Simplified Learning Series, which are brief booklets on different diabetes-related topics.

**Joslin Diabetes Center**
One Joslin Place
Boston, MA 02215
Tel: (617) 732-2695
Fax: (617) 732-2500
Website: http://www.joslin.harvard.edu

**Mission:** To provide medical treatment for people with diabetes; to do research related to all facets of diabetes; and to provide medical education.

**Materials:** Joslin Diabetes Center publishes books for people with diabetes and professionals, videotapes, and other educational materials. They also publish *Joslin*, a quarterly newsletter.

# Index

# Index

Page numbers followed by 'n' indicate a footnote. Page numbers in *italics* indicate a table or illustration

## B

## E

## F

## G

## H

## J



## K

## N

## O

## P

## S

## Diabetes Sourcebook, 2nd Edition

*Basic Information about Insulin-Dependent Diabetes, Noninsulin-Dependent Diabetes, Gestational Diabetes, and Related Disorders, Including Diabetes Prevalence Data, Management Issues, the Role of Diet and Exercise in Controlling Diabetes, Insulin and Other Diabetes Medicines, and Complications of Diabetes Such as Eye Diseases, Digestive Disorders, Periodontal Disease, Amputation, and End-Stage Renal Disease; Along with Reports on Current Research Initiatives, a Glossary, and Resource Listings for Further Help and Information*

Edited by Karen Bellenir. 800 pages. 1998. 0-7808-0224-1. $78.

■

## Diet & Nutrition Sourcebook, 1st Edition

*Basic Information about Nutrition, Including the Dietary Guidelines for Americans, the Food Guide Pyramid, and Their Applications in Daily Diet, Nutritional Advice for Specific Age Groups, Current Nutritional Issues and Controversies, the New Food Label and How to Use It to Promote Healthy Eating, and Recent Developments in Nutritional Research*

Edited by Dan R. Harris. 662 pages. 1996. 0-7808-0084-2. $78.

**"Useful reference as a food and nutrition sourcebook for the general consumer."**

— *Booklist Health Sciences Supplement, Oct '97*

**"Recommended for public libraries and medical libraries that receive general information requests on nutrition. It is readable and will appeal to those interested in learning more about healthy dietary practices."**

— *Medical Reference Services Quarterly, Fall '97*

**"An abundance of medical and social statistics is translated into readable information geared toward the general reader."** — *Bookwatch, Mar '97*

**"With dozens of questionable diet books on the market, it is so refreshing to find a reliable and factual reference book. Recommended to aspiring professionals, librarians, and others seeking and giving reliable dietary advice. An excellent compilation."** — *Choice, Feb '97*

■

## Diet & Nutrition Sourcebook, 2nd Edition

*Basic Information about Nutrition, Including General Nutritional Recommendations, Recommendations for People with Specific Medical Concerns, Dieting for Weight Control, Nutritional Supplements, Food Safety Issues, the Relationship between Nutrition and Disease Development, and Other Nutritional Research Reports; Along with Statistical and Demographic Data, Lifestyle Modification Recommendations, and Sources of Additional Help and Information*

*Edited by Karen Bellenir. 600 pages. 1998. 0-7808-0228-4. $78.*

■

## Ear, Nose & Throat Disorders Sourcebook

*Basic Information about Disorders of the Ears, Nose, Sinus Cavities, Pharynx, and Larynx, Including Ear Infections, Tinnitus, Vestibular Disorders, Allergic and Non-Allergic Rhinitis, Sore Throats, Tonsillitis, and Cancers That Affect the Ears, Nose, Sinuses, and Throat, Along with Reports on Current Research Initiatives, a Glossary of Related Medical Terms, and a Directory of Sources for Further Help and Information*

Edited by Karen Bellenir and Linda M. Shin. 592 pages. 1998. 0-7808-0206-3. $78.

■

## Endocrine & Metabolic Disorders Sourcebook

*Basic Information for the Layperson about Pancreatic and Insulin-Related Disorders Such as Pancreatitis, Diabetes, and Hypoglycemia; Adrenal Gland Disorders Such as Cushing's Syndrome, Addison's Disease, and Congenital Adrenal Hyperplasia; Pituitary Gland Disorders Such as Growth Hormone Deficiency, Acromegaly, and Pituitary Tumors; Thyroid Disorders Such as Hypothyroidism, Graves' Disease, Hashimoto's Disease, and Goiter; Hyperparathyroidism; and Other Diseases and Syndromes of Hormone Imbalance or Metabolic Dysfunction, Along with Reports on Current Research Initiatives*

Edited by Linda M. Shin. 632 pages. 1998. 0-7808-0207-1. $78.

■

## Environmentally Induced Disorders Sourcebook

*Basic Information about Diseases and Syndromes Linked to Exposure to Pollutants and Other Substances in Outdoor and Indoor Environments Such as Lead, Asbestos, Formaldehyde, Mercury, Emissions, Noise, and More*

Edited by Allan R. Cook. 620 pages. 1997. 0-7808-0083-4. $78.

**". . . a good survey of numerous environmentally induced physical disorders . . . a useful addition to anyone's library ."**

— *Doody's Health Science Book Reviews, Jan '98*

**". . . provide[s] introductory information from the best authorities around. Since this volume covers topics that potentially affect everyone, it will surely be one of the most frequently consulted volumes in the *Health Reference Series*."** — *Rettig on Reference, Nov '97*

**"Recommended reference source."**

— *Booklist, Oct '97*

■

## Fitness & Exercise Sourcebook

*Basic Information on Fitness and Exercise, Including Fitness Activities for Specific Age Groups, Exercise for People with Specific Medical Conditions, How to Begin a Fitness Program in Running, Walking, Swimming, Cycling, and Other Athletic Activities, and Recent Research in Fitness and Exercise*

Edited by Dan R. Harris. 663 pages. 1996. 0-7808-0186-5. $78.

**"A good resource for general readers."**

— *Choice, Nov '97*

**"The perennial popularity of the topic . . . make this an appealing selection for public libraries."**

— *Rettig on Reference, Jun/Jul '97*

## Food & Animal Borne Diseases Sourcebook

*Basic Information about Diseases That Can Be Spread to Humans through the Ingestion of Contaminated Food or Water or by Contact with Infected Animals and Insects, Such as Botulism, E. Coli, Hepatitis A, Trichinosis, Lyme Disease, and Rabies, Along with Information Regarding Prevention and Treatment Methods, and a Special Section for International Travelers Describing Diseases Such as Cholera, Malaria, Travelers' Diarrhea, and Yellow Fever, and Offering Recommendations for Avoiding Illness*

Edited by Karen Bellenir and Peter D. Dresser. 535 pages. 1995. 0-7808-0033-8. $78.

**"Targeting general readers and providing them with a single, comprehensive source of information on selected topics, this book continues, with the excellent caliber of its predecessors, to catalog topical information on health matters of general interest. Readable and thorough, this valuable resource is highly recommended for all libraries."**

— *Academic Library Book Review, Summer '96*

**"A comprehensive collection of authoritative information."** — *Emergency Medical Services, Oct '95*

## Gastrointestinal Diseases & Disorders Sourcebook

*Basic Information about Gastroesophageal Reflux Disease (Heartburn), Ulcers, Diverticulosis, Irritable Bowel Syndrome, Crohn's Disease, Ulcerative Colitis, Diarrhea, Constipation, Lactose Intolerance, Hemorrhoids, Hepatitis, Cirrhosis, and Other Digestive Problems, Featuring Statistics, Descriptions of Symptoms, and Current Treatment Methods of Interest for Persons Living with Upper and Lower Gastrointestinal Maladies*

Edited by Linda M. Ross. 413 pages. 1996. 0-7808-0078-8. $78.

**". . . very readable form. The successful editorial work that brought this material together into a useful and understandable reference makes accessible to all readers information that can help them more effectively understand and obtain help for digestive tract problems."** — *Choice, Feb '97*

## Genetic Disorders Sourcebook

*Basic Information about Heritable Diseases and Disorders Such as Down Syndrome, PKU, Hemophilia, Von Willebrand Disease, Gaucher Disease, Tay-Sachs Disease, and Sickle-Cell Disease, Along with Information about Genetic Screening, Gene Therapy, Home Care, and Including Source Listings for Further Help and Information on More Than 300 Disorders*

Edited by Karen Bellenir. 642 pages. 1996. 0-7808-0034-6. $78.

**"Provides essential medical information to both the general public and those diagnosed with a serious or fatal genetic disease or disorder."** — *Choice, Jan '97*

**". . . geared toward the lay public. It would be well placed in all public libraries and in those hospital and medical libraries in which access to genetic references is limited."**

— *Doody's Health Sciences Book Review, Oct '96*

## Head Trauma Sourcebook

*Basic Information for the Layperson about Open-Head and Closed-Head Injuries, Treatment Advances, Recovery, and Rehabilitation, Along with Reports on Current Research Initiatives*

Edited by Karen Bellenir. 414 pages. 1997. 0-7808-0208-X. $78.

## Health Insurance Sourcebook

*Basic Information about Managed Care Organizations, Traditional Fee-for-Service Insurance, Insurance Portability and Pre-Existing Conditions Clauses, Medicare, Medicaid, Social Security, and Military Health Care, Along with Information about Insurance Fraud*

Edited by Wendy Wilcox. 530 pages. 1997. 0-7808-0222-5. $78.

**"The layout of the book is particularly helpful as it provides easy access to reference material. A most useful addition to the vast amount of information about health insurance. The use of data from U.S. government agencies is most commendable. Useful in a library or learning center for healthcare professional students."**

— *Doody's Health Sciences Book Reviews, Nov '97*

## Immune System Disorders Sourcebook

*Basic Information about Lupus, Multiple Sclerosis, Guillain-Barré Syndrome, Chronic Granulomatous Disease, and More, Along with Statistical and Demographic Data and Reports on Current Research Initiatives*

Edited by Allan R. Cook. 608 pages. 1997. 0-7808-0209-8. $78.

## Kidney & Urinary Tract Diseases & Disorders Sourcebook

*Basic Information about Kidney Stones, Urinary Incontinence, Bladder Disease, End Stage Renal Disease, Dialysis, and More, Along with Statistical and Demographic Data and Reports on Current Research Initiatives*

Edited by Linda M. Ross. 602 pages. 1997. 0-7808-0079-6. $78.

## Learning Disabilities Sourcebook

*Basic Information about Disorders Such as Dyslexia, Visual and Auditory Processing Deficits, Attention Deficit/Hyperactivity Disorder, and Autism, Along with Statistical and Demographic Data, Reports on Current Research Initiatives, an Explanation of the Assessment Process, and a Special Section for Adults with Learning Disabilities*

Edited by Linda M. Shin. 579 pages. 1998. 0-7808-0210-1. $78.

## Men's Health Concerns Sourcebook

*Basic Information about Health Issues That Affect Men, Featuring Facts about the Top Causes of Death in Men, Including Heart Disease, Stroke, Cancers, Prostate Disorders, Chronic Obstructive Pulmonary Disease, Pneumonia and Influenza, Human Immunodeficiency Virus and Acquired Immune Deficiency Syndrome, Diabetes Mellitus, Stress, Suicide, Accidents and Homicides; and Facts about Common Concerns for Men, Including Impotence, Contraception, Circumcision, Sleep Disorders, Snoring, Hair Loss, Diet, Nutrition, Exercise, Kidney and Urological Disorders, and Backaches*

Edited by Allan R. Cook. 760 pages. 1998. 0-7808-0212-8. $78.

## Mental Health Disorders Sourcebook

*Basic Information about Schizophrenia, Depression, Bipolar Disorder, Panic Disorder, Obsessive-Compulsive Disorder, Phobias and Other Anxiety Disorders, Paranoia and Other Personality Disorders, Eating Disorders, and Sleep Disorders, Along with Information about Treatment and Therapies*

Edited by Karen Bellenir. 548 pages. 1995. 0-7808-0040-0. $78.

**"This is an excellent new book . . . written in easy-to-understand language."**
— *Booklist Health Science Supplement, Oct '97*

**". . . useful for public and academic libraries and consumer health collections."**
— *Medical Reference Services Quarterly, Spring '97*

**"The great strengths of the book are its readability and its inclusion of places to find more information. Especially recommended."** — *RQ, Winter '96*

**". . . a good resource for a consumer health library."**
— *Bulletin of the MLA, Oct '96*

**"The information is data-based and couched in brief, concise language that avoids jargon. . . . a useful reference source."** — *Readings, Sept '96*

**"The text is well organized and adequately written for its target audience."** — *Choice, Jun '96*

**". . . provides information on a wide range of mental disorders, presented in nontechnical language."**
— *Exceptional Child Education Resources, Spring '96*

**"Recommended for public and academic libraries."**
— *Reference Book Review, '96*

## Ophthalmic Disorders Sourcebook

*Basic Information about Glaucoma, Cataracts, Macular Degeneration, Strabismus, Refractive Disorders, and More, Along with Statistical and Demographic Data and Reports on Current Research Initiatives*

Edited by Linda M. Ross. 631 pages. 1996. 0-7808-0081-8. $78.

## Oral Health Sourcebook

*Basic Information about Diseases and Conditions Affecting Oral Health, Including Cavities, Gum Disease, Dry Mouth, Oral Cancers, Fever Blisters, Canker Sores, Oral Thrush, Bad Breath, Temporomandibular Disorders, and other Craniofacial Syndromes, Along with Statistical Data on the Oral Health of Americans, Oral Hygiene, Emergency First Aid, Information on Treatment Procedures and Methods of Replacing Lost Teeth*

Edited by Allan R. Cook. 558 pages. 1997. 0-7808-0082-6. $78.

**"Recommended reference source."** — *Booklist, Dec '97*

## Pain Sourcebook

*Basic Information about Specific Forms of Acute and Chronic Pain, Including Headaches, Back Pain, Muscular Pain, Neuralgia, Surgical Pain, and Cancer Pain, Along with Pain Relief Options Such as Analgesics, Narcotics, Nerve Blocks, Transcutaneous Nerve Stimulation, and Alternative Forms of Pain Control, Including Biofeedback, Imaging, Behavior Modification, and Relaxation Techniques*

Edited by Allan R. Cook. 667 pages. 1997. 0-7808-0213-6. $78.

**"The information is basic in terms of scholarship and is appropriate for general readers. Written in journalistic style . . . intended for non-professionals. Quite thorough in its coverage of different pain conditions and summarizes the latest clinical information regarding pain treatment."** — *Choice, Jun '98*

**"Recommended reference source."**

— *Booklist, Mar '98*

## Pregnancy & Birth Sourcebook

*Basic Information about Planning for Pregnancy, Maternal Health, Fetal Growth and Development, Labor and Delivery, Postpartum and Perinatal Care, Pregnancy in Mothers with Special Concerns, and Disorders of Pregnancy, Including Genetic Counseling, Nutrition and Exercise, Obstetrical Tests, Pregnancy Discomfort, Multiple Births, Cesarean Sections, Medical Testing of Newborns, Breastfeeding, Gestational Diabetes, and Ectopic Pregnancy*

Edited by Heather E. Aldred. 737 pages. 1997. 0-7808-0216-0. $78.

**". . . for the layperson. A well-organized handbook. Recommended for college libraries . . . general readers."**

— *Choice, Apr '98*

**"Recommended reference source."**

— *Booklist, Mar '98*

**"This resource is recommended for public libraries to have on hand."**

— *American Reference Books Annual, '98*

## Public Health Sourcebook

*Basic Information about Government Health Agencies, Including National Health Statistics and Trends, Healthy People 2000 Program Goals and Objectives, the Centers for Disease Control and Prevention, the Food and Drug Administration, and the National Institutes of Health, Along with Full Contact Information for Each Agency*

Edited by Wendy Wilcox. 698 pages. 1998. 0-7808-0220-9. $78.

## Rehabilitation Sourcebook

*Basic Information for the Layperson about Physical Medicine (Physiatry) and Rehabilitative Therapies, Including Physical, Occupational, Recreational, Speech, and Vocational Therapy; Along with Descriptions of Devices and Equipment Such as Orthotics, Gait Aids, Prostheses, and Adaptive Systems Used during Rehabilitation and for Activities of Daily Living, and Featuring a Glossary and Source Listings for Further Help and Information*

Edited by Theresa K. Murray. 600 pages. 1998. 0-7808-0236-5. $78.

## Respiratory Diseases & Disorders Sourcebook

*Basic Information about Respiratory Diseases and Disorders, Including Asthma, Cystic Fibrosis, Pneumonia, the Common Cold, Influenza, and Others, Featuring Facts about the Respiratory System, Statistical and Demographic Data, Treatments, Self-Help Management Suggestions, and Current Research Initiatives*

Edited by Allan R. Cook and Peter D. Dresser. 771 pages. 1995. 0-7808-0037-0. $78.

**"Designed for the layperson and for patients and their families coping with respiratory illness. . . . an extensive array of information on diagnosis, treatment, management, and prevention of respiratory illnesses for the general reader."**

— *Choice, Jun '96*

**"A highly recommended text for all collections. It is a comforting reminder of the power of knowledge that good books carry between their covers."**

— *Academic Library Book Review, Spring '96*

**"This sourcebook offers a comprehensive collection of authoritative information presented in a nontechnical, humanitarian style for patients, families, and caregivers."**

— *Association of Operating Room Nurses, Sept/Oct '95*

## Sexually Transmitted Diseases Sourcebook

*Basic Information about Herpes, Chlamydia, Gonorrhea, Hepatitis, Nongonoccocal Urethritis, Pelvic Inflammatory Disease, Syphilis, AIDS, and More, Along with Current Data on Treatments and Preventions*

Edited by Linda M. Ross. 550 pages. 1997. 0-7808-0217-9. $78.